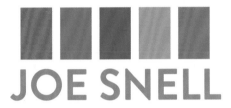

JOE SNELL

YOUR BEST HOME

5 SPACES x 5 DESIGN STEPS = A BETTER LIFE

MURDOCH BOOKS

SYDNEY · LONDON

CONTENTS

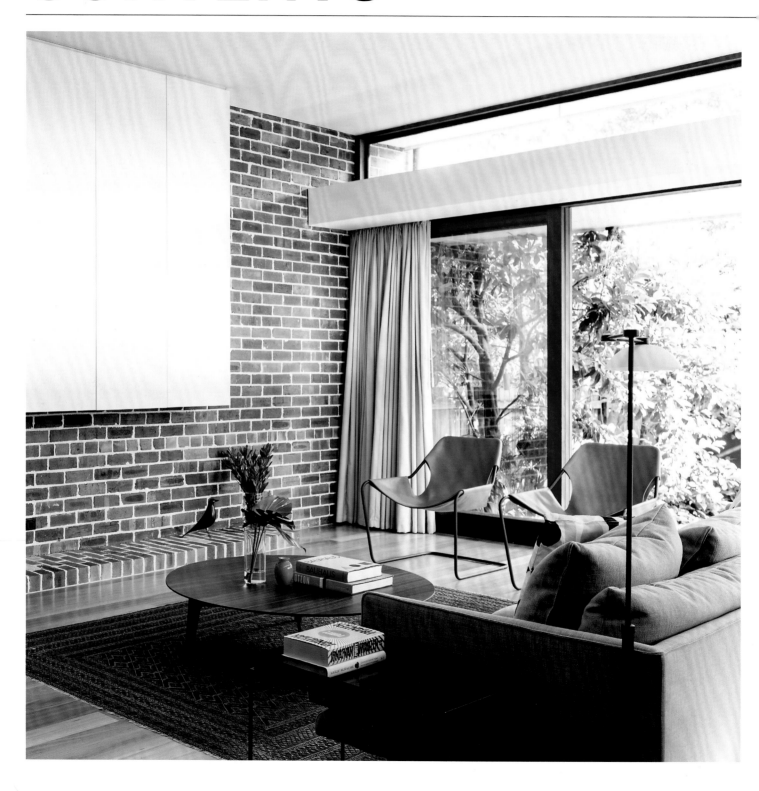

THE 5X5 PREMISE

FOR A BETTER LIFE AT HOME, THE 5 DESIGN STEPS NEED TO BE FOLLOWED – OTHERWISE YOUR STYLING, COLOUR AND CUSHIONS END UP JUST PAPERING OVER THE CRACKS.

ONCE YOU HAVE THE 5 DESIGN STEPS RIGHT, THE DECISIONS AND CHOICES YOU MAKE IN STYLING, COLOUR AND CUSHIONS WILL NOT ONLY BE BETTER, BUT ALSO EASIER.

A HOME THAT HAS YOUR STYLING, COLOUR AND CUSHIONS, BUILT ON THE STRONG FOUNDATIONS OF THE 5 DESIGN STEPS WILL BE THE BEST IT CAN BE, AND CAN GIVE YOU AND YOUR FAMILY A BETTER LIFE.

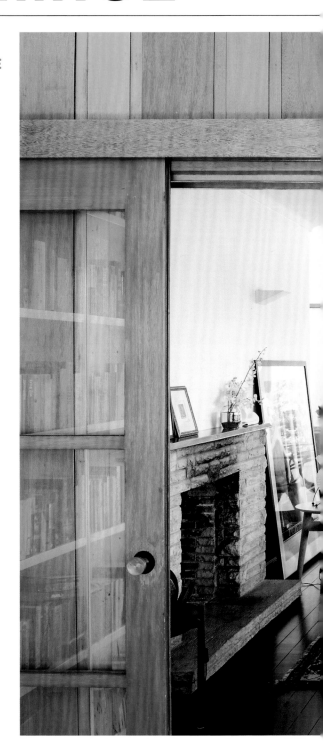

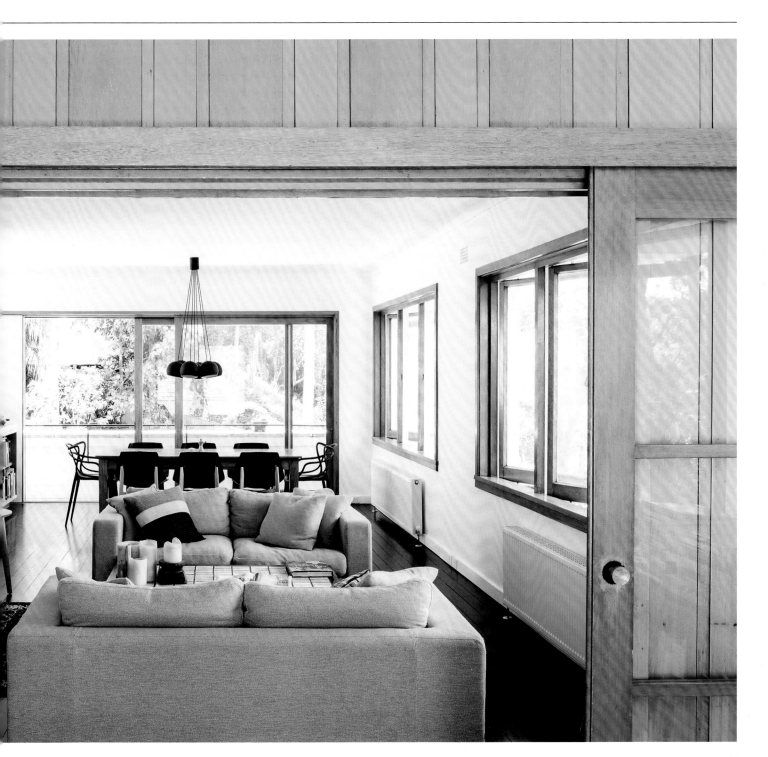

5 STEPS X 5 ROOMS

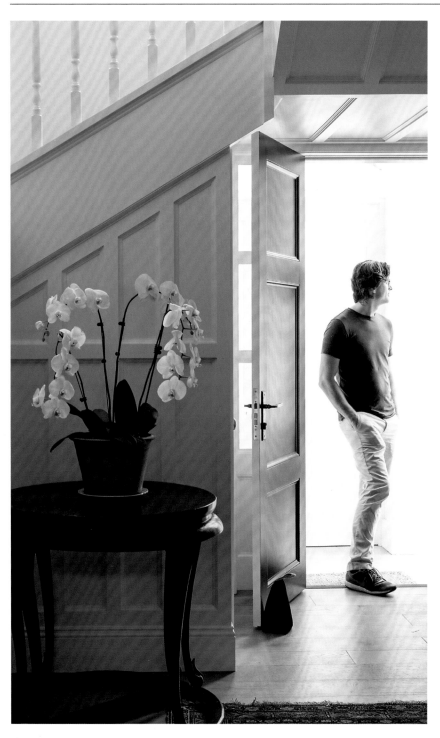

It doesn't matter how big or small your home, if its basic design elements are right it will be a wonderful place to live and grow.

Sometimes, despite beautiful styling, colours and cushions, a home doesn't feel good; it just doesn't feel right. We often don't have the fundamentals correct. All the money and effort spent on superficial styling are just papering over the cracks. It seems that our society often tells us to just 'fix it' with the next layer of style, the next layer of trend, when the true answer is to dig deeper and get the basics, the bones, right.

And that is what this book is about. Whether you are looking to redecorate your home with some easy fixes, to renovate, or to build your dream house, this book will advise and guide you on how to implement the 5 design steps that I apply to every home before doing anything else.

THE HOMES IN THIS BOOK

This book is not a portfolio of my work – these design fundamentals are being applied in many homes; we just need more of them!

Here is a reference to the homes featured and the architects who designed them.

Apartment renovation by **Tribe Studio** (page 127). Lead design architect: Hannah Tribe.

House renovation by **Daniel Boddam** (left). Lead design architect: Daniel Boddam.

House renovation by **Snell Architects** (page 135). Lead design architect: Kevin Snell.

Semi-detached house renovation by **Downie North Architects** (page 111). Lead design architects: Daniel North and Catherine Downie.

House renovation by **Daniel Boddam** (page 156). Lead design architect: Daniel Boddam.

New house by **Snell Architects** (page 106). Lead design architect: Kevin Snell.

Bungalow renovation by **Tribe Studio** (page 99). Lead design architect: Hannah Tribe.

Terrace renovation by **Snell Architects** (page 116). Lead design architect: Joe Snell.

These are the building blocks of good home design and the secret weapons to creating wonderful spaces for us to inhabit. It's not rocket science and it's not complicated, but it is vital to apply them if you want a home to flourish in.

Space, light, air, sound and view are the absolute fundamentals. In every home I work on, I systematically consider these elements to ensure a high quality of shelter and, as you will discover, they are interconnected. Together, the 5 design steps create a fantastic home; leave one out and your home will not be all it could be.

STEP 1: **SPACE**
DESIGN AND PLAN YOUR SPACE IN 3D
It's all around you. It involves planning and thinking in all three dimensions.

STEP 2: **LIGHT**
HARNESS THIS TO ENLIGHTEN YOUR HOME
Both natural and artificial lights need to be harnessed and controlled.

STEP 3: **AIR**
CONTROL AND DIRECT THE FLOW OF AIR THROUGH YOUR HOME
It is what you breathe and smell and it is the temperature that you feel.

STEP 4: **SOUND**
TUNE YOUR HOME TO SOUND LIKE THE HOME YOU WANT IT TO BE
It's what you hear and feel and is often the most forgotten of our senses in the home.

STEP 5: **VIEW**
CAPTURE AND FRAME THE VIEWS AROUND AND WITHIN YOUR HOME
It's what you see and it is how you interpret your home and your surroundings.

In this book I apply the 5 design steps to the 5 most important rooms of your home, whether that home is a one-bedroom apartment or an 18-bedroom mansion. You can implement the steps in your home today, as part of a renovation tomorrow, or as a vision of your new dream build of the future. By following them you will be able to make the important changes necessary to create the bones of a wonderful home.

ROOM 1: **ENTRY**

ROOM 2: **LIVING ROOM**

ROOM 3: **KITCHEN**

ROOM 4: **BEDROOM**

ROOM 5: **BATHROOM**

◁ From the black-painted door, to the double-height stairwell, to the side-light window, to the rug on the floor and the orchid on the table, the 5 design steps have been applied to this entry.

MY STORY

I am husband to Laura and father to three boys: Asger, Bjorn and Peter. I am a Registered Architect and so is my father; I grew up in an architect household. By the time I was 20 years old I had lived in 17 different houses; my family would buy a house, renovate it, and then do so again, and again... and again. After school I studied architecture at the University of Sydney, gaining first a Bachelor of Science, majoring in Architecture, and then a Bachelor of Architecture. During my second degree I took a wonderful student exchange programme with *Det Kongelige Danske Kunstakademi* (The Royal Danish Academy of Fine Arts) in Copenhagen. It was my first overseas trip and it changed my outlook on design, architecture and the home. I also met a Danish lady by the name of Laura and, as they say, the rest is history.

Living in Copenhagen was an amazing education – I saw a society that appreciated the value of good design in a grassroots way. Danish design is not just for elites who can afford architects, but for the every-person. I started to formulate the idea that our society in Australia is lacking in knowledge about good home design. It became my cause and passion: I wanted to know what people saw in a home.

Having grown up in an architect household, and studied architecture for seven years, I felt I was stuck in an echo chamber, talking only to those with a similar outlook. I wanted to ask non-architects how they felt about their homes, and I decided to go to London, where I surprised my architecture friends by not looking for a job in architecture, but instead in real estate. This was my way of finding out at the frontline what people really valued when they were choosing a home.

Of course, no London estate agents had the slightest interest in taking me on. So I worked two bar jobs while I kept looking. Finally, I met a recruiter who took the time to sit down to have a coffee and wasn't put off by my architecture education. He decided that it could, in fact, be an asset, although he did advise me to change my grey tie to pink. I went out and bought a pink tie, and got a job at my first interview. I still have that pink tie.

I started work at Andrew's Estate Agents in Putney and had the time of my life. Andrew's was started by Cecil Jackson-Cole, who also founded the charity Oxfam, and the company had a philanthropic basis — interesting for an estate agency! He believed commercial success should benefit society and so a percentage of every sale went to charity.

In the 18 months I was there I became one of Andrew's highest selling agents, but what I really learnt was that when people buy a home they don't look at style. They look beyond the items in the room to the bones of the building. They go back to basics, with observations such as: 'This is a sunny room'; 'I love how this room feels'; or 'This place has such good bones'.

They looked past the style, colours and cushions and saw the basics of the space. They were interested in the quality of the shelter. They tended to look down their noses at the styling, often seeing it as 'not for them'. They implicitly knew the styling was superficial to the 'bones' of the house.

Why, then, is so much of our literature focused on improving the home through styling, colour and accessories? For too long we have been unashamedly sold the latest 'new fad' of decorating that we are expected to go out and buy. To make real change we must ensure the home has good bones; then, and only then, should we apply the style.

My mission became to teach the community that we have the power to change our fundamental environment: the home. It can be done in stages, over time, and the good news is, it doesn't need to be expensive. I returned to Sydney and joined Snell Architects, where I work with a passionate team, including my father, Kevin, across a range of work for homes, offices, bars, cafes, restaurants, shops, showrooms, exhibitions and art installations.

It is fantastic applying my design knowledge to different types of architecture, but for me the place that holds the most emotion is, and always will be, the humble home.

On average, homes garner the least attention of designers and architects: less than five per cent are planned by architects. So what happens with the rest? Well, they are in the hands of the public, so the public needs to have the knowledge and tools to affect change in its own environment.

That is what this book is about, and also why I worked on a television show like *House Rules*. To be in living rooms around Australia, explaining the positives and negatives of space and how to make them better, was a great opportunity and privilege. I received so many requests from viewers for advice on how to 'fix' homes, that it led me to write this book.

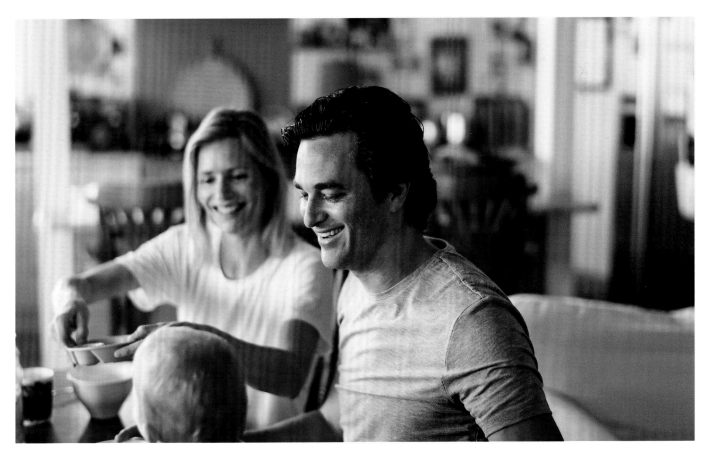

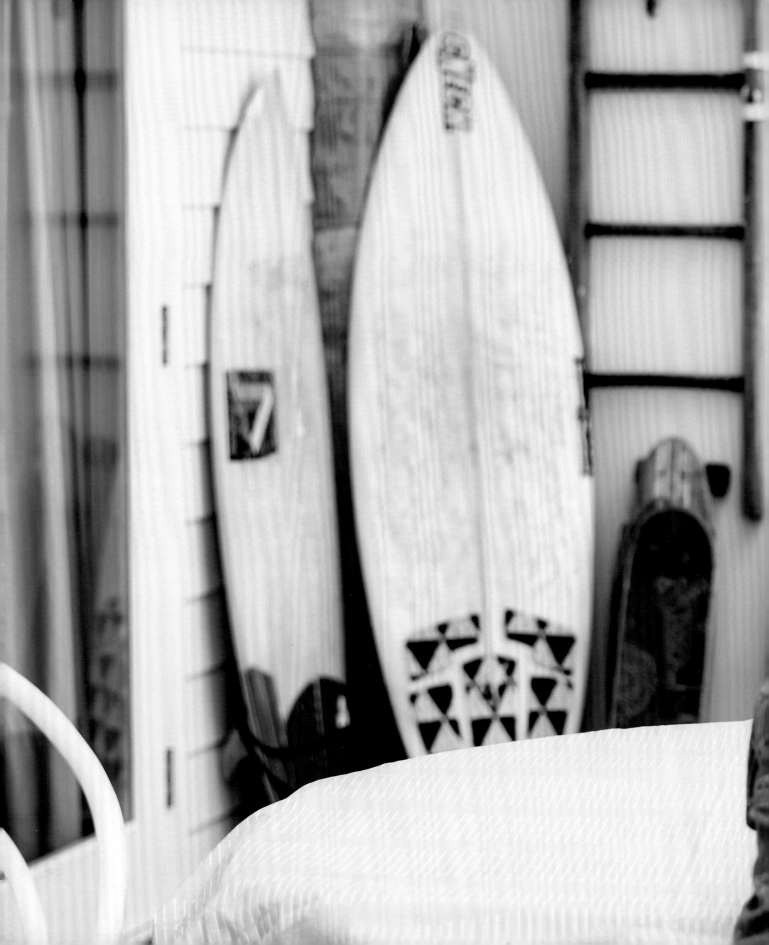

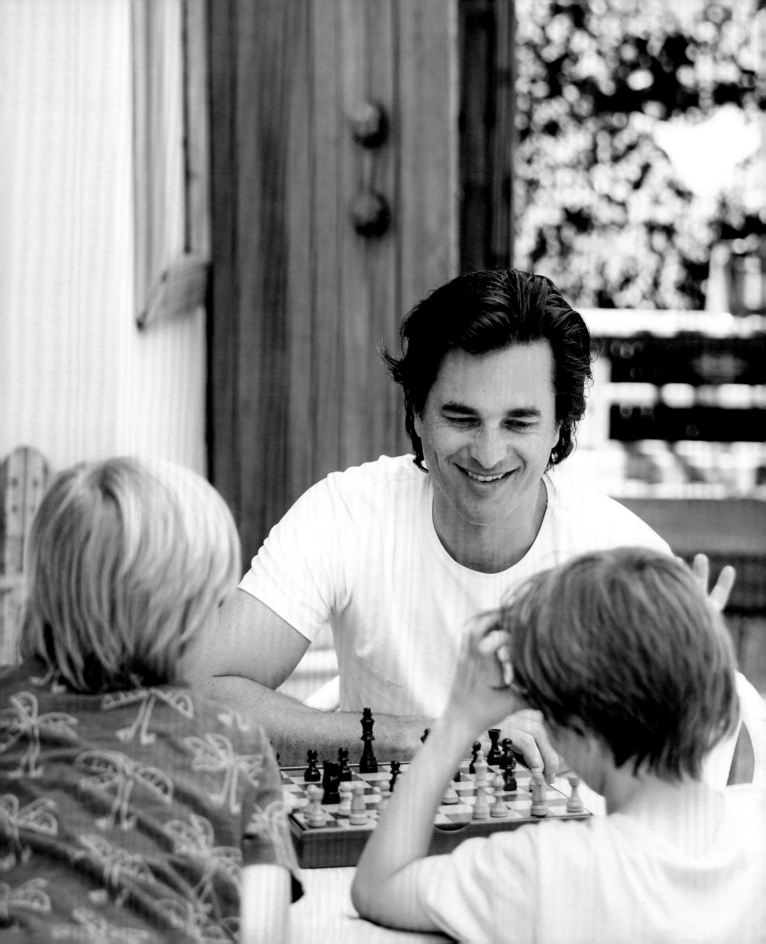

A FEW THOUGHTS BEFORE WE GET STARTED

SHELTER

'All architecture is shelter, all great architecture is the design of space that contains, cuddles, exalts, or stimulates the persons in that space.'

PHILIP JOHNSON, AMERICAN ARCHITECT

We all live inside. By 'inside' we mean a shelter from the external environment. This can take many forms, but in every one of those forms humans strive to make a home, a nest, a place for their family and themselves to retreat, nourish, rejuvenate, flourish and grow. Whether you are renting an apartment, renovating a bungalow or building a dream home, this book focuses on the fundamental must-do's of creating a wonderful inside. It is about getting back to the basics of shelter and comfort, well before you even consider style, colour and cushions. It is about informing you on the basic design principles of creating a home where you and your family will have a better life, rather than focusing on short-term trends. And how to not only build or renovate a home, but also how to use it, how to manage it, and how to get the most out of it.

SUBSTANCE BEFORE STYLE

TWO THOUGHTS...

I bet you have walked into a home where you don't like the styling of the space, but the home itself just feels right. It has good bones.

On the other hand, I bet you have walked into a home that has everything, all the styling, all the mod cons, yet it just doesn't feel good, just doesn't feel right.

Those two thoughts are what I heard time and time again when I worked as an estate agent. The essence is that you can't truly cover up bad bones, no matter how good your styling. The answer is to get the bones of your house right; then your styling will follow on and truly sing.

For too long the conversation has started at decoration, style, colour and cushions. We need to go back to the basics of home design so that the decoration, style, colour and cushions actually work. When you get the design elements correct, you have the foundation that informs your decoration and make your choices much easier. The right home design will create a classic that lasts, also saving you the money that is sometimes spent in constantly changing the style of a home that never feels 'quite right'.

GOOD DESIGN AND YOUR ENVIRONMENT

Good design makes your day easier to get through; therefore, it makes you feel better. My dad has always said: if the building wins, we all win.

Good design, by its very definition, means that it is sustainable. If a design isn't sustainable then it can't be good. The most sustainable design is one that understands and responds to its environment.

It has been found that office workers are happier and more productive if they have control over their environment. By simply getting up and opening or closing a window, office workers feel able to manipulate their setting, have a sense of control and are invigorated by the action – far more invigorated and stimulated than when sitting in a static temperature-controlled

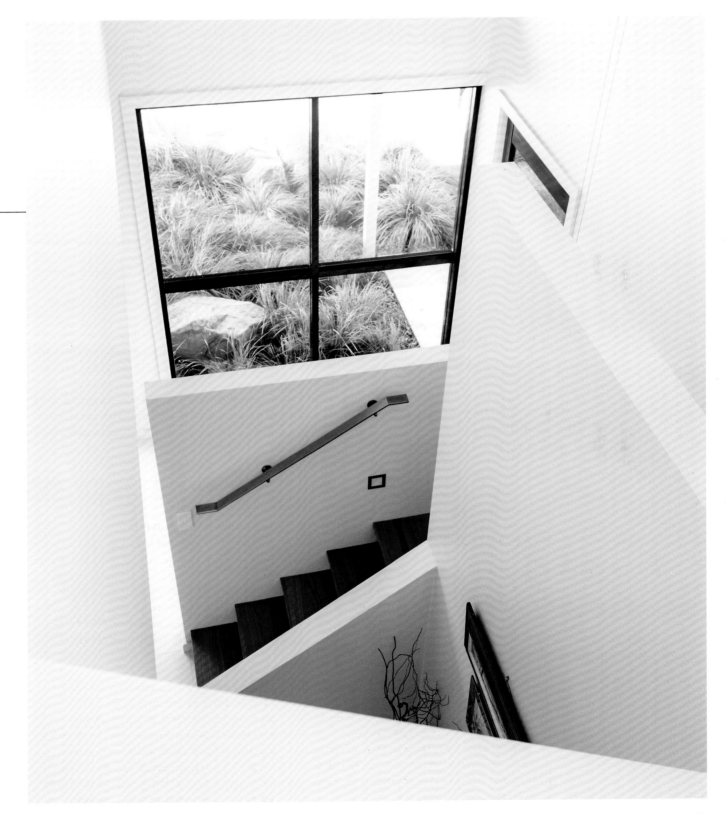

environment where they are dictated to by the room. Biologically we have been designed to respond to our environment, and we become dull and insensitive if we don't have stimuli to respond to. This is no different to what happens in the home. Static is boring. Don't lock yourself out of the environment around you in a dull sealed box for 24 hours a day 365 days a year, otherwise it will make you dull too. Instead, learn to manage your home so that you can experience the change in the day and seasons of the year, and you will feel invigorated and that you are really living. What a wonderful thing to teach your children, rather than sealing them off from Planet Earth.

STYLE

Style is so, so important. Style is what inspires me, excites me and, when it is beautiful and perfect, makes me feel great joy; it should be led by and add to the delight of the architecture. However, attempts at style and colour sometimes don't work because the design basics, the design steps, of the home are simply not right. Every quality designer will tell you that if the bones are good, if the design basics of the space are excellent, then the style will always have a better chance. The best homes are those that have these design steps perfected, with style, colour and cushions all built upon those foundations.

I don't care what your style is: it is your home. You can indulge your love of purple and velvet for all I care. It is not my business. What I do care about is the quality of your home; its health and happiness. To make your home truly healthy and happy you need to get the basic elements right.

The best homes are those that have these basics and then build their style, colour and cushions on them. The style accentuates the space, the colours enhance the light, and the cushions manipulate the sound. Suddenly all the facets are working in tandem, in harmony, and a truly great home has been created.

I do feel that styling should spring from the fundamentals of your home and its location in the world. It is not an accident that the white and light-timbered Scandinavian look came from a part of the world where there is relatively little daylight – the style comes from trying to capture limited light. Similarly the deep dark rich timbers used in Balinese styling are to create deep cool shade in the height of a tropical summer. So I can't help but feel a little cold and ridiculous when I come across Balinese styling in a cool temperate climate like England, or feel hot and bothered in a stark white unshaded Scandinavian-style space in northern Queensland.

TASTE AND STYLE: IT'S ONLY RIGHT IF IT'S ALL ABOUT YOU

People are wonderful. We are all so varied and different, and so unexpected. I love visiting people's homes because you gain an insight into who they are, what they enjoy, and what they stand for.

The exception is when you enter a home and know instantly that it has been 'done'. The homes with the least soul are those that have had someone come in and impose their priorities, their taste, their style over the top of the people who actually live there. (And it is funny that often, despite all the show and perfection, the people who live there don't seem that comfortable.)

This is not a style- or taste-led book. Instead it is about implementing the basics of how we live, so that you can then reveal your taste and style on that foundation. I know that it is sometimes hard to have the confidence to create a home, but understand that what actually makes a great home is not style and colour and taste, but getting the basics right.

After many years of working as an architect and an estate agent I have come to understand that we all have different tastes and styles, and that is OK. Actually, it is more than OK: it is bloody marvellous, otherwise life would be oh-so-boring.

As an architect, my goal is to create a home that harnesses the 5 design steps to encourage a family to flourish. This book is about giving you the confidence to apply those steps to make a great home. Remember, it will still be a great home no matter how you dress it up afterwards, because the bones are right. With that knowledge, you will have the confidence to explore your own style, your own sense of colour and your own taste in cushions. Do what makes you happy; not what someone down the road thinks is the right thing to do. The great thing about style and fashion is that you can change them, if you get the basics right first. Sometimes we forget that.

So, don't rush in when you move into a home, or finish building/renovating one, and employ a stylist to make it 'done'. Instead, spend time there; learn its qualities, its opportunities, and then furnish your home with the things that you cherish, that you deeply understand, that represent your past and your future. Over time this place, this shelter, will become your home. A place you love. And, interestingly enough, it will also be a place that your friends and guests love too, because it is you.

EMOTION

You will see that I use a lot of emotional words — such as lonely, happy, sad — about inanimate objects in the home. I do this because, although they are inanimate, your response to them is not. So, when I say that the little chair in the corner is 'lonely', of course it doesn't feel loneliness, but you as an observer respond to the way that chair looks in the overall room. Its size and placement give off a sense of loneliness; the chair just doesn't look comfortable with its position. Trust these emotions – they are one of your strongest guides in creating a comfortable home. Treat your home as a living thing, as it is what you are alive in. A comfortable home will give you a good life.

HERMIT CRAB OR SEA SNAIL?

Most homes we live in were designed for someone else, yet we still make a home in them. We can make a home anywhere. Home is a metaphor for self. Home is the storehouse of memory. Home is made by, and makes us, what we are. Home is where we can be ourselves.

The hermit crab makes its home in another creature's discarded shell, usually a sea snail's. The sea snail builds its own home shell and eventually moves on from it, only for the shell to be gratefully picked up by the hermit crab. We are experts at taking a home and making it ours – we seem to have an amazing ability to take complete ownership with not a thought in the world to the previous occupants. Very few of us will ever have the opportunity to be a sea snail and build our own home, so it's important we embrace the idea of being the best hermit crabs we can be.

THINK LIKE A CHILD

Children have a wonderful understanding of scale: something that we tend to lose, as we take on the baggage of adulthood. The tents and cubby houses that kids make are always to a perfect scale for their size and shape. When we go back to basics it can sometimes be a good idea to be more childlike in our thinking, drop some of that baggage and just be in the moment of asking: what do I really need?

The tiny house movement is all about creating 'just enough' house for your life, and being more sustainable is part of this thought change. Maybe that extra bedroom, bathroom or excessively large room is just not necessary?

FLEXIBILITY IN SPACE

Sometimes in the course of my design work, I will be faced with a site that only has one good aspect. For whatever reason: the rest of the house is overshadowed by other buildings, or faces due south and is exposed to cold winds, or is on a major polluted and noisy road, or is an apartment with only one external wall. I have to make the most of the good, but limited, aspect of the home. And this is where flexibility of space comes in. Through clever design, I need to make this one good aspect the breakfast room, the living room, dining room and movie room. The key is to make the elements in the room moveable or expandable. Find a table that can be pushed against a wall or moved into the middle of the room, and make sure it can change from a 4-seater into an 8-seater. This will be the breakfast table in the morning, study during the day and entertaining table in the evening . Find a lounge setting that can be transformed into a number of shapes: straight along a wall, two facing sofas, or at a right-angle to form an 'L shape'. Make sure that the flooring is robust enough (but not too 'grippy') to move furniture around easily. Now you have about a hundred configurations to suit any occasion or gathering. Over time, you will find the three furniture configurations that suit your main activities: perhaps day to day, friends over for dinner, and movie night? Once you have these down pat, you will be able to make the transition in about 5 minutes. All our spaces need to be flexible to take on the merging of work and home and also the fact that we are living in increasingly small spaces. Design is key to making this a pleasant experience, rather than a ghetto experience.

BETTER HOME = BETTER LIFE

A home is a place where we are nurtured and where we grow. It is the place we retreat to, to recharge and to regroup. We need to invest our thinking into ensuring it serves our family and ourselves as best it can. If you get things right at home then you have more chance of getting things right everywhere else. A better home really can lead to a better life.

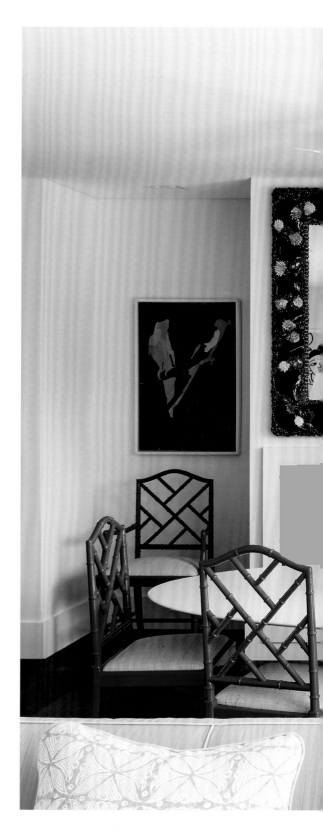

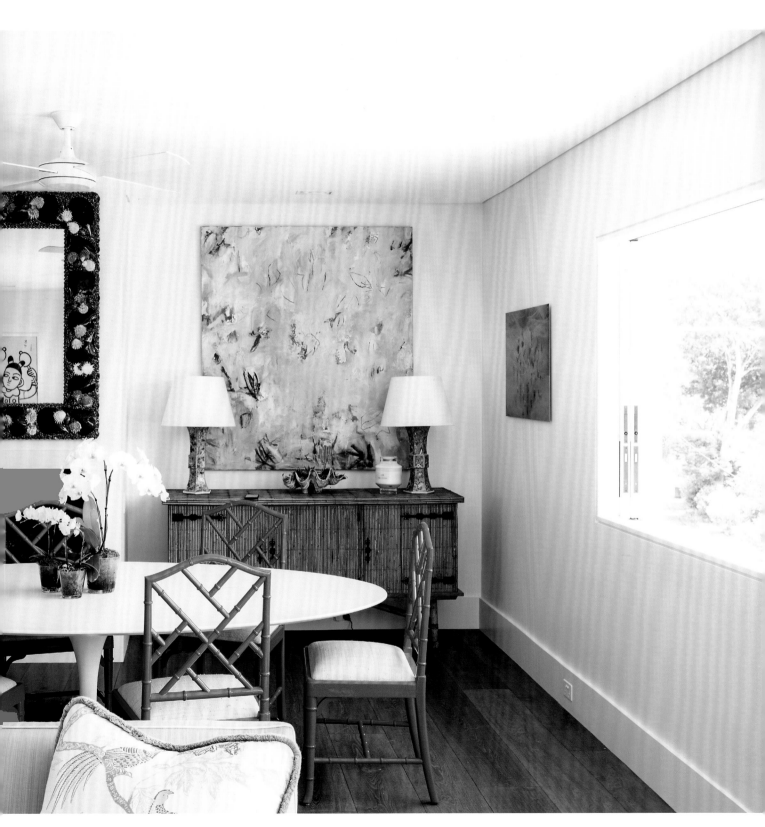

THE 5 DESIGN STEPS

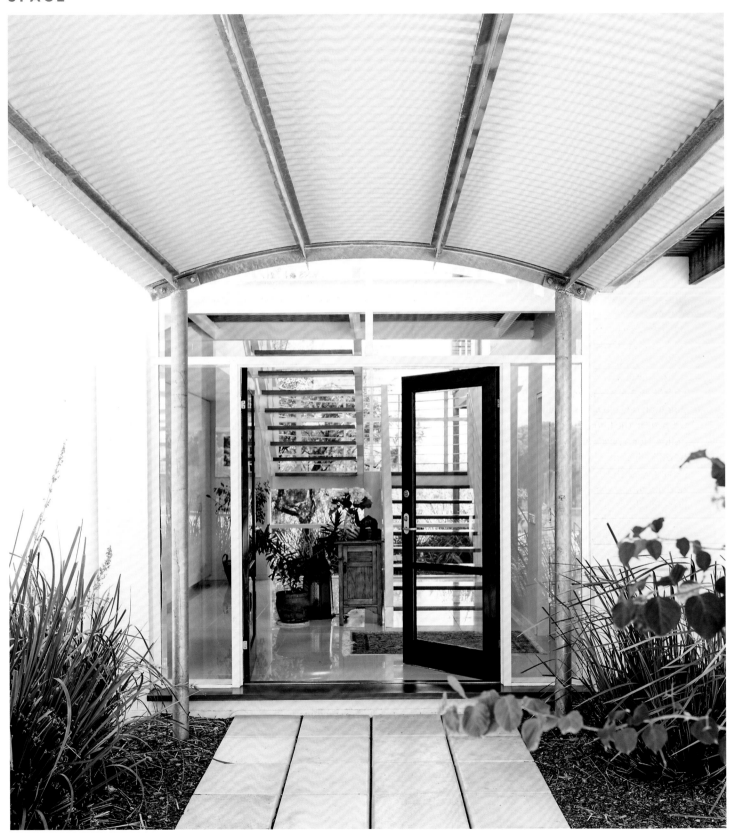

1 SPACE

*'The reality of the building does not consist of the roof and walls,
but the space within to be lived.'*

LAO TZU, PHILOSOPHER, AS QUOTED BY FRANK LLOYD WRIGHT, ARCHITECT

Space is any form of enclosure, and the quality of space is what makes a home good or bad. A house's first purpose is to form and contain spaces in which we shelter and make our home.

Everyone understands that a small room feels different to a large room; therefore everyone understands the basics of space. However, what is not as well understood are the techniques at our disposal to make one room seem different to another room of the same size, simply by manipulating elements that affect us spatially.

Space in the home is the sense of an area defined for a particular use. This can sometimes be difficult to identify... A kitchen space, for example, can be defined from a dining space, yet both might sit within an overall open-plan living area. On the other hand, a room with four solid walls and a door is easily identified as, say, a bedroom. Making sure the space you create is a quality space is essential for how you and your family will feel living in it. As you will see, the other design steps also play a large role in the quality of a space.

When I am designing a home I spend a huge amount of time thinking about how the space is going to work and feel. I always think in 3D. Even when I'm drawing a two-dimensional plan, I picture the space in three dimensions at all times. It's crucial to think in both the horizontal and the vertical, not to mention the diagonal! We generally move horizontally, due to gravity, but we are incredibly agile in how we see and perceive a space. We constantly move our line of sight and have a wide peripheral vision. Our natural tendency when moving is to have our gaze directed at some form of diagonal, up, down or sideways.

Some homes have spaces that feel very much as if they've been extruded from two-dimensional plans: 'Yep, the layout's right, now all we have to do is hit this button – the walls come up 2.5 metres and, hey presto, we have a home!' Well, it doesn't work like that, and such homes can feel bland.

Good-quality space relies on good-quality planning in all dimensions. Imagine a ceiling that opens upwards to capture a sky view; or a TV room where you go down a few steps into a cosy lowered couch; or climbing into a window seat in a wall to read a book. All these examples are about playing with the form of your space. Space can dramatically change how you feel. A high ceiling can be uplifting, or it can be cold. A low ceiling can be cosy, or it can be claustrophobic. It is good design that determines whether a space has good qualities or bad, and there are several key elements to consider.

FUNCTION

Function is the reason that something exists. A tap exists to deliver water: it does not have another job. When designing, we should always try to understand things in their most basic form. Once we understand the true function of the objects in our homes, we have a clearer idea of what to do with them, how to elaborate them, or even question whether we need them.

'Form follows function' is a famous principle usually associated with the Modernist school of architecture and design in the twentieth century. For example, a tap should deliver water and do nothing more, and thus should have no ornamentation whatsoever, only perform its primary function.

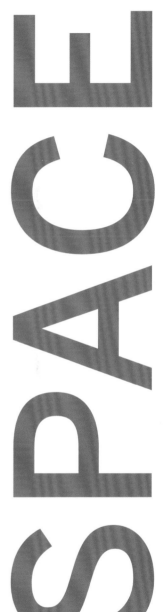

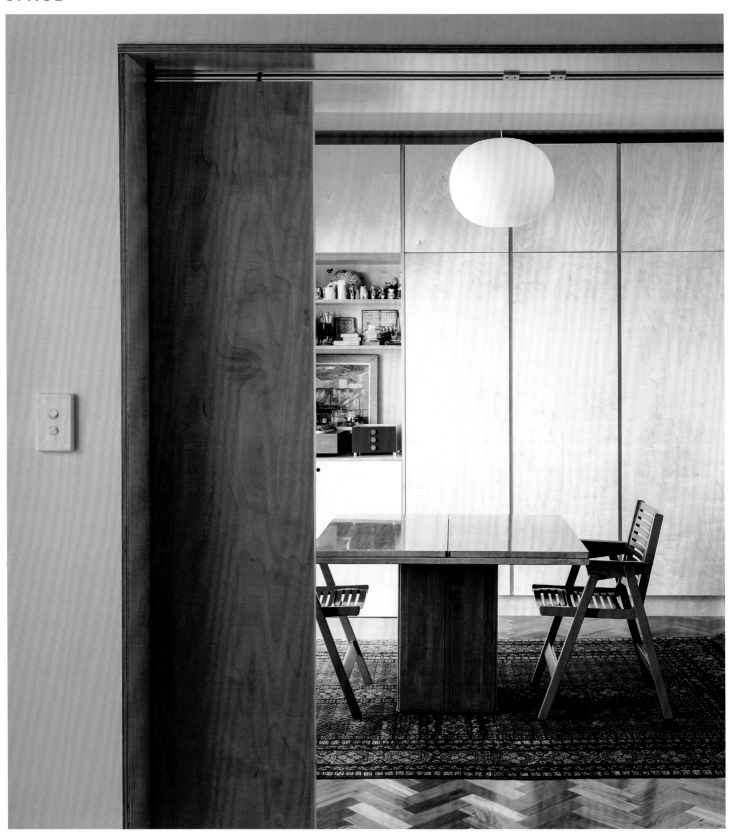

FLOW

Flow is how we move through our home. Does the design encourage or inhibit people's movement in the house? Does it create high-flow zones through spaces that should really be slower? For example, it is not great to have a high-traffic thoroughfare flowing between the TV and sofa, or the cooking area and the fridge.

ZONES

Zones are areas of a home that have a particular identity or function. They might be separated by walls, or they could be different spaces in a room, and they might even overlap. For example, a bedroom is a zone in itself, while an open-plan living area might have a number of zones, such as sofas, dining area and kitchen. These zones can be delineated by different floors, ceilings, finishes and furniture, but can also often overlap.

SYMMETRY

Symmetry is when a room or space is balanced as you look at it; when the elements that make up the room are similar parts facing each other or arranged equidistant on an axis. For example, noticing that two identical windows in a room are not positioned symmetrically can feel uncomfortable. We are basically (but not perfectly) symmetrical and so are many elements of nature, and thus we find symmetry comforting. However, sometimes going into a space that is too symmetrical can feel bland or 'too perfect'. Once you become confident in design, messing with symmetry can be great fun and very rewarding. (Or a disaster!)

PROPORTION

Proportion is one of the most important principles of good design. It is all about the visual relationship of objects and spaces: if something is too big or too small in relation to the overall space, then it feels uncomfortable and just 'looks wrong'. An example might be a huge front door on the front of an otherwise small house, or a really small rug in a large lounge room with big sofas and furniture. The door and the rug are out of proportion with the whole.

BALANCE

Nothing is comfortable when it is off balance, and the same goes for the home. This is not so much about symmetry as about weighting. So, if there is a heavy, dense-looking sofa on one side of a room, you might add some darker coloured built-in joinery on the other side, so that the space doesn't feel uncomfortably heavy and weighed down along one particular wall.

SCALE

Scale is all about the relative size of objects next to each other. The skyscraper rising up in a neighbourhood of single-storey homes is not in scale. Scale can be put to use to create impact. It is not an accident that cathedrals are gigantic spaces completely out of scale with human size: their vastness was intended to create a sense of awe and it works very effectively.

HERITAGE

Heritage in the home refers to the building or the objects within having some particular historical significance. Some buildings are protected by law to be preserved for the knowledge, record and enjoyment of future generations. Often, though, we use the term 'heritage' in design to refer to a certain period: for example, cornicing in a Victorian design would be considered a heritage look (even if it weren't original) compared to a square-set ceiling in a modern design.

It is always important to consider movement when designing spaces. How are spaces connected, how do we move through them, what is the journey, and how does that journey feel as we move through a home? So, when 'space' is referred to in this book, I am talking about the three-dimensional space of the room, and that can run in any direction.

You will see as we move through the five rooms in this book that we have some incredible inventions in our homes that help us enhance and control space, such as stairs, lifts, ramps, dormer windows, window seats, skylights, bifolds, sliding doors, screens, colour and light.

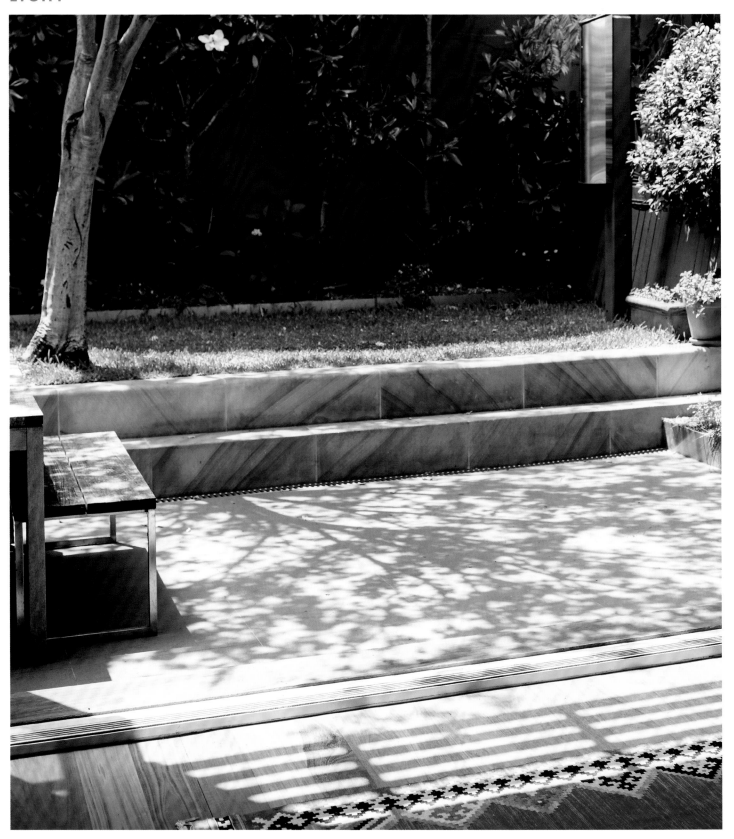

2 LIGHT

No matter how good your planning, materials and furniture, if your lighting is not good then you have nothing. One of the imperatives of human nature is to seek daylight. We need to capture and control daylight within the family home to promote health, happiness and joy.

The American architect Louis Kahn said 'a room is not a room without natural light'. Light is fundamental to our existence and our perception of the world. Natural light invigorates and sustains us, giving vital energy through the day.

Before artificial light technology, firelight was our only night option. We primarily wrapped our time around daylight hours, and early shelters reflected that: they were always open to the morning light to get us up and into the outdoors.

With the advent of the light bulb, human activities changed and now our days run well into the night. While that has been a boon for progress, increasingly we see related health issues around the world, and not only from lack of sleep: sometimes artificial light can be bad for us. We are creatures who have evolved under the best overhead light there is: the sun. The sun gives a full visual spectrum of light and our bodies' chemistry is geared to its cycle: our circadian rhythm. Not getting the right type of light at the right time can affect our health.

Unfortunately, in some jobs people are stuck under artificial light for very long periods. New high-quality LED technology is developing light sources with an increased spectrum of light and technologies that can reset the circadian rhythms of night-shift workers so that they can be productive even though there is no sun. This technology is spilling out into the consumer world, often accessed through smart phones.

Knowing that sunlight and artificial light is connected to our circadian rhythms and increasingly linked to our health, it is imperative that we get it right at home. If you have healthy lighting in your home, you will find that it is more lovely and liveable. It is about getting the right quality of light in the right spot, from ensuring there is sun on the breakfast table in the morning, to checking that your child has the right lighting to do their homework. Too much light can be an issue as well. Studies show that the darker your room is at night, the better your quality of sleep. So controlling light is the key.

Right now, we are lucky to have clever artificial lighting technology such as LED: a highly efficient light source, which is also able to produce literally millions of colours. It gives off next to no heat and, when coupled with a smart phone, can be a powerful asset in creating different environments and effects in your home. I use this technology in my home to let me create different moods and effects, as well as downloadable apps which turn my lights into disco lights for parties!

The three types of lighting you will read about in this book are:

AMBIENT LIGHTING which brings definition to the overall room.

ACCENT LIGHTING which can highlight an element of a room or create a particular effect – such as a spotlight on an artwork in the bathroom or an under-cupboard pelmet strip light to accentuate the kitchen splashback. It can be directional, or it can be decorative.

TASK LIGHTING is good-quality focused light that enables you to do jobs such as chopping vegetables in the kitchen, or applying makeup in the bathroom.

There are many clever technologies that can help with light in your home, such as windows, skylights, louvres, vegetation, shade, LED, mirror, sun tubes, diffusers and screens.

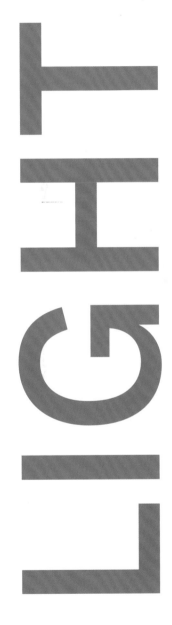

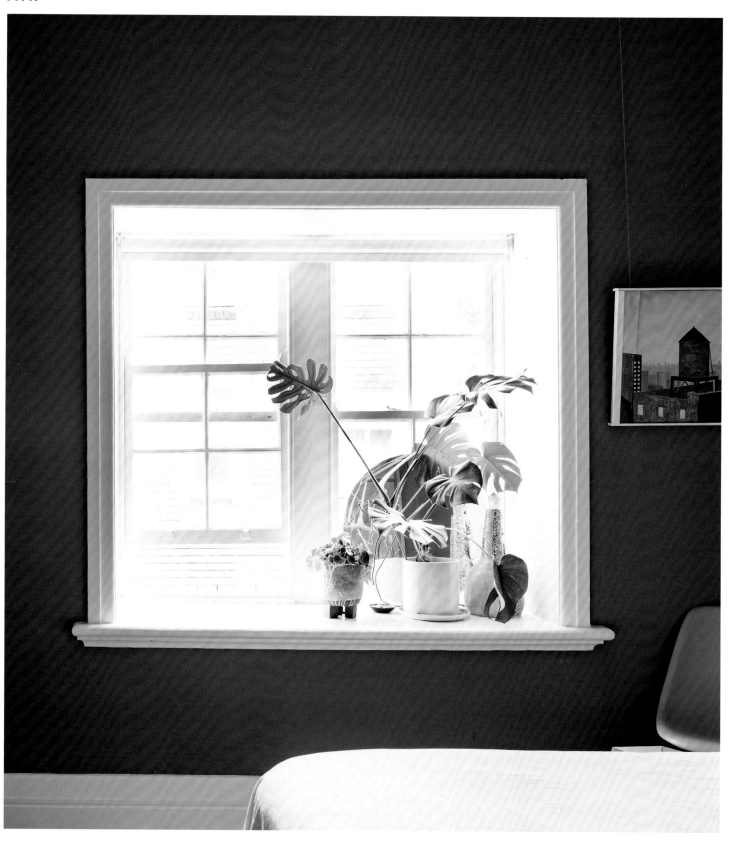

3 AIR

Air is one of the foundations of life and its quality is imperative for a healthy home. Stale air is to be avoided; keeping air fresh and moving is key to maintaining a comfortable home. The secret to good air quality is making sure that external air can pass through your home.

Cross-flow ventilation sounds complicated – but it isn't. It just means getting a breeze through your house. What's good about a breeze? Well, it cools you down in summer and freshens the air in the house, getting stale air out and fresh air in. Cool air prevents the need for an air-conditioner. If you want to save money on energy bills, design your home to take advantage of natural airflow.

Air flows in much the same way as water. If you let air in and want it to move, you have to ensure it has a place to exit. Air will move between entry and exit points as a positive and a negative.

It is easy to control air movement to make your day better. First, research the prevailing breezes of your neighbourhood. In Australia we tend to get summer breezes from the north to north east, and winter winds blow from south to south west. But, depending on the geography of your site and buildings, this might apply less than you assume.

Heating and cooling are also intrinsically linked to air, not only in terms of temperature but also in cooling effects, such as evaporation from air movement. The temperature of the air around us generally determines whether we feel warm or cold. The relatively temperate climate of some countries (such as here in Australia, where I'm writing) can be a blessing; however, in terms of our homes it has also been a curse. It has made us lazy. And it has made many of our buildings lazy. So many Europeans and North Americans have moved to 'sunny Australia' and never felt colder in their lives, because we don't build our homes to create proper shelter. In colder climates there would never be gaps under doors and around windows. There would never be large areas of single-glazed glass windows and doors, one of the worst places for temperature transfer. Walls and ceilings would be insulated and there would be central heating throughout the home. There is no point heating or cooling a home if the heat or cool escapes through porous walls. Australia is one of the biggest users of energy in heating and cooling homes because many haven't been built to capture the natural amenity of the location, namely sun and wind. Many homes are sieves that let the outside in and the inside out all too easily.

Hot air rises and cool air falls – and in some ways we need to protect against this and harness and use it. Consider installing skylights that can be opened to allow rising hot air to escape. This is sometimes referred to as an 'air chimney'. If you are clever you can use this rising hot air in the house to then draw cool air from a shaded spot into the house at a lower level. This is called the 'stack effect'. You can even create pools of cool water as an aesthetic device around the outside of the house – these create cool air that you draw inside by the stack effect, and then up and out of skylights in a sort of vertical cross-ventilation.

The skinnier a house, the easier it is to cool with cross-ventilation: air will cross the space easily without leaving any 'dead air' spots. The wider a house gets (fat house) the more difficult it is to cool, as more and more dead spots of air in the centre of the house are not pushed out and replaced with fresh air. In winter there will be a similar problem with cold and darkness, because the sun never gets far enough to warm the innermost areas. So, the slimmer your house, the easier it is to use elements of nature to heat and cool it. One reason air-conditioners are an absolute requirement for poorly designed project homes (sometimes called McMansions) is that they are large fat houses in every direction – this makes them impossible to heat and cool naturally.

There are many clever technologies to improve air in your home, such as windows, vents, skylights, louvres, air-conditioners, fans, deodorisers, heaters, coolers, pools, vegetation, shade and underfloor heating.

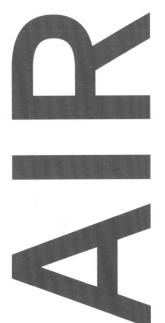

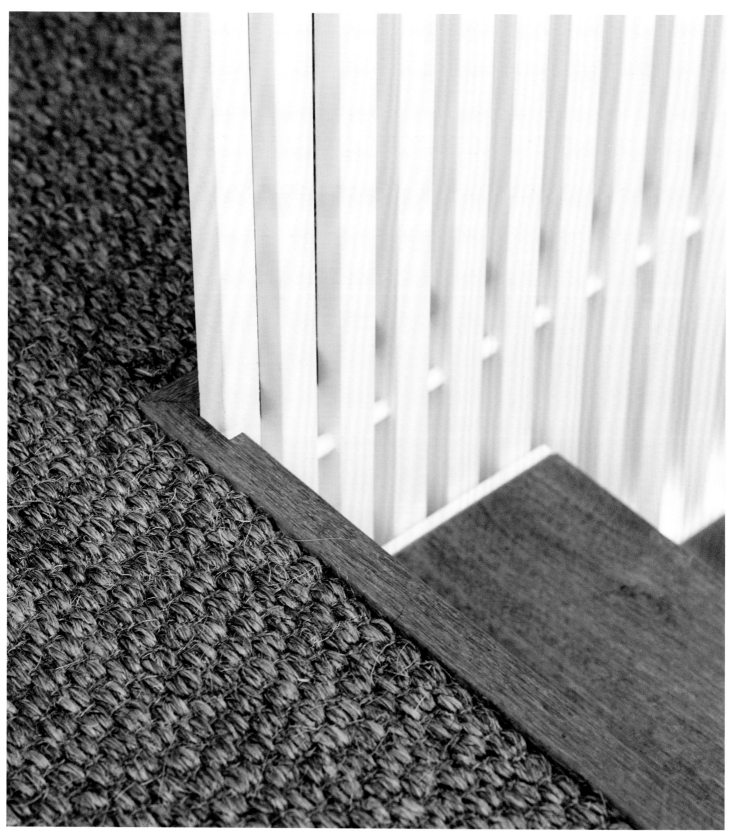

4 SOUND

Sound is often the most forgotten aspect of home design. Hearing is a crucial sense and it deeply affects how we perceive and enjoy a space. We often talk about how noisy a restaurant is, but rarely about how uncomfortably loud some spaces in our homes are. Ever been to a house where the only thing you can hear are the click-clack of shoes echoing on the floors? I remember taking off my shoes in some houses because I felt self-conscious about how much noise I was making.

When you have spent time in a space that you considered to be sophisticated, I guarantee that a big part of that experience is that it sounded good. If a space echoes badly and is full of clatter it will feel unsophisticated. A lot of time is spent on hospitality projects ensuring the acoustics create a comforting sound. We are now bringing that same concern into the home. Clever use of acoustic materials can radically change how sophisticated your home feels — how cosy, and how welcoming. Also, when we are thinking about sound, we consider separation and connection, depending on how much we want a space to be public or private. Private for the bathroom, for example – but public for the kids' play area that we want to hear from the kitchen.

We will talk about the many clever technologies that can help with the sound quality of a home, such as acoustic materials, sound systems, baffles, acoustic walls, ceilings, upholstery, books and fabrics.

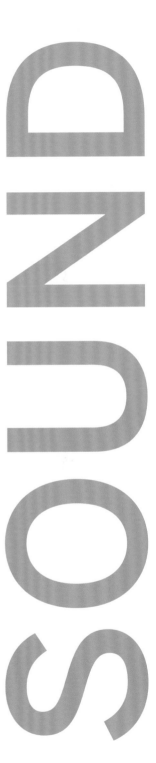

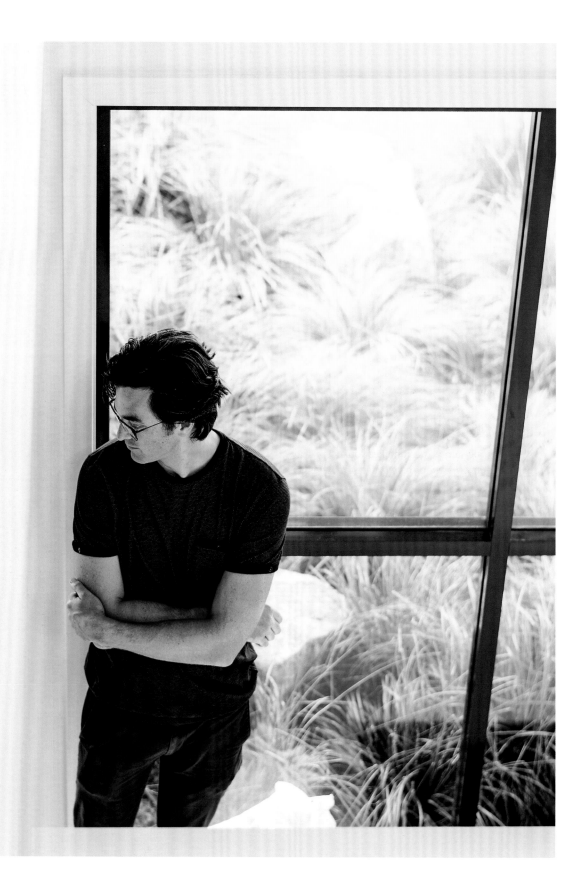

5 VIEW

The pace of life is so rapid today that we need refuge more than ever, and our homes have to provide that. The famous British geographer Jay Appleton wrote about the concept of 'refuge' and 'prospect', discussing the theory that humans feel most comfortable in a space that is a 'refuge', overlooking a view that is 'prospect'. An example is a cave on a hill overlooking a plain, or a shelter at the edge of woodland overlooking a meadow. In both these examples, humans are nestled into a contained space with protection from the sides and rear, and with an uninhibited view across a large landscape that allows them to see any potential incoming threats.

It sounds primitive, but what it really means in a home is relaxation and privacy. You can relax better when you can easily see and take stock of your surroundings, while feeling protected and safe at the same time. It makes you feel private and in control when you can see someone approaching your home, yet they can't see you.

This theory has focused on the internal to the external view; however, I would like to extend it inside the home as well. There are many instances when we create views in the home for privacy and control, but also for enjoyment. You might not have a million-dollar view but it is remarkably easy to create a quality view with clever design that uplifts and makes you feel like the king or queen of your particular castle. A sheltered nook to overview your space? A dining room chair that has the best view in the house – over the table, across the lounge, through the window, into the garden and to the lush frangipani and sky beyond? Now that is a view; compared to a dining room chair that has you contemplating a wall.

We will talk about the many clever technologies that can help you with the view in your home, such as windows, doorways, skylights, louvres, mirrors, screens, pools, vegetation and shade.

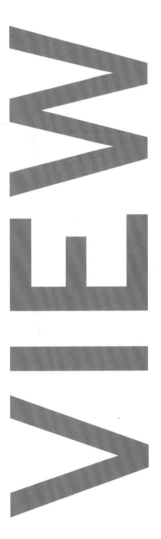

THE 5
ROOMS

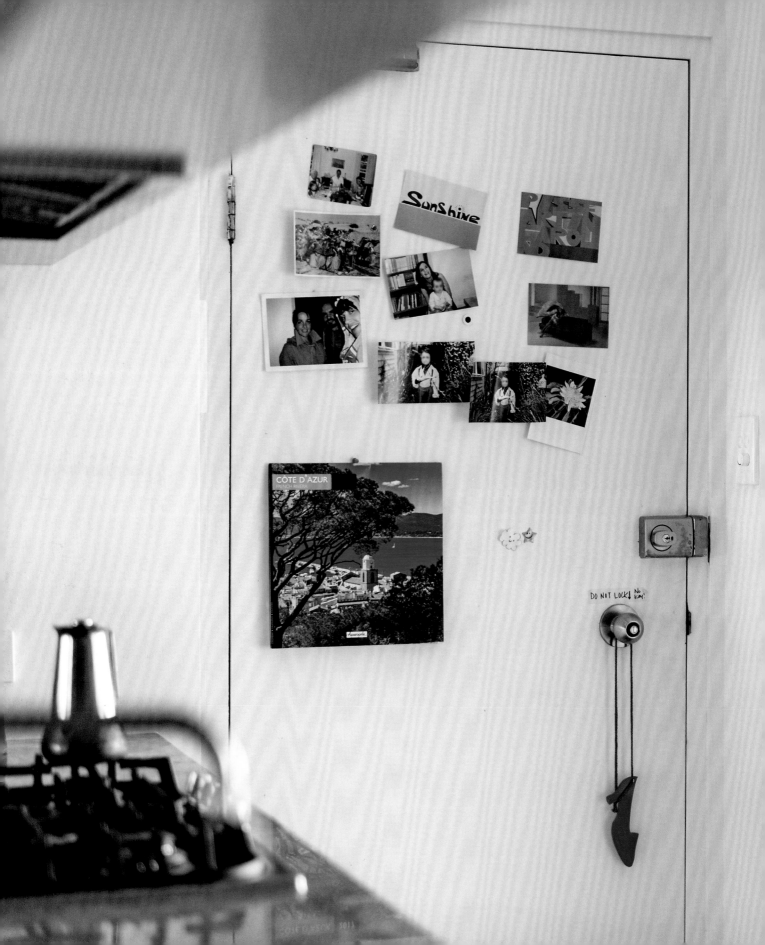

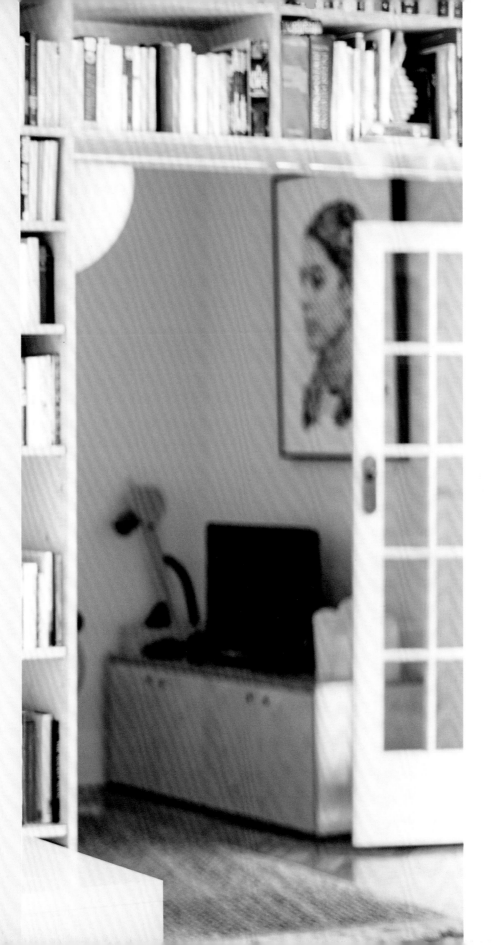

CHAPTER ONE

ENTRY

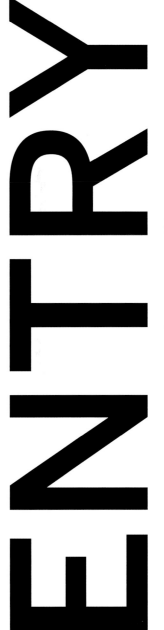

THE ENTRY TO YOUR HOME sets the tone for the whole house, for your guests and also for you and your family. They say you never get a second chance to make a first impression and it is the same for your entry. How the entry space welcomes you is an opportunity to control the introduction to the next series of spaces and experiences in your home.

An entry is primarily about shelter. It is about the transition from outside to inside. It is the point where we cross the threshold from a tough exterior world into the safety, shelter and comfort of the home; the place where we are protected from external elements, such as weather and predators. Finding a place of shelter is deep within our evolutionary make up, and in popular culture we often use that primeval need to trigger emotion. Think of all the movies that have an entry sequence into a house, which foreshadows the quality of the home and the expected welcome beyond. Is there a guiding light, escape from a snowy blizzard, the hanging up of coats and the taking off of boots? Now you're in a safe place. Or is it a cold dark entry, where there is no answer to the bell that echoes inside, and no welcome? The future is not looking safe or bright, and we all know what's coming.

Once we have the shelter aspect of entry sorted, then we can consider the aesthetic and how we introduce the rest of the home. No one will be enjoying your coastal shell collection in the hall if they are stuck battling with a flimsy front door that's being blown around by the afternoon southerly wind.

Interestingly, an entry is one of the few spaces in a house where no one is invited to spend an extended period of time. It is a transition space. The two key roles of the entry are to be a place of welcome and to be highly functional. The following space, light, air, sound and view steps will systematically show you how to achieve these two key roles, whether your project is a new build, a renovation or an easy fix.

SPACE

In Europe there is always allowance on house plans for an entry, with space to remove jackets and hang them, and to remove shoes and stow them away; and not only for the inhabitants of the house, but also for guests. It is very welcoming to have a clear space to stow your belongings when you're visiting someone's house; you're then able to move into the rest of the home unburdened and ready to engage in hellos and conversation.

In apartments the primary entry is often straight off the street and is a shared space. An important part of apartment design today is to get the communal entry right, and an ever-increasing percentage of the budget is given to the apartment lobby. Developers know that this entry space sets the tone for the whole building, particularly for potential buyers, who are greatly influenced by the entry that will greet them and

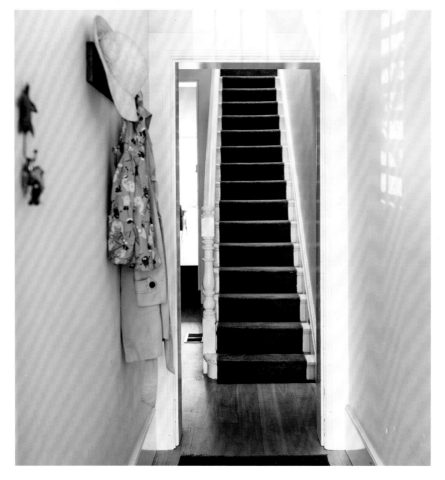

▼ Even in a small entry, some simple coat hooks are practical, while also making a difference to the sense of home. The rug here is welcoming and ties in with the stair carpet beyond.

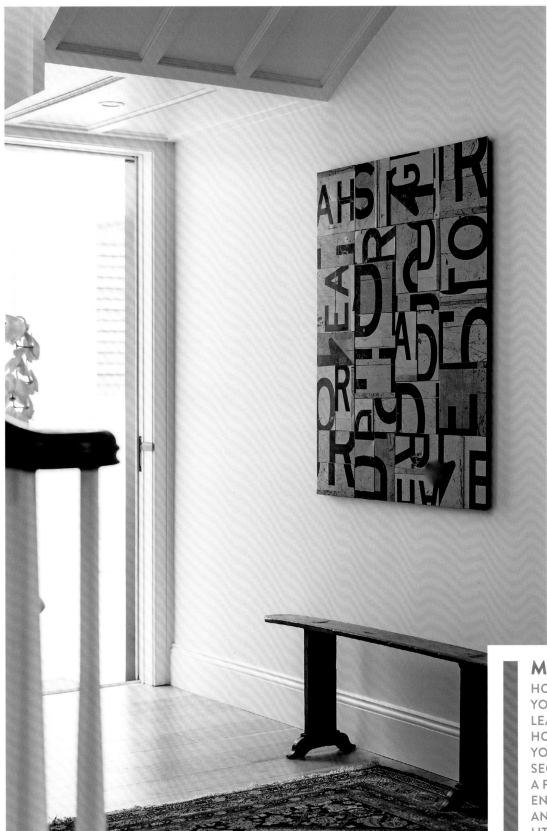

◁ This combination of artwork and bench is a lovely gesture. The bench is a courtesy — somewhere to put on or take off shoes, or just set down your bags. The artwork is a statement to the taste and character of the home owners.

MUST DON'T

HOWEVER MINIMALIST YOUR LIFESTYLE, TRY NOT TO LEAVE THE ENTRY OF YOUR HOME BARE AND SOULLESS. YOU DON'T EVER GET A SECOND CHANCE TO MAKE A FIRST IMPRESSION. YOUR ENTRY IS THE PLACE TO GIVE AN INTRODUCTION TO – A LITTLE PEEK INTO – YOUR HOME AND PERSONALITY.

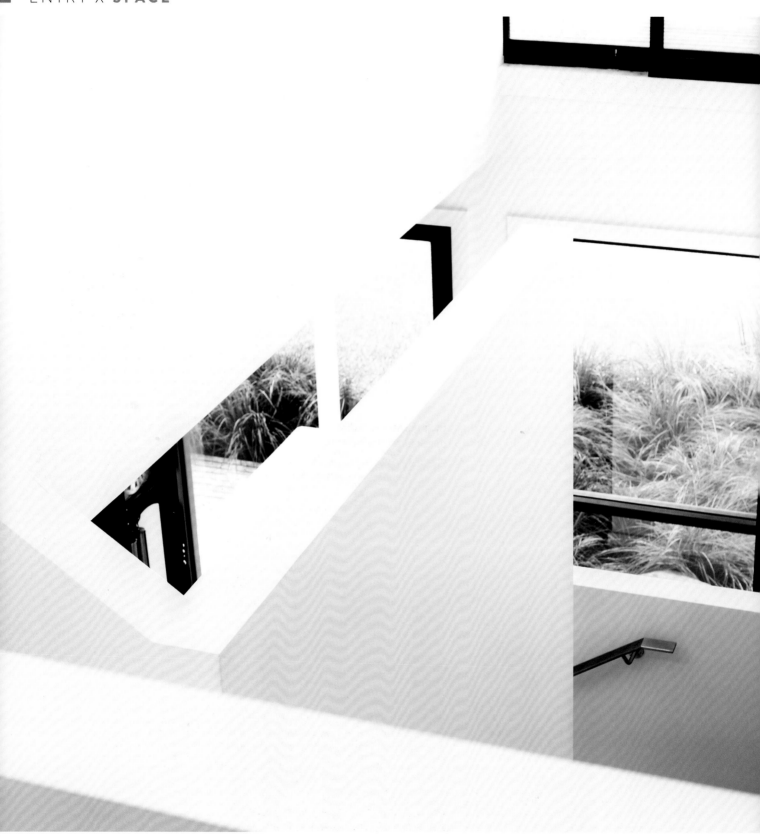

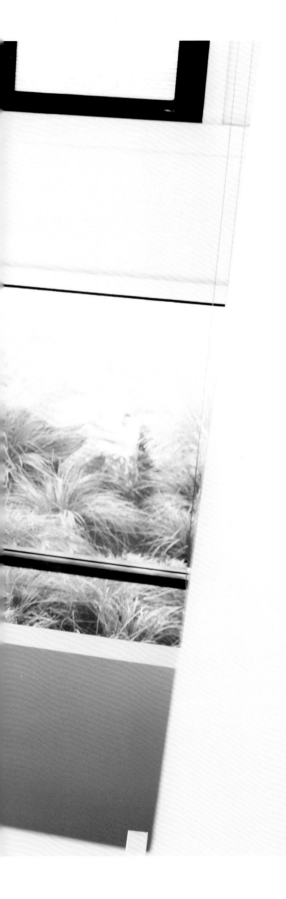

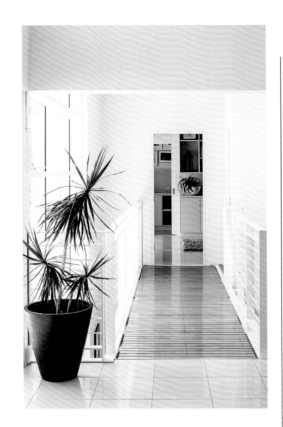

◀◀ In your entry, think in three dimensions. If you have the chance, invite people to look up as they come in. Incorporating a stairwell can be an excellent device to create a dynamic entry, as well as a piece of practical planning. Added bonuses in this home are light and airflow, as well as the opportunity to easily look down and connect with people in the entry.

◀ This home has a bridge leading from the entry stairs, which enhances the light and sense of space. Always more interesting than a hallway, a bridge is a great connector between areas of the home.

their guests every day. We should bring that developers' discovery to our house plans. The entry is crucial in setting the tone, and planning this first impression is important. The interesting thing about the entry to an apartment is that it is semi-private; you only have real privacy once you are in the apartment. In a house the entry is only public in as much as it is seen from the street.

DEDICATED ENTRY SPACE

A dedicated entry space allows control. The key principle is to allow entry into the home but not expose the home unnecessarily. At the moment of entry, privacy is a two-way street: the occupant doesn't want to be unexpectedly revealed lying on the sofa in their night-time finest; and the person arriving is not ready to be seen either, perhaps laden with shopping bags, coats and windswept hair. It is pleasant to unload in privacy rather than become visual entertainment for the occupants as you struggle out of your coat. For the guest, it is simply bad manners to put them in a position where they feel they are intruding, when they have no intention of doing so. Some form of privacy is required, in particular visual privacy. Acoustic privacy is often not as important.

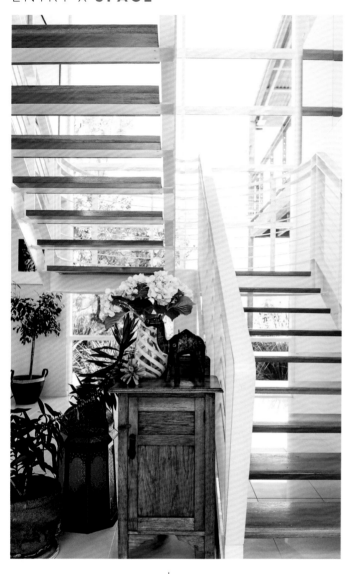

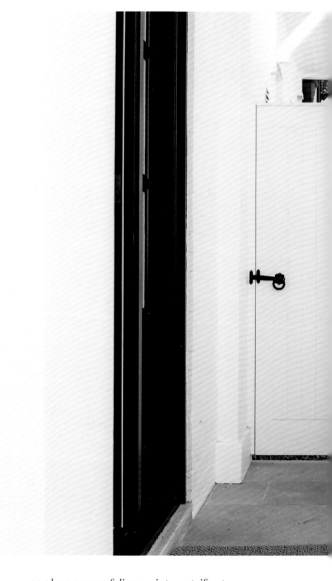

I would definitely class this as an 'uplifting' entry, with its two-storey, light-filled space that draws the eye upwards. The open-tread stairs are perfect for emphasising the light.

PERFECT PROPORTIONS

By its very definition, an entry is leading to somewhere else and therefore it is never an island. It must relate to the spaces beyond both in terms of style and proportion. It would feel mean if the entry to a large spacious home were too small, and ridiculous if the entry to a compact home were bloated and inefficient compared to the rest of the house. Similarly, if you have a heritage home, it would not be comfortable to arrive through an uber-minimalist and modern entry. Your entry should reflect not only your character and the first impression you want to give to guests, but also the proportion of the home beyond. Some homes I have visited seem to have gone too far in making a grand entry: there

can be a sense of disappointment, if not incredulity, as you move into the rest of the house. We humans are very good at picking up on false grandiosity, so don't set off on the wrong foot. It is far more interesting to gain an insight into the occupants of the house through simple charm rather than big statements, and it makes for a more friendly welcome.

UPLIFTING OR COSY?

Once you have considered the proportion of your home, imagine how you want to feel as you enter. I like to define an entry as either 'uplifting' or 'cosy'. If you want to feel uplifted and have the room, then consider a two-storey space; maybe include the stairwell of the house to create a

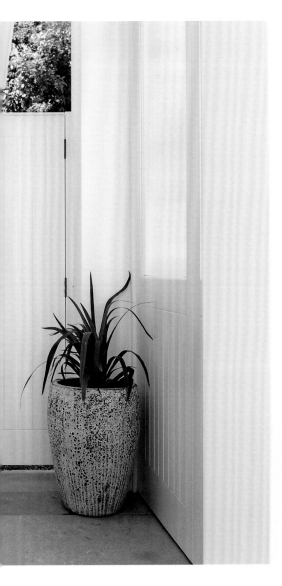

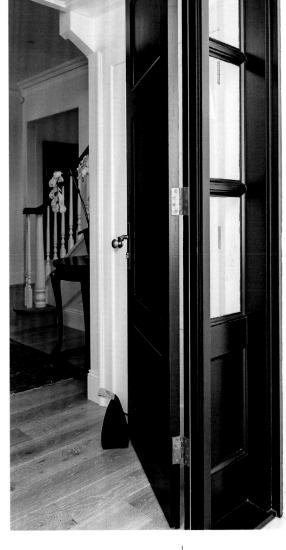

functional sculpture that signals vertical movement through to the house beyond. Decorate in lighter, refreshing tones; ensure the upper reaches, in particular, are clean and white.

If you prefer a cosier entry, think horizontally, with a single-storey entry and the introduction of skirting boards, dado rails, picture rails and cornices. Between the skirting and dado rail, add wallpaper or other textures, such as painted pressed metal, to add pattern and charm to the cosiness of the space – and to 'earth' it.

FIRST IMPRESSIONS

You, and your family, use your entry more than anyone else. You should feel happy walking through the door, as if you were arriving to a friendly embrace. Impressing a visitor must always come second to that. Familiarity is the key. When you arrive at the entry it needs to feel like home, not like an emotionless vestibule before you get to the real thing.

Your entry space is the interface, the threshold, between the outside world and your private home. Think of it as a space to commence your journey, an opportunity to introduce the personality of you and your home. If you are a mad fan of cacti, then why not introduce that passion into your entry. Or a wonderful singular piece of art? Don't overdo it – give your visitors a taste but don't overload them. While you want to set the mood, your entry is a first impression not only for your guest but also for you – every day.

◀◀ The entry of your home is the face it presents to the outside world. Interestingly, it is one of the few spaces in a house where no one is expected to spend an extended period of time. It is a transition space.

▲ The two key roles of an entry are to be a place of welcome — both for the home owners and for visitors — and to be highly functional.

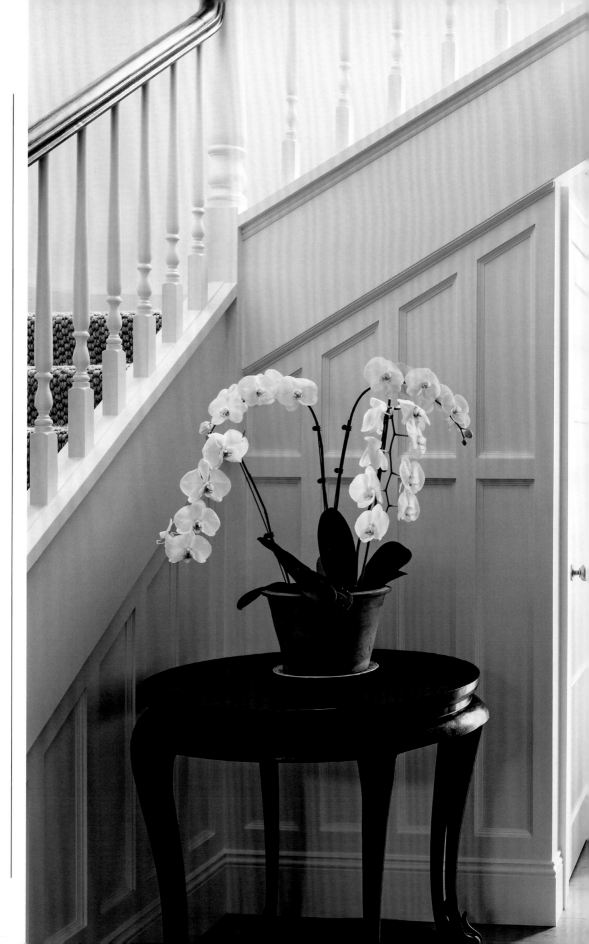

▶ This classic entry combines a stairwell with the main hallway of the house. Not only is this practical in a planning sense, but it gives an opportunity for a sense of grandeur in the entry, through the combination of sculptural stairs, a two-storey space and the resulting light and airflow.

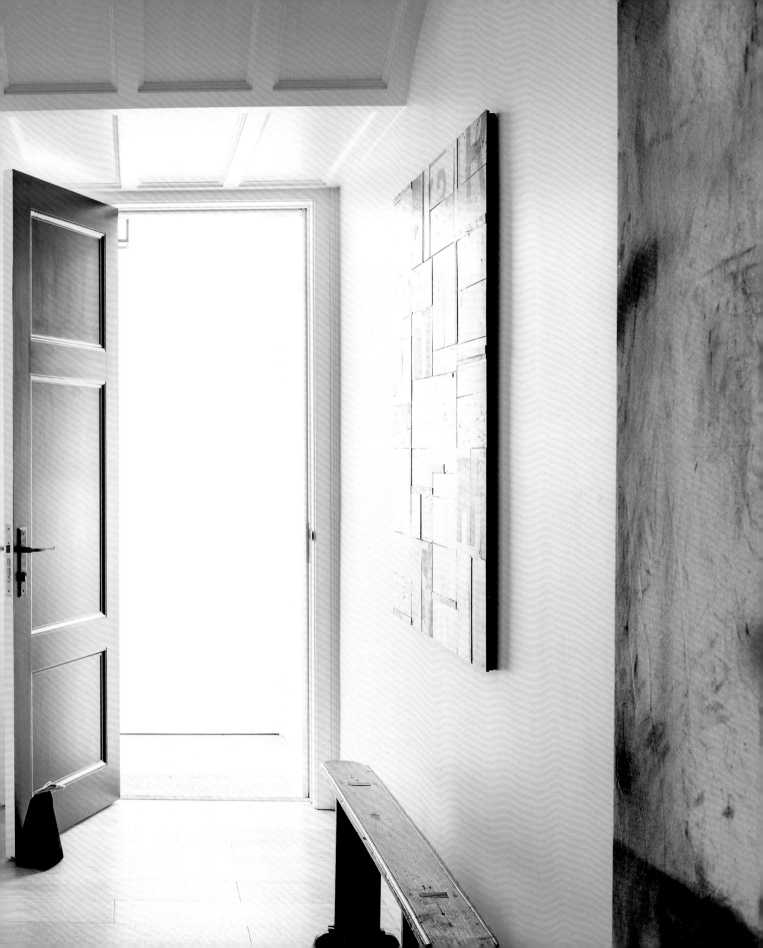

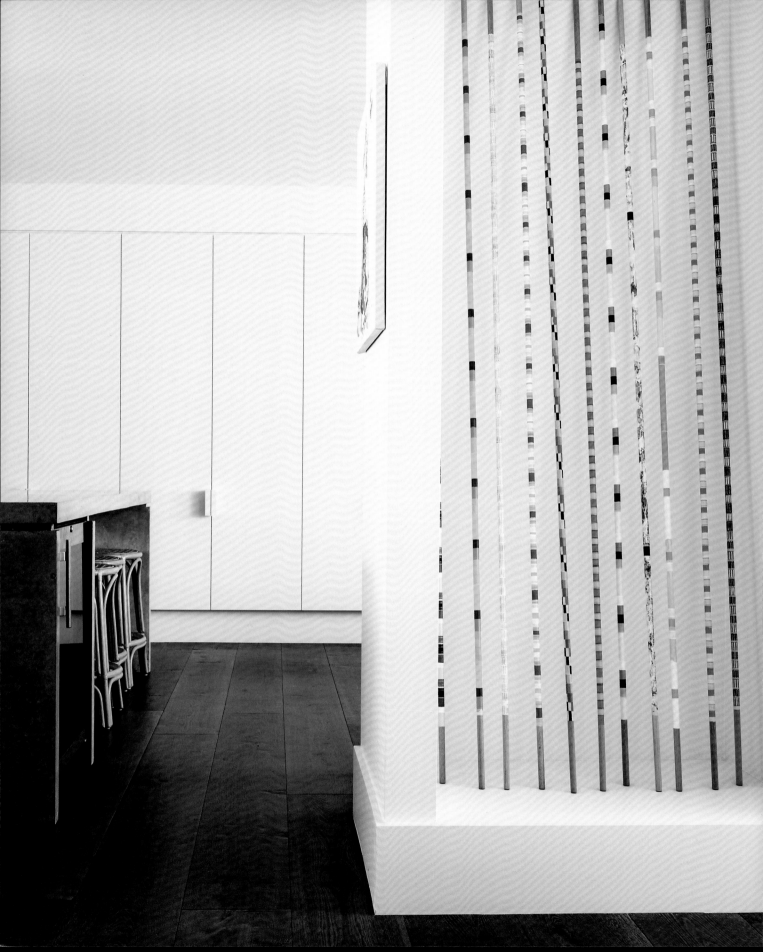

So, don't clutter the space – you don't want to feel and appear disorganised and dysfunctional – and you don't want to walk into chaos every night!

An entry space is an opportunity to show items that have been or will be passed down through the generations. Start a tradition: find something that will be in the entries of your family's homes in the future. Hang a family portrait, or a favourite artwork or heirloom. My grandmother had an ornate drawing room console from her mother's home. It was always a piece of history I enjoyed as I entered her home, and it meant a lot. An entry should be a little bit inspiring and tell a story.

ROOMS OFF THE ENTRY

If I have the opportunity, I include a mud room off the entry: this is important in a farmhouse or a country house with a larger garden and allows you to be rid of muddy boots, dirty shoes and wet coats before going into the clean part of the house. You can store all your outdoor gear, including coats, gumboots and even tools, in a mud room. A sink is always a great addition.

If you are locating a study or home office, it makes good sense to have this leading off the entry. The entry is often quite a quiet part of the house: no one spends any time there, so there are no TVs or radios playing. It has good access to couriers, and if you have meetings or staff it allows them to come and go without entering the main part of the house.

A guest powder room also works well off the entry, as it is a public part of the house but relatively private as most activity is occurring elsewhere. It is an easy place to locate for guests, as they have already passed through the entry on the way in, and means they don't have to go into the private parts of your house. Also I have found that if the powder room is located near the entry it is often used a lot more by the occupants of the house, either leaving or coming home from work or school, or simply as the nearest loo if they are gardening or playing soccer in the front yard.

CREATING AN ENTRY FROM PART OF AN EXISTING ROOM

While having a separate entry room is the ideal situation, if you are in an existing house or apartment where this isn't possible, there are other design options available to you. If you have a front door that opens directly into the living room, what are your options?

SMALL-SCALE BUILDING TO MAKE AN ENTRANCE

You can create, in effect, a short hallway by partially enclosing the area around the front door on two sides. The key here is to create enough space to allow for storage and the practicality of unloading as you enter your home. There needs to be room for a console and coat racks or hooks.

If you have an in-wall hall closet near the front door, consider removing this and using the space to form an entry alcove to support your dedicated entry. Embellish the newly formed alcove with shelves, practical compartments and racks, as well as a burst of colour to define the entry.

◀ This specially designed raised gallery space was created to house a bright artwork. It greets everyone when they reach the top of the entry stairs.

▼ White timber slats travel vertically through the house to veil the staircase. This is a clever aesthetic device that also allows for good transfer of light and air.

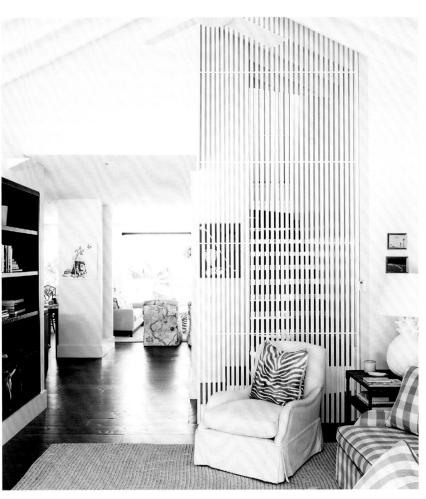

▷ An entry can be small — no more than just a door. This one has been defined by a collection of postcards (a metaphorical window to the world beyond) and an adjacent column of practical storage.

▷▷ The white timber slats connect the entry across three floors, linking even to the spaces at the top of the house.

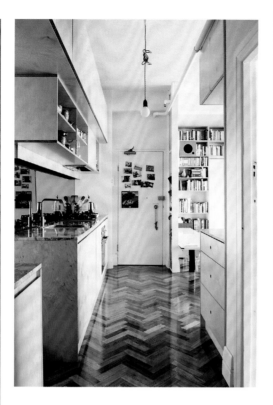

If putting in full-height walls to create an entry space will encroach too much on the living area, consider a half-height wall. The key here is to make sure the half wall is not flimsy, or it won't ever truly feel like part of the house. Consider building a column up to the ceiling at the end of the half-height wall; this gives a feeling of stability and also creates a 'window' from the living room, which will create the sense of an entry. This is also a great opportunity to add some architectural ornamentation to the entry area, with cornicing and fenestration (installing a window). This will ensure that the half wall feels as if it's meant to be there.

For a less walled-in solution, consider installing floor-to-ceiling or half-height joinery shelves. The joinery can form an entry area and can be as private or see-through as you like. Fill it with books and ornaments and allow gaps for some connection between the two spaces. You can even design the joinery to be accessed from both the entry area and the living room. This solution can be less overbearing than a solid wall and there is also something very friendly about a wall of books at the front door.

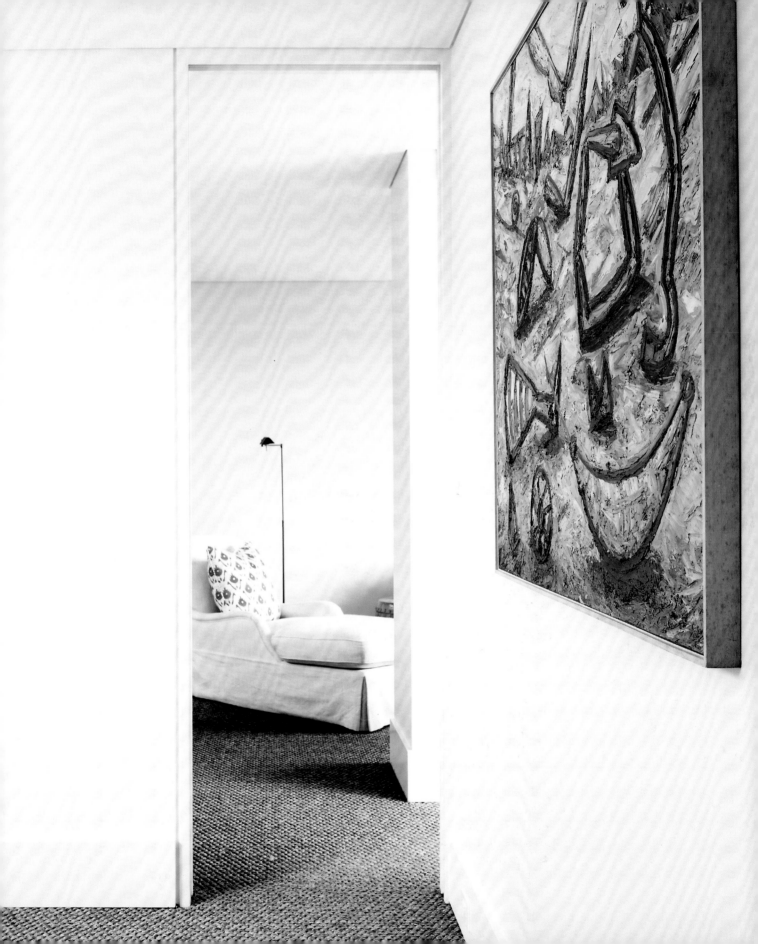

SMART HOME

TODAY'S HOME CAN BE PROGRAMMED WITH A 'COMING HOME' EVENT TO SENSE YOUR APPROACH, UNLOCK THE FRONT DOOR, TURN ON THE LIGHTS AND HEATING, AND SWITCH ON THE TV TO YOUR FAVOURITE EVENING NEWS! IF YOU ARE IN THE CAR IT WILL OPEN THE GARAGE DOOR.

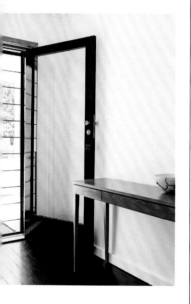

▲ A clear-glazed black framed door with a steel security gate is a good combination that allows for vision, airflow and safety, as well as sleek good looks. The lovely console desk sets the aesthetic tone for the home.

MAKING AN ENTRANCE WITH FURNITURE

If there is simply no opportunity in your room to fit in a wall or joinery, then you can use your furniture to create a sense of a separated entry. Position the back of a long sofa or two armchairs to form an entry area. Even better, run a slim sideboard/sofa table along the back of the furniture on the entry side. This instantly becomes an entry console and a practical solution for keys and shoes, as well as an opportunity to show off some ornaments.

Find a special piece of storage furniture that is designed to accompany the front door only and it will form a sense of entry, and, of course, it is useful for all your things as you arrive home. Add a clock and mirror on the wall and a free-standing coat rack inside the corner of your door and you have a dedicated space.

At the very least, hinge the front door so that it swings into the living room, giving some privacy as the door swings open. This also blocks sight lines into the room when you open the door to someone outside.

MAKING AN ENTRANCE WITH FLOORING

To further define the entry space, consider using a different floor finish to the rest of the living room. This is practical, too, as the floor finish to an entry needs to be easy to clean. Hard surfaces are the way to go – carpet is not. Consider tiles, timber or polished concrete. Practically speaking, people need to wipe their shoes as they enter; I find myself doing this as a gesture of courtesy even if I don't feel that my shoes are dirty. Consider installing a recessed door mat inside the front door; there is something very practical about a mat and just by its material it defines the entry space.

A quick fix to creating a sense of entry is a floor rug at the front door. It can have a very positive effect of defining the space but also make a friendly gesture of welcome. Depending on the floor plan, consider a longer runner; this can give a sense of creating a hall, even when the 'hall' is not defined by walls. A runner is also directional and helps to channel people where you want them to travel. A guest will rarely depart from the direction of a hall runner and will follow its lead. By its direct connection with the outside world, an entry will receive more dirt than other rooms; it would be disappointing if your rug or runner became the surrogate door mat that everyone wiped their feet on – another reason to have a good stiff welcome mat either inside or outside the front door. Store a secret dustpan and brush in the area for quick clean-ups.

FUNCTIONAL ENTRY FURNITURE

Arriving home is a transition from the outside world to the inside. The entry becomes the space for that transition. As it is one of the few spaces in the home where no one is expected to spend any extended time, it can afford to be more practical than anything else. There are generally three types of arrivals – the house occupants coming home, guests arriving for a visit and those who are not going to move beyond the entry, such as couriers or service people.

For the residents, a sequence of zoning is very important to allow a comfortable welcome home. You need to be able to unload all your 'stuff of the day' and not trudge it through the house. Shedding the items of the day and walking into the rest of the house with a literal weight off your shoulders is a great feeling.

Make a comprehensive list of what each householder does as they arrive home. For me, it would be to drop the keys, then the bag, then the jacket, then shoes and then I go into the rest of the house. If you don't provide space for each of these items, you are going to find a big pile of stuff at your front door – especially when the kids get home from school. Any good entry needs to cater for all these items, so design into your entry a tray or shelf for keys, phones and wallets, a series of lower level hooks or a large deep shelf for bags, a series of hooks or a cupboard for coats, hats and scarves, and a low rack for outdoor shoes.

Provide somewhere for umbrellas and raincoats too; it is always embarrassing to place a dripping umbrella in a corner and then see the puddle it has formed when you come back to it.

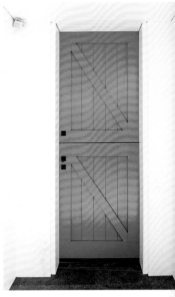

△ These bright orange stable doors can be fully opened or half opened, giving flexibility and character to this home. With the top half of the door open, the house has a great connection to the outdoors, while still being secure for small children.

◁ White vertical panelling runs down the wall and then projects out to take in a practical bench and set of storage drawers. Importantly for this clean, white, uncluttered aesthetic, there are no handles on the drawers, which instead use push–catch latches. The beach artworks speak of the location of the home and taste of the owners.

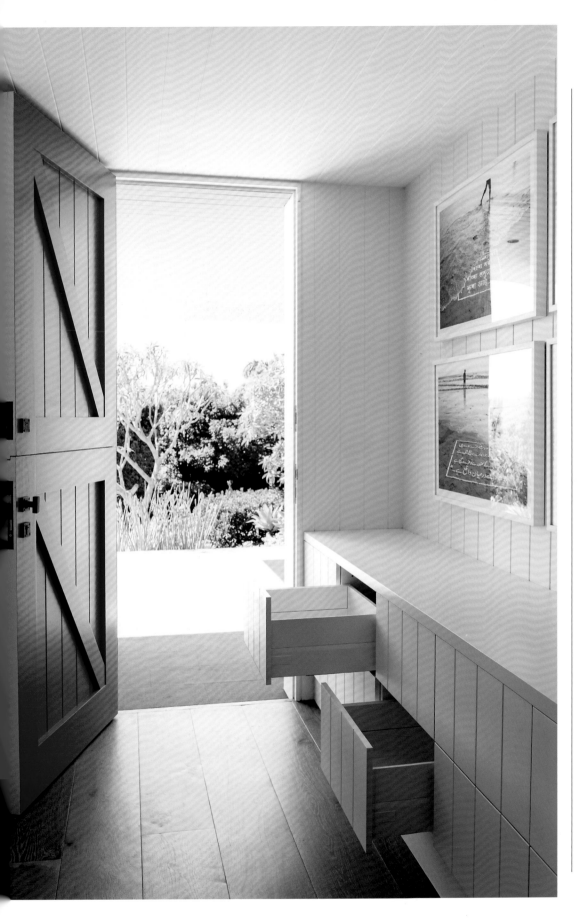

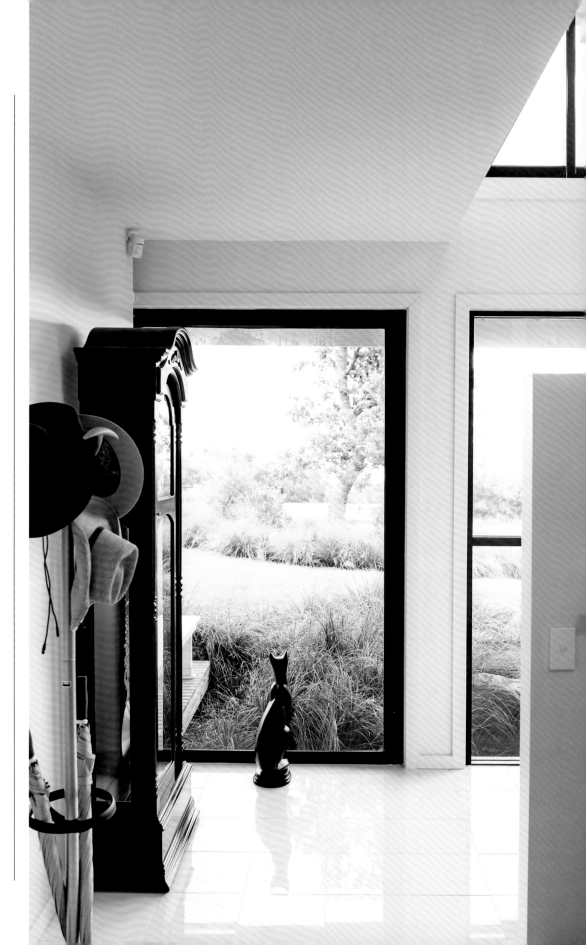

▶ This entry houses a family
heirloom — the grandfather
clock — and sets the scene for
those who enter. The window
frames the outside world. (And
the quirky, elegant cat seems
to be enjoying the view.)

A shoe rack is also great – especially if it is muddy or wet outside – to lift shoes off the entry floor, so you don't feel you are making the floor dirty.

When I'm designing a new home, I create an alcove for all these items – the placement of each needs to reflect the entry sequence of coming home. Each has their own space – a series of cupboards, shelves, hooks and racks, designed around what the family is happy to have on show or prefers to keep hidden. We are usually happy to see coats and scarves hanging up, but prefer to hide away untidy piles of family shoes.

Do be careful where you keep your keys! When I was living in London there was a spate of burglaries where fishing rods were poked through letterboxes to hook keys that were traditionally on a hook near the front door. That tradition went out the door pretty quickly (along with all the other household goods). Store your keys out of sight.

COAT HOOKS

One of the lovely things about arriving home is to see whose coats are already hanging on the coat hooks. You automatically look along the rack and mentally note who is home, then, as you move into the rest of the house, you are already formulating your conversations with those inside. This feeling is quintessential to the sensation of arriving home, and something I am very conscious of when I design entry spaces.

Ensure that you allow for your guests to feel welcome and comfortable, too: dedicate a couple of coat hooks and some space on the shoe rack – hanging your coat on top of someone else's can feel uncomfortable if you aren't a member of the family or close friend.

If you find someone is consistently leaving a bag or other item on the floor in the same spot every day, then put a hook there. It solves a problem and sometimes it is easier to follow the nature of your home and the people within it.

BENCH SEAT

If you expect visitors to take off their shoes when they enter the house (which I think is a good idea) then you must provide a seat or bench so that they can do so with some elegance. A top-notch entry would never be without a bench to sit on;

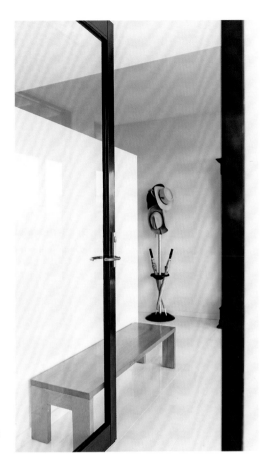

The unfussy bench and hat stand match the clean feel of this space, while adding a practical touch of welcome.

at the end of the day it is just good manners to provide that. It is embarrassing, and sometimes difficult for older people, to hop around an entry space battling with a shoe. If you are not hopping, then you are bent over or crouched – all inelegant and all uncomfortable. Then again, you could sit on the floor...

A bench seat in the entry hall is simply a friendly gesture; it literally invites the person arriving to have a seat and take a load off their feet. It also gives you a great opportunity to inject some personal style into the space. A cushioned bench can add colour and a sense of sophistication. While a rough timber bench has a rustic charm.

CONSOLE TABLE

A console table is often one of the first pieces that you or a guest encounters when entering a home.

MUST DO

SEE YOUR COAT AND BAG HOOKS AS MORE THAN JUST STORAGE; INSTEAD, DESIGN THEM AS A VISIBLE CALLING CARD OF WHO IN THE FAMILY IS ALREADY HOME. IT IS ALL PART OF THE COMFORTING FEELING OF ARRIVING HOME.

With a console table I always say, if you are going to have one, then make sure it's worth presenting to the world. This is an opportunity to present style, character and a bit of your story, and could be a period piece or something modern and finely crafted. You have the opportunity to decorate it with a vase, fresh flowers, or some elegant stationery. But don't put too many things on it – remember it is also a practical place to sign for parcels and papers or courier forms and put down the post.

This is the place where you have mini-meetings, with couriers or delivery people, and it is less confronting to have a table to work on when engaging with a stranger (it is less 'front on'). If you don't want these meetings to intrude into your private space, the entry is the most comfortable place to conduct them. In many houses, especially for those who are particularly concerned with security, we design a door separating the entry from the rest of the home. That way you can secure your home behind you as you answer the front door.

You might even want to put a small meeting table and chairs in the entry for a more formal short conversation. This happens in larger entries and can be a great asset if you have a home office. It is also an opportunity to bring some lovely pieces of furniture and style into the space. If you have the room, a table, chairs, vase with flowers and a rug will create a generous welcome in the entry of your home, even if they are not used by every arrival.

COURTESY MIRROR

A mirror can be a lovely and practical addition to an entry space. It creates a courteous opportunity for those arriving or leaving to give themselves a

▼ A table with an arrangement of flowers will create a generous welcome.

▶ The large mirror here offers a courteous opportunity to check your appearance as you enter or leave the home. It also bounces light around and gives a great relection of the stairs.

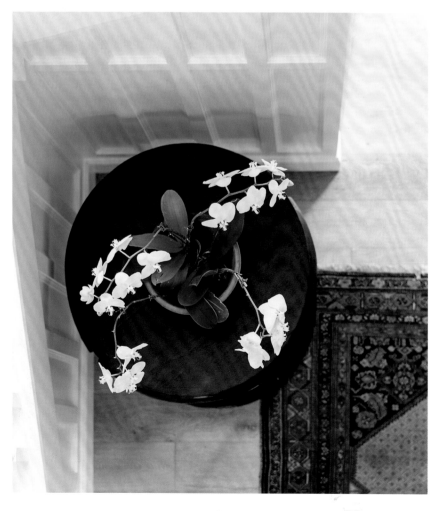

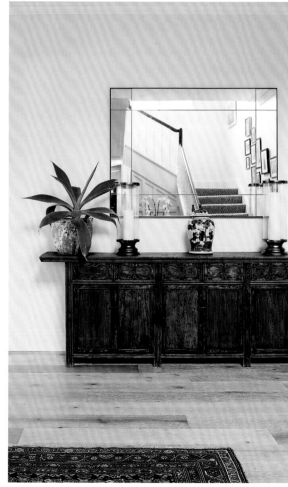

quick cautionary glance before they go further into the home or into the outside world. It is often coupled with a console table that lets you put down a handbag or other items. Knowing they've had an opportunity to check their appearance makes visitors more comfortable to proceed into the house. (In apartments the mirror in the lift is often used for this, as it's more private than checking yourself out in the public lobby.)

STORAGE SPACE

Very quickly an entry area can become the dumping ground for all the items in your house that don't have a home, and it is not a good look. Think of your entry as a place where nothing is permanently stored. Everything in that space should be 'of the season' and in use at least every month, if not every week. So, in summer your winter coats should be put away in storage and not left hanging in the entry. If they are to remain in the entry, then put them away in cupboards. A seasonal clean-out is a cathartic opportunity to give your entry a facelift. Consider creating high storage to hold your non-seasonal items, behind doors preferably, or at the very least in baskets.

If you have a big family with many belongings requiring day to day storage in the entry, then consider buying a range of good-looking baskets or containers to hold items in an accessible but screened way. Some discreet labelling can keep the kids on the straight and narrow.

THE FRONT DOOR

A front door says a lot. I always specify a solid-feeling door. Arriving at a home and finding a flimsy cheap door doesn't make a great first impression. Keep in mind that solid does not always mean opaque; a clear glass door can feel heavy and secure even though it is see-through. Your door can be timber, metal, glass or a mix of all – but most of all it needs to feel solid in your hands. The feel of that door in your hands forms the sensory background to your experience as you step into the entry space.

MAKING A STATEMENT

The front door is the first statement of the quality and status of the house. The doorbell and the handle begin to distinguish the character of the

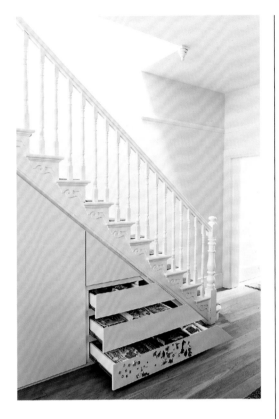

people that occupy this home; they are the first comments on their style – is it antique or modern, trendy or traditional?

A quick fix to change the impression of your home is to change its front door. If you intend to do this, make sure you understand the period and style of the house. I remember in one *House Rules* episode a door was changed on a beautiful period Queenslander, but the contestants chose a very modern timber door. Not only was its style, and the type of timber, out of kilter, but also it was proportionally too big. It felt ridiculous in your hands as you entered what was overall quite a petite house.

And watch out for unusual shapes often found in modern doors. I remember one that had a large, curved, inlaid glass panel. It was supposed to be a feature, but a glass banana in the front door is probably not the first impression the owners were trying to give.

An even quicker fix is to not change the door but just change the hardware. By changing the handle and lock and introducing a door knocker, you can completely change the feel of your entry.

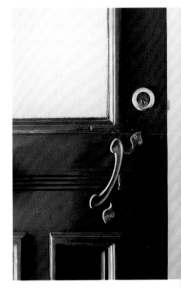

◀ Make use of the space under your stairs for storage. These clever drawers can be custom made to fit any size.

▲ Your front door handle should look good and feel great in the hand. It would be a shame to have a flimsy handle give a poor first impression of your home.

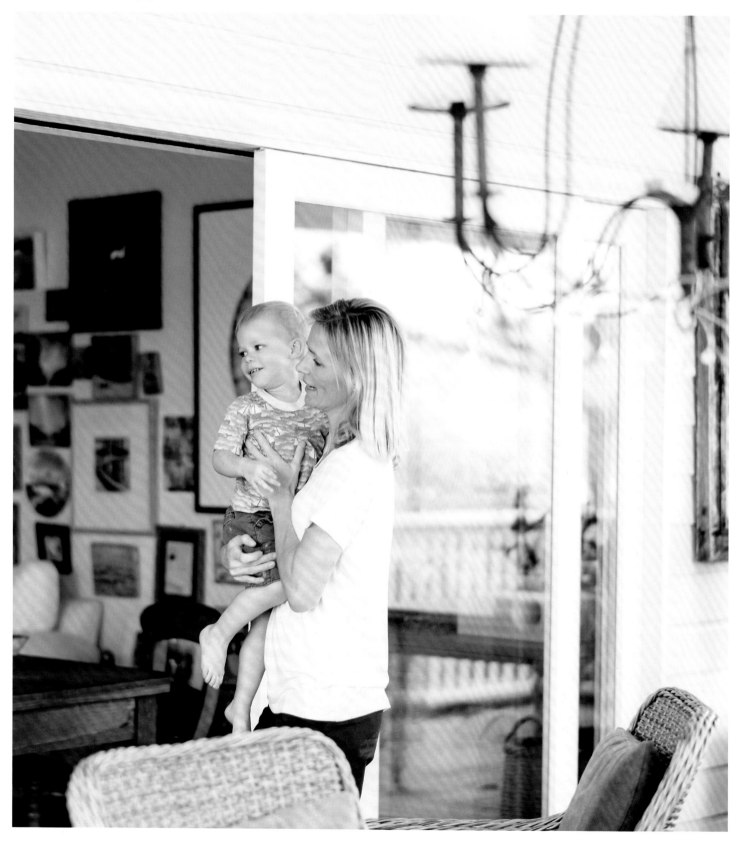

For example, if you paint the door dark charcoal and replace the door hardware with brass fittings, you will greatly change the first impression of your home. Just make sure the fittings are proportionally correct for the door: they need to appear big enough to move the door, but not so big that they look as if the door can't support them.

The trick with a door is to ensure it gives a sense of security while at the same time appearing welcoming. One of the best and easiest ways to do that is to take a big solid door and paint it a bright colour, such as red or yellow. Just by standing out, the door is saying 'notice me, and come inside'.

The front door is one area where there is a focus on the outside, as well as the inside, environment. Make sure you provide some shelter for those outside, such as an awning, so they don't get rained on as they search for keys or wait for someone to open the door. A simple awning is a simple courtesy.

ENTRY SECURITY

Security in the home can be an important factor for some people when they are designing their entry space. We have occasionally installed two sets of doors with different levels of vision through them, simply for security reasons. This actually mirrors the security door sequence found in apartments, which is different because the doors are positioned further apart. There is no doubt that a good intercom system is worth the investment, whether you live in an apartment or a house. They are not as expensive as they once were and give you a chance to check out who has arrived, and whether they are welcome. And that's not just about 'baddies' but also about unwanted spruikers. Often just seeing an intercom system can be a deterrent to cold-callers, as they know that no easy access is available. Barring an intercom, good vision is crucial before you open the door, and the old chain-lock still works.

NOT THE FRONT DOOR?

Most homes these days are not accessed by the front door! What? Can that be true? In the suburbs, where most homes are accessed by car

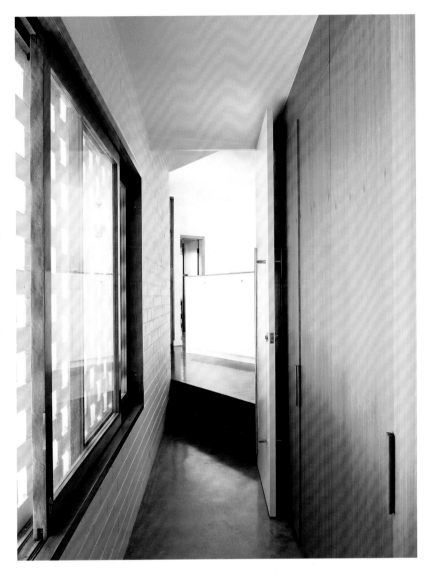

and work is via a car commute, it makes sense that the primary entry to the home is often not the front door but actually the garage door. If that is the case for you, then I always recommend to put some love into that space and make it more of a welcome into your home.

Create an entry vestibule at the door that enters the house from the garage, place some hooks for coats, make a shelf for bags and a low shelf for shoes. Do all the things you would do for an entry at a conventional front door. Of course, if you're building a new house, you have an opportunity to design it to allow both the street and garage to enter the home in the same space.

A veil of brickwork creates a visual screen here, giving privacy while allowing the occupant to see out as anyone approaches. It also creates a beautiful dappled light that just raises the spirits.

In a warm climate there is no excuse for not having a seamless connection between indoor and outdoor areas during much of the year.

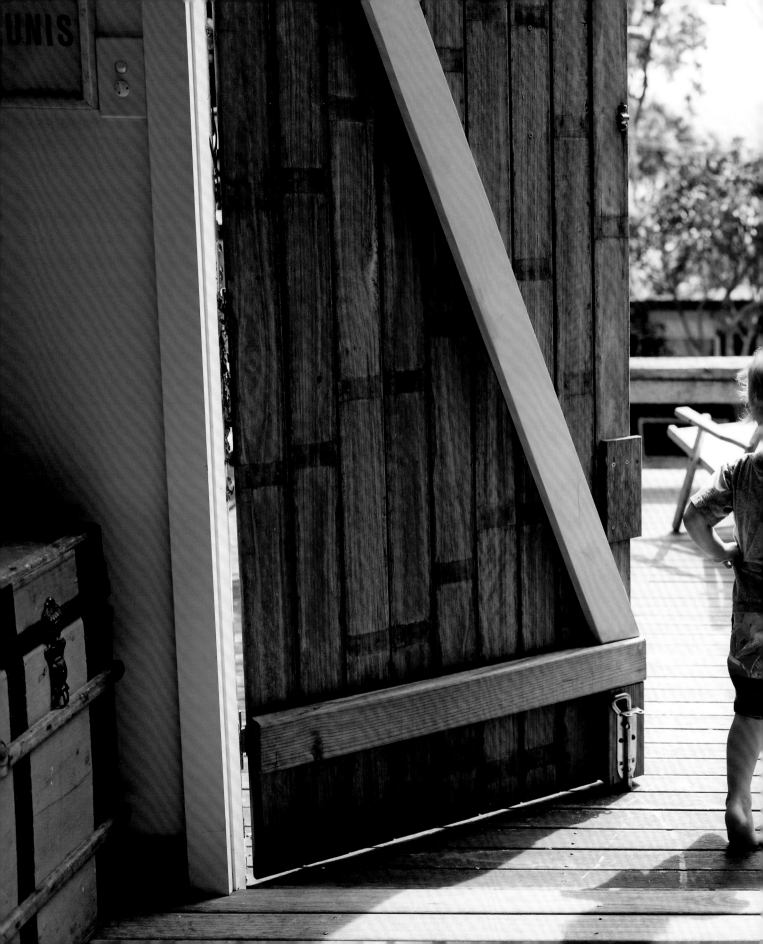

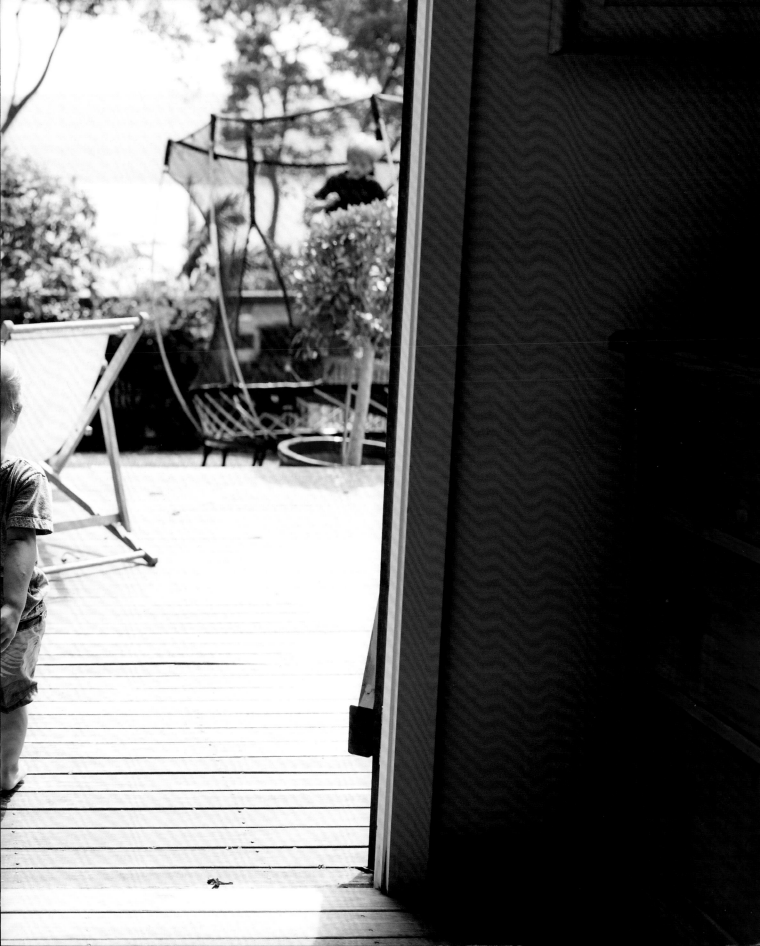

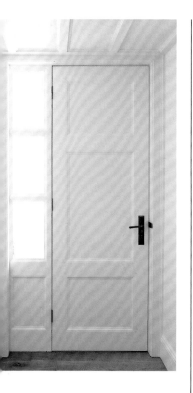

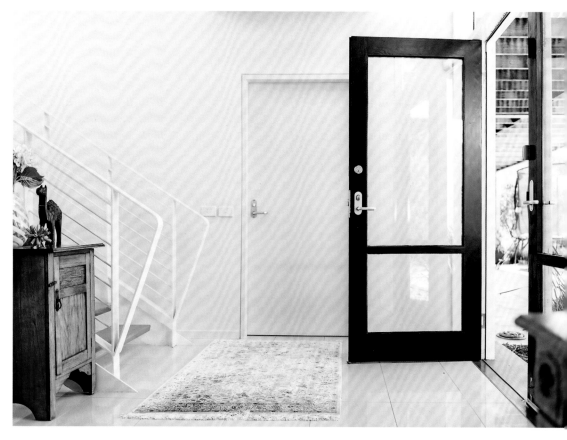

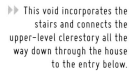

A side window provides light into the hall even when the door is closed — as well as giving the chance to see who is at the door before you open it.

Light is a great asset in creating atmosphere. If you have the chance to build or renovate, I would suggest creating a two-storey entry space that can let in daylight from above during the day.

This void incorporates the stairs and connects the upper-level clerestory all the way down through the house to the entry below.

LIGHT

'I'll leave the light on' is a lovely thing to hear when you are going to arrive home late. And this is the sentiment to bear in mind as you design your entry lighting – not only for your loved ones, but also for yourself and the neighbourhood.

Movies and novels often depict a garden path leading to a warm and welcoming entry, usually at night, where beyond that glowing front door is the promise of an embrace and hot cocoa.

Creating a dedicated entry gives you an opportunity to light that space so that it is a visual and welcoming beacon from the street. The front door opens into it, creating a lovely, warmly lit, welcome home.

When we go for a walk at night in our own neighbourhood, we notice people's front doors and their welcoming entry from the street. Those that have warm light spilling from the interior feel friendly and attractive. Then there are the homes that appear cold and dark, with no friendly

contribution to the street, and therefore no sense of community. Light at your entry also has natural security benefits, preventing any strangers lurking. Good design will allow vision into the entry but not into the house beyond.

GUIDING THE WAY

It is good manners to clearly identify the entry to your home through the lighting of the front door and the garden path. It makes a contribution to the friendliness of the street and also prevents your guests stumbling around in the dark looking for the front door.

AMBIENT LIGHT

Cold white light is definitely not the way to go for an entry; while the glare is noticeable from afar, it is not attractive, except maybe to a moth. A soft, warm diffuse light is the best way to light an entry, so head for lamps that are around 2700 Kelvin – a nice warm-coloured light. Because at night it is generally dark outside, the entry space should be designed as a transition in terms of light. Ideally, it should be lit so that you are not blinking from the transition as you come in through the door. Don't be afraid to have less light in the entry than in the main part of the house. For a soft diffuse light use wall washers (lights that are mounted to the wall and shine up or down the wall, rather than giving off a direct glare) and ceiling uplighters, to achieve a reflected light (the ceiling must be white). And it is always a friendlier scene when a desk or floor lamp is involved. If you already have downlights, make sure the bulbs are warm white and have dimmers fitted.

TASK LIGHT

Light is a very practical feature of an entry; you want to be able to see who is arriving at the front door. It makes sense that the exterior is well lit so that you can clearly see if it's friend or foe. I prefer to soften the lighting within the entry and increase the lighting outside the entry, so that the person approaching the house is more on show than the person answering the door.

Inside the entry space there should be enough light for you to be able to go through the process of unloading bags, jacket and keys etc. Give the option of a task light, such as a directed downlight, to light up the storage area, much as you would light up a wardrobe.

A desk lamp on the entry console, or a well-positioned floor lamp, is practical if you are signing documents or courier forms, as well as adding to the ambience of the space.

EYES UP

Light is a great asset in creating atmosphere. During the day let daylight in from above; if you have the opportunity to create a two-storey space, then take it. You will find that you, and your guests, look up as you arrive at the door; it's a technique used in cathedrals and, psychologically, just the very action of raising the head is uplifting. Further inspired by cathedrals, I often design a feature of glass louvres or coloured glass to be seen and enjoyed as you look up in the entry. During the evening this can be up-lit to enhance the experience. If you have some glass at a higher level, you can make quite the statement with a soft beacon of welcoming light to the street, much like a lighthouse.

If you are working with an existing building and can't create a two-storey space, then you still have options to help create a sense of uplift with light. In a dark terraced house I have created a

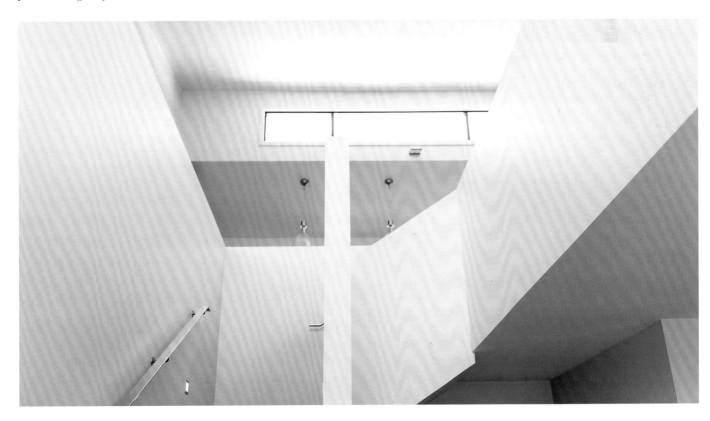

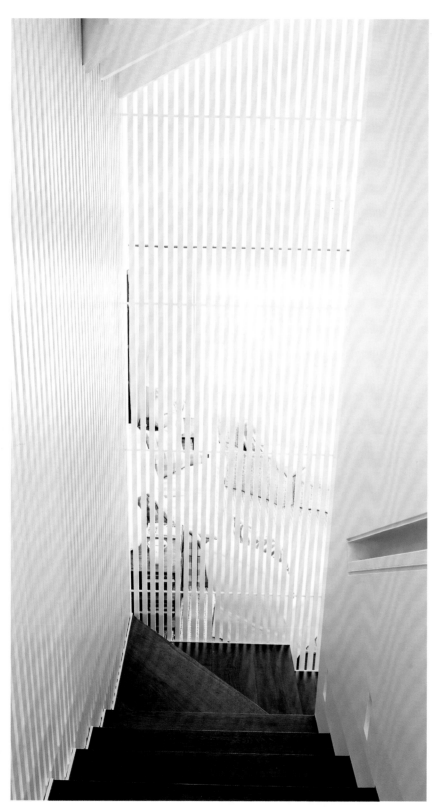

recessed ceiling and painted it white inside. I then lined the surround of the recess with upward-facing dimmable LED strips, keeping the light source concealed from the person looking up below. Then I added a diffuser of opal acrylic to the recess, flush with the ceiling. This gave the effect of a skylight in the entry area with diffuse light illuminating the space; a little like creating a halo in the entry. Importantly, the dimmable nature of the lighting means you can control the strength of the light so you can make sure it is at a comfortable level. Ensure that you use a warmer light at between 2700 and 3000 Kelvin, otherwise you risk that the feature becomes too glary.

Another option to create a sense of uplift is to use silver mirror on the ceiling (silver mirror is standard mirror, as opposed to more exotic versions, such as bronze or smoke mirror). This will give a sense of depth and add movement and life as people travel through the entry. Do make sure the mirror is professionally fixed, as it can be quite heavy.

OR COSY?

For a cosy space the key is a 'less is more' approach with lighting. Absolutely no downlights are allowed! Instead, use a series of desk lamps, wall lamps with shades, and floor lamps. Add mirror for some reflection of light in the space, but consider using smoke or bronze mirror on a wall so that any light bouncing around takes on its more sultry, more cosy, reflection of light.

LIGHT AND COLOUR

Traditionally, light was often brought into the entry in an aesthetic way by the use of stained glass, either in the front door itself or window surrounds. This style was used a great deal in Australian bungalows and terraces, so is familiar to us, and it can be an ornate and elegant way to bring colour and character into the space. Of course, it offers visual privacy to the inhabitants, as well as allowing for light. A modern interpretation of the stained glass window can really set the scene for the beginning of a journey into a lovely home.

A note to remember if you are considering using a coloured light at your front door or entry, is that light colours have been used traditionally

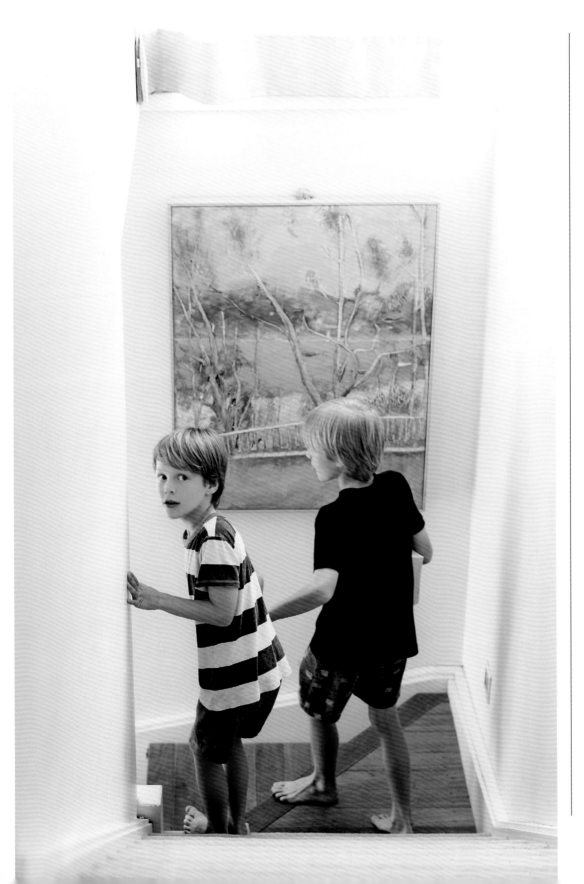

◀◀ Create views from your entry that connect to other parts of the house. Stairs offer a good opportunity to connect visually and acoustically between the different levels of your home.

◀ Bjørn and Asger passing a landscape on the stairs. Interestingly, this painting is probably the most viewed artwork in the whole house. The real quality of the space, however, comes from the window above.

▽ A desk in the entry, for short meetings and signing papers, is a great inclusion.

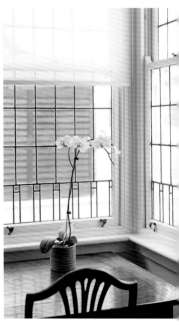

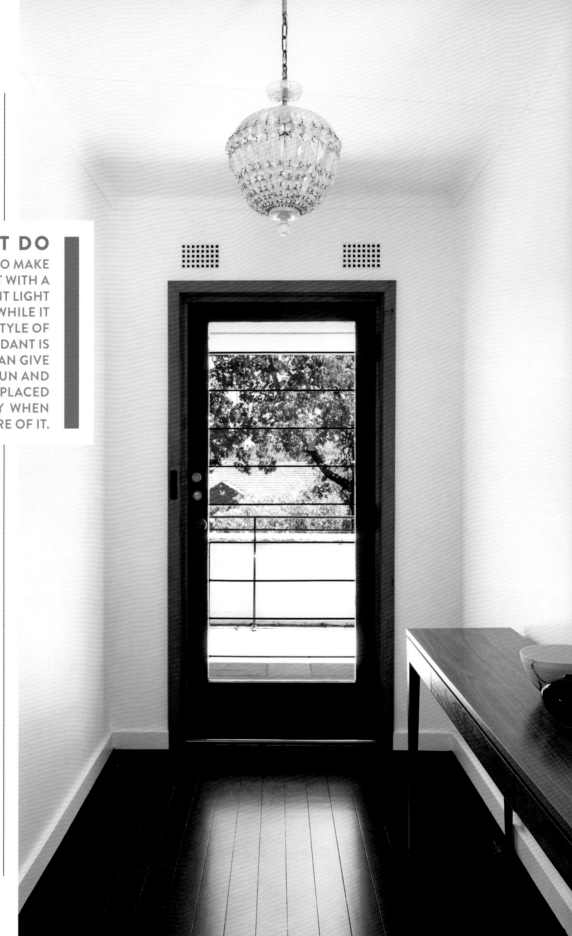

MUST DO

DON'T BE AFRAID TO MAKE A STATEMENT WITH A BEAUTIFUL PENDANT LIGHT IN THE ENTRY. WHILE IT SHOULD FIT THE STYLE OF THE HOUSE, A PENDANT IS SOMETHING THAT CAN GIVE AN ELEMENT OF FUN AND SURPRISE AND BE REPLACED FAIRLY EASILY WHEN YOU TIRE OF IT.

▶ This entry has a natural symmetry with the door, vents and central chandelier. Only the door handle and console table sit outside this symmetry. Notice how the console table is positioned on the same side that the door swings open to, leaving plenty of space to walk into. The door glazing, framed in black, speaks to the glass chandelier, while the black framing speaks to the dark timber floor. The chandelier will come into its own in the evening.

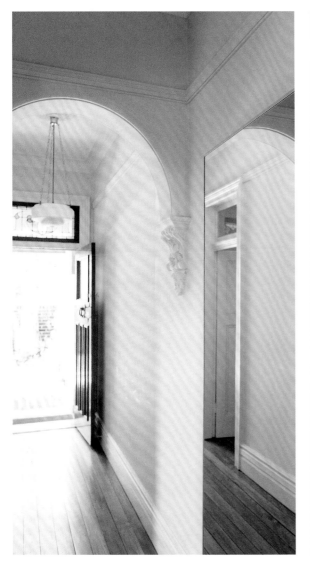

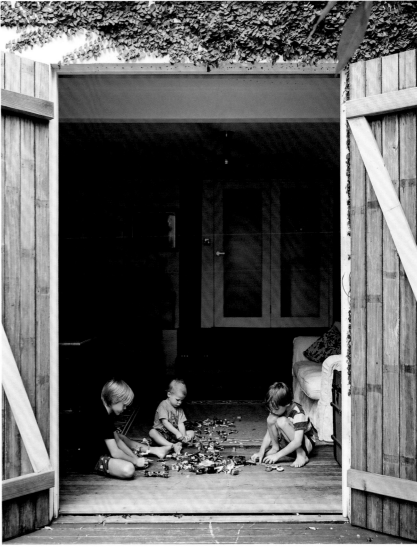

to signal occupations. A red light signifies a doctor's surgery and, at the other end of the spectrum, a brothel... A bright neon light represents an open business. Unless you are a doctor or running a business then your home is probably not best lit this way. A warm white to yellow light is the way to go. Although Christmas lights are an exception.

A STATEMENT LIGHT

Finally, don't be afraid to make a splash in the entry. It is always fun to enter a home and be surprised by a sparkling chandelier. Be careful, though; the novelty can wear off quickly! The room needs to be able to support the size and scale of the chandelier, so choose its size carefully. A pendant light is also a great option: it can help define the entry, uplight the ceiling and give a soft ambient glow. A pendant can be modern or heritage so there are plenty of options to support the style of any home.

Do remember practicalities, though; if your front door is the main entry to your house and where furniture deliveries are made, and large parcels, bikes and surfboards are taken in and out, then be careful not to obstruct the doorway with a low-hanging pendant.

◀◀ The large mirror here reflects the light and bounces it around what could have felt like a confined space.

▲ When there is little opportunity to bring light into an entry, a pair of over-large barn doors, opening to the world, will allow in plenty of light from the outside.

AIR

I often worry that Australians have forgotten the importance and ceremony of entry, perhaps because of our relatively temperate climate. The temperature transition between outside and inside is not as great as in other parts of the world, but the reality is that we do have cold days, and hot days, and we need to cater for both when we are making our entry a welcoming place.

ENTRY AS A CLIMATE BUFFER

On a practical level your entry should be a buffer between the outside world and the inside of your home. In colder climates the entry becomes a vestibule and is a thermal barrier between the outside and the inside. I often design sealable entry spaces so that they become a thermal barrier from hot weather as well as the cold. The best way to do this is obviously with walls and doors; however, if an enclosed entry space is not an option then ensure that your front door is well sealed and offers a barrier to the outside temperature and wind – in winter a draught is your enemy.

If you don't have an enclosed space to create a thermal barrier and you are considering renovating, then a good option can be to enclose a front entry porch. This also gives you an opportunity to add some charm to the front of your house and make a contribution to the street. At the very least and for maximum efficiency use double glazing in your windows and any glass doors to create a thermal barrier that will protect the internal temperature.

▼ In a two-storey house it is lovely to design an entry that incorporates the stairs. This can become a vertical chimney that draws hot air up from the living areas and ventilates it out through a roof vent or upstairs clerestory.

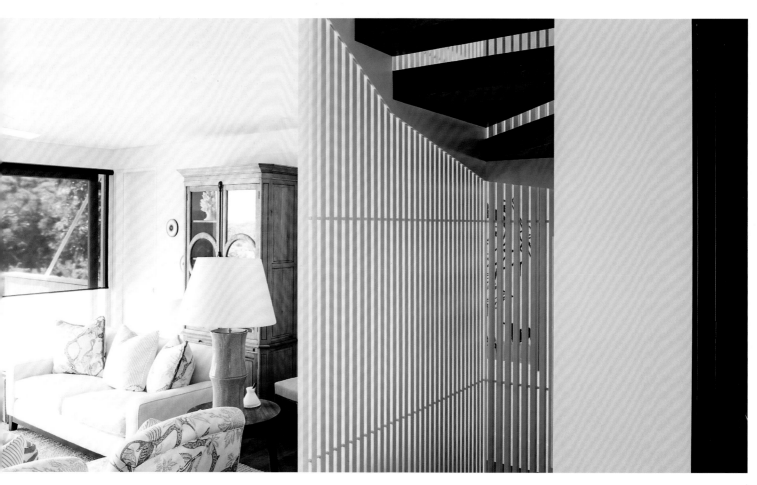

ENTRY AS A BREEZEWAY

Controlling the air into your house through your entry will help filter out fumes from the street if you live in an area of air pollution. If you are lucky enough to live in an area with fresh air, your entry can be a ventilated space that captures a cooling breeze and cools down a house. A breezeway is a classic way to form an entry. Use a bank of louvre windows up high, or simply windows that can be opened. Depending on the orientation of your building, a well-designed entry can often be a living, breathing air-conditioner attached to your home.

If you have a two-storey entry, then it can become a vertical chimney that draws hot air up from within the house and ventilates it out through a roof vent or clerestory... A roof vent is a device that allows air flow from inside the house to the outside without letting in other elements, such as rain. Some examples are 'whirlybirds', which are powered by a motor or the passing wind and suck warm air out of a house or roof cavity. A clerestory is an area of the roof that is raised above the rest of the roof; the area of wall between the roofs is glazed to let in light as well as allow for airflow through louvres or vents.

In a two-storey house I often design an entry that incorporates the stairs. In this way the vertical space is doing many jobs at once, including vertical transportation, efficient access to the upstairs floor without passing through the downstairs area, making a feature of the stairs in an atrium space and providing an air chimney for the house. In winter you can close the ventilation windows at the top of the air chimney and add some slow-moving ceiling fans to push and circulate the warm air that gathers there back down into the living spaces.

SCENT OF AN ENTRY

Scent sets the sensory scene of how your home is perceived, and is also an important part of forming memories. Many of us will remember the smell of Grandma's home; for instance, for me, it was dried flowers in the form of potpourri. Consider planting something fragrant near the front door, such as a well located gardenia, frangipani or jasmine. That smell will always make you think of arriving home. In the same way you could always have some flowers on the entry table, or a scented candle on cold nights.

As the entry is the first line of defence to outside dirt, use high-quality natural cleaning products but be aware that you don't want to come home to the scent of antiseptic and a front entry that smells like a hospital.

The traditional clerestory window above an internal door is perfect for maintaining airflow, even when the door is closed.

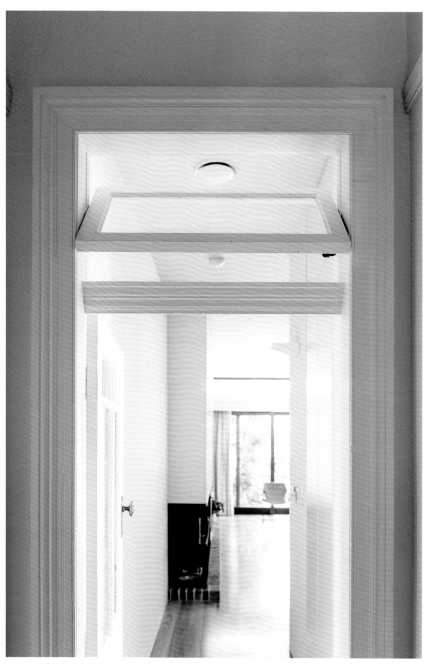

▶ If you have the opportunity for a large amount of glazing, then make sure you build in a number of different window designs to allow for different types of airflow. Sliding doors create large openings, which give a sense of the outdoors; however, when you leave home you generally need to close them. Louvres can be left open and still be secure. They are also perfect to leave open just a little, during colder times of year.

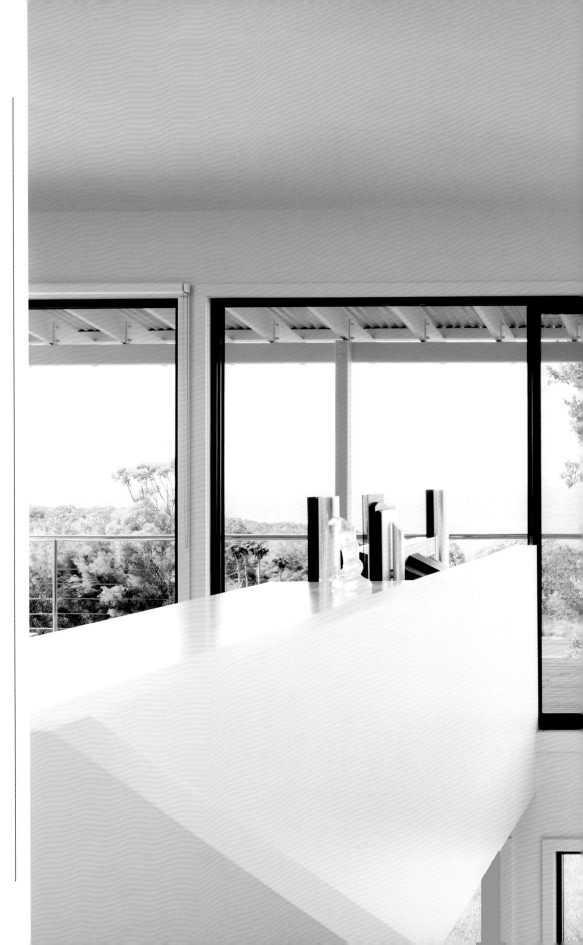

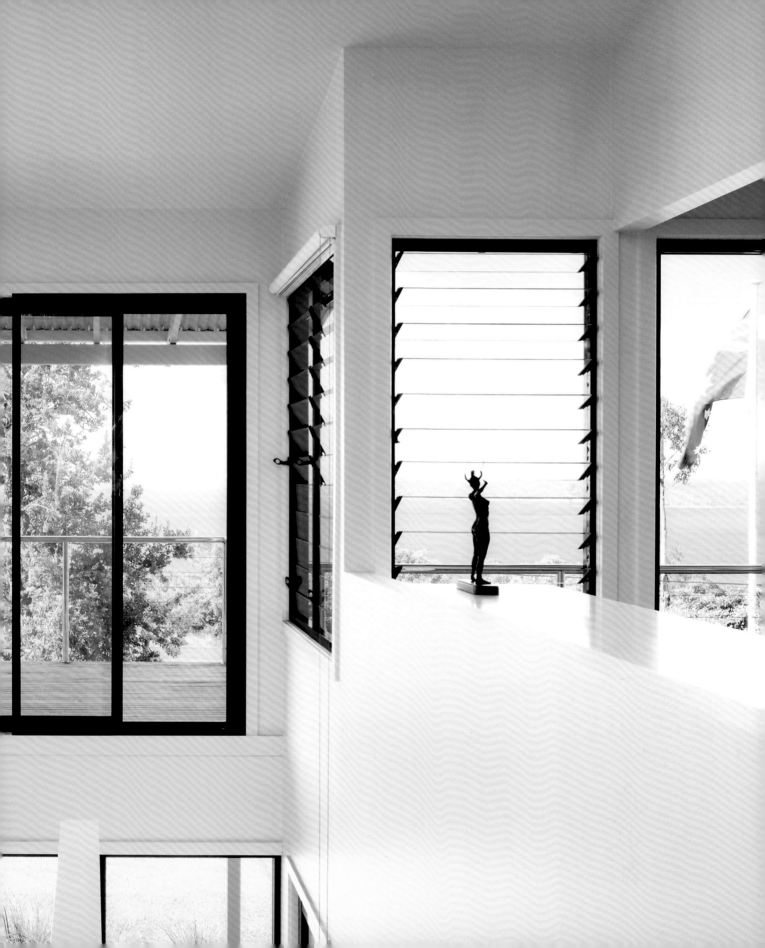

SOUND

If you live on a busy street, then your entry needs to shut out the noise of traffic or passers-by. A solid, well-sealed door is key to this: it not only gives a quality feel and shuts out the outside temperature, it also becomes a good sound barrier. If you use glass in your front door or beside it, then double glaze: the cushion of air between the two layers of glass will prevent the transmission of sound, as well as being a thermal barrier. You should then create an instant feeling of calm and relaxation as you close the door to your home and shut out the world.

If you have the opportunity to create a dedicated entry space, then another set of doors leading into the main house will go a long way to blocking out any noise pollution from the outside. The entry itself becomes a larger version of double glazing.

ENTRY ECHO

In many houses the entry, with its hard floor surface, can be an echoing and harsh-sounding place where the clip clop of shoes dominates. If this is so, I often introduce an acoustic ceiling, such as a perforated plasterboard or an acoustic baffle. An entry rug can also help dampen the sound. Even an in-built coir welcome mat can reduce the bouncing around of sound in the space. Another option is to use an acoustic material on at least one wall; I have used soft panels that are actually pinboard material and are designed to absorb sound. This comes in a range of colours and its texture is lovely and unexpected in an entry space. It can be quite fun as well to use as a giant pinboard to leave messages on the wall for loved ones coming in and out of the house.

Oh, and that lovely solid and heavy front door? Put a soft closure on it so it doesn't slam and wake up the whole household.

SOUND CONNECTIONS

While you don't want a noisily slamming front door, an acoustic connection to the entry of your home is a good thing to have. It is nice to have an ear out as someone comes through the front door; you can't see them, but you can hear them, identify who it is in your mind, listen to them drop their bags and keys and enjoy the emotion that comes with knowing they are home safely.

And, if we are putting a sound system with speakers throughout a house, then I always include one in the entry. It is a nice touch to arrive in a house filled with music: it can change your mood instantly and help you forget the troubles of the day.

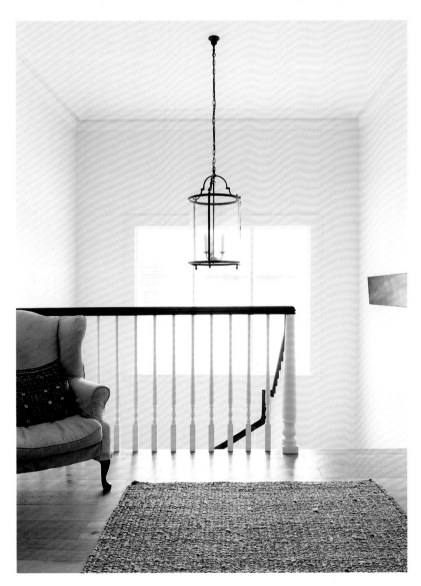

▽ Just a rug and some soft furnishings will help soak up echo and dampen noise.

Adding a hall runner will change the sound of the entry by absorbing the noise of shoes clacking on a hard floor.

SMART HOME

AS WELL AS PLAYING MUSIC FROM YOUR COLLECTION, YOUR SMART SYSTEM CAN BE PROGRAMMED TO NOTIFY YOU IF THERE IS SEVERE WEATHER COMING, OR IF A MOTION DETECTOR OR FIRE ALARM HAS BEEN TRIGGERED. IT CAN LOCK OR UNLOCK ALL DOORS AND WINDOWS AUTOMATICALLY. IT WILL ALSO LET YOU KNOW REMOTELY WHEN YOUR CHILDREN HAVE ARRIVED HOME FROM SCHOOL.

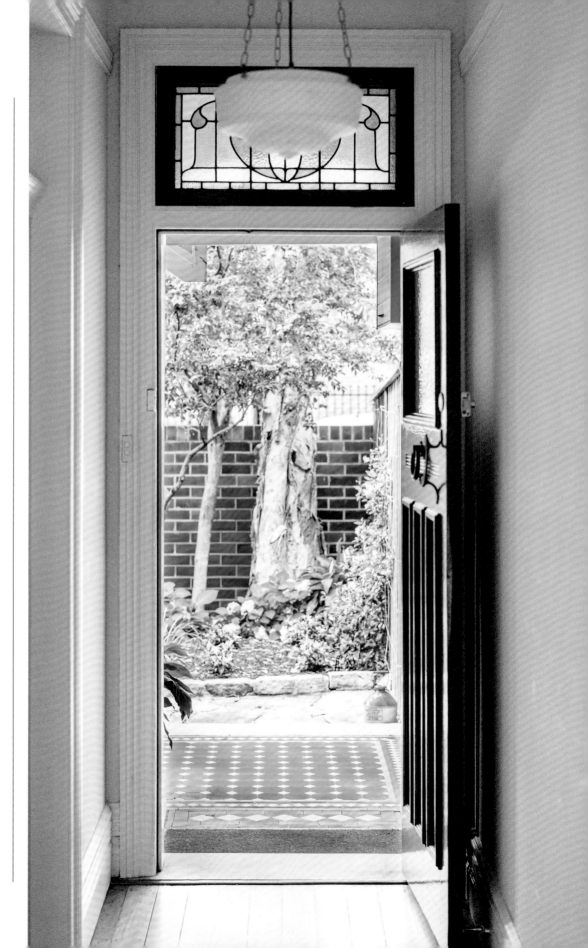

▷ The entry that your home shows to the street can contribute to the community, making it an even lovelier place to live. Here the colourful tiles of the verandah and the stained glass clerestory window give a welcoming atmosphere.

VIEW

An entry to a home must be welcoming and we should broadcast that feeling to the street. In fact, by displaying an openness to the street, to and from, you are doing a public service to your community. By allowing vision into your entry (no need for any further than that) you are offering a gesture in both directions. To the street and the neighbourhood, you are saying hello and that you are happy to be part of this community; you are saying that if a child is hurt or lost they can knock on the door and you will make sure they are all right and get them back home safely.

By having an open entry, you are also saying to any potential wrong-doers that you are watching the street, you care what is going on and you are part of the community. There has been much research showing that creating safe areas is very much about passive surveillance by the local community. Public spaces with a lot of overlooking windows are much safer than areas without. It is the idea of the traditional Italian piazza – check out how many windows overlook those spaces. Any trouble and it doesn't take long for the whole town to know! The best streets you ever live in are those that feel safe, and the safest ones are those watched by the community.

PRIVACY, OR COMMUNITY?

For those who like privacy, it is extremely easy to provide. However, try not to design a home that turns its back on the street: it is not good for the neighbourhood. At the very least, make an open and friendly entry as a contribution to the street. It doesn't have to be much... I remember a house I used to walk past almost daily. It was a simple house with a normal front door, but next to that door was a pane of glass around 600 mm wide and the same height as the door. Behind the window was where a pram was stored. Most days it was there, other days it wasn't, and I found it a lovely thing to notice every day. It spoke a little of the life of the house. It told a story and was friendly and open, making me feel I knew the owners a little bit even though I had never actually

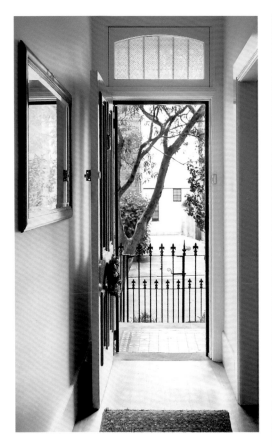

This perfectly placed mirror is a dynamic asset here. It reflects the view from outside, making this a more interesting and attractive space.

seen them. That small gesture to the street was like shaking someone's hand. I often wonder what is in that entry window today: possibly a couple of kids' bikes, or maybe a table and a vase of flowers. Whatever it is, it will always be better than a blank wall or a high fence.

At the other end of the scale, I remember walking in the streets of Copenhagen at dusk and being surprised that I could see not only into the entry, but actually into the living room of nearly every house. It created a wonderful sense of community because it spoke of trust and respect. The people inside were happy to allow the street to have some insight into their homes, and vice versa the people on the street drew comfort that the public space was a safe place and was not isolated, but actually flowed into people's homes and their living rooms. Walking the streets that evening, as a foreigner, I felt that I was not alone; I felt that I was receiving a proverbial hug from these people, from this community. I have never felt safer walking a street. The architecture made me feel secure. All our streets should have this sense of security. We must ensure that new housing developments have excellent connection to the streets, with homes brought right down to the street level. It can feel frightening to walk around the barren base of an apartment block with no humans in sight when trying to get to your refuge in the sky. We need to heed the lessons learnt from the tower block ghettos created last century and, instead, activate the streets with residences at ground level. Retail and commercial buildings are not the answer, as they are often empty in evenings and at weekends. A human scale is important; a scale that invites connection and encourages community. We should all fight for this connection.

There are many opportunities for providing privacy beyond the entry, and ways of introducing security through good design without making your home look like a jail. Entries with good vision shouldn't need bars and grilles. There is no need for high walls and gated compounds; we have seen where that has led other communities. You can deter by using unobtrusive technology and security systems (most of us don't notice them but would-be criminals are looking for them). So when you come to design your entry make it a welcome gesture to the street – the neighbourhood's safety is your safety.

If you can't provide a view into your entry but would like to contribute a friendly presence to the street, then simply paint your front door a bright, happy colour. I remember passing many houses in London and couldn't help but crack a smile when suddenly a bright yellow door popped up. Londoners often dress their door with some form of vegetation or decoration, as well, and this creates a friendly impression for the passer-by. Anything is better than drab.

VIEW TO THE STREET

Just because you have allowed a view into your entry from the street doesn't mean you can't control your level of privacy. For most people, a natural and safe position is to be able to view the street without being seen. If you don't want the street to see into your living room, then make sure they can't. Vegetation is a lovely way to do this. Not only does vegetation form a lovely view from inside your house to outside, but it also provides a filtered view through natural screening. Inside, you are close to the vegetation so you are able to see out through it far better than anyone who is trying to look in. It is perfectly natural to not want to be observed at night. Investing in some hedging or a well-placed crop of foliage is a win-win solution.

Shutters are also a good form of privacy screening that allow a view out. By partly opening them you have good vision out but allow very limited vision into the house from afar. When someone is approaching you have a clear view of them, but they don't have a view inside your home. Aside from screens, you can use your superior knowledge of your building. You can design your

If you can, provide a view specifically for the person who has just entered the home. Here the gaze is drawn naturally down the hallway to the garden.

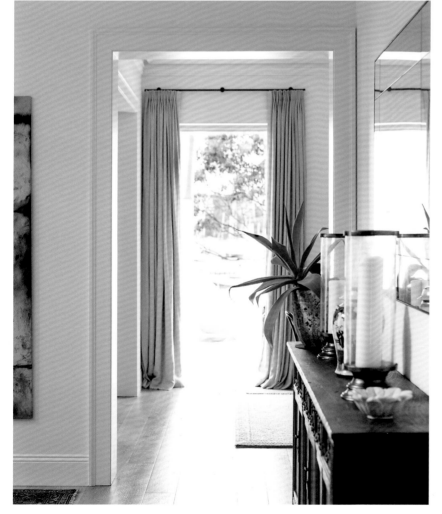

entry space so that you are able to observe who is at the front door through a side window where they would not expect you to see them. If you are really concerned, use mirror glass that you can see through from your side but on the other side it is just a reflection – it's not very friendly but it controls the view. And, finally, there is intercom. A clear necessity for apartments, these are becoming more common than door bells. Now, through smart home technology, you can answer your front door, not only from anywhere in the house, but from anywhere in the world.

Just like the window with the pram, a window from the entry is a great way to capture a view back to the street. Install a feature window – oval, round, perfectly square, or tall and slim. Make it charming with a lovely architrave that frames the view and maybe even embellish it with ornamental or textured glass, or perhaps stained coloured glass.

Often there is not an opportunity to create a new window next to the entry door; however, many front doors, especially in terraces, have a clerestory or narrow side windows. I have often placed a mirror directly next to these openings on the adjacent wall – it creates lovely reflections and views in an unexpected way.

VIEW INTO THE HOME

Once you have accepted someone into your home you have the opportunity to provide them with a view. I have created homes that have a multiple staging: into the entry, and then over a bridge over a pool, and then down the stairs to the view and then into the welcoming living room. See the entering of your home as a series of views that tell a story and give an experience. It will certainly be a conversation starter.

I try to provide a view that is specifically to be enjoyed from the entry, such as into an internal garden, down a heritage hallway or to a spot-lit featured artwork. It is lovely to come into a space that provides some hint of what is to come but does not reveal all. It is not ideal to have a view into a bedroom or a bathroom, or even, if you can avoid it, directly into the living room. If there is no opportunity to use length for a view, then I will go up and create an atrium to encourage the person arriving to look up.

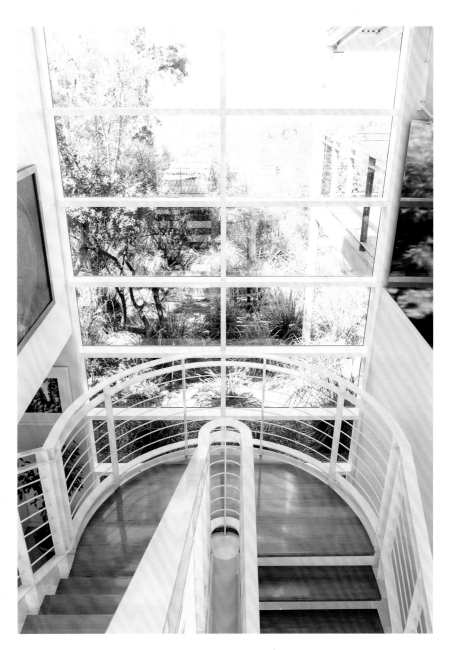

Consider your entry as the beginning of a journey and make the rest of your house a slower revelation. Welcome a guest, get them to take off their jacket and store their bags, and then say 'come through'. Then take them from the entry around a corner to reveal your home. On the smallest scale, just by creating an entry sequence from a relatively small entry into the larger form of your living room, you will be creating a lovely experience for a guest.

▲ If you have the opportunity to open up an entry wall to the view, then do consider it. Walking up or down stairs is one of the few times we have a moment to contemplate a view, as we are moving relatively slowly and automatically.

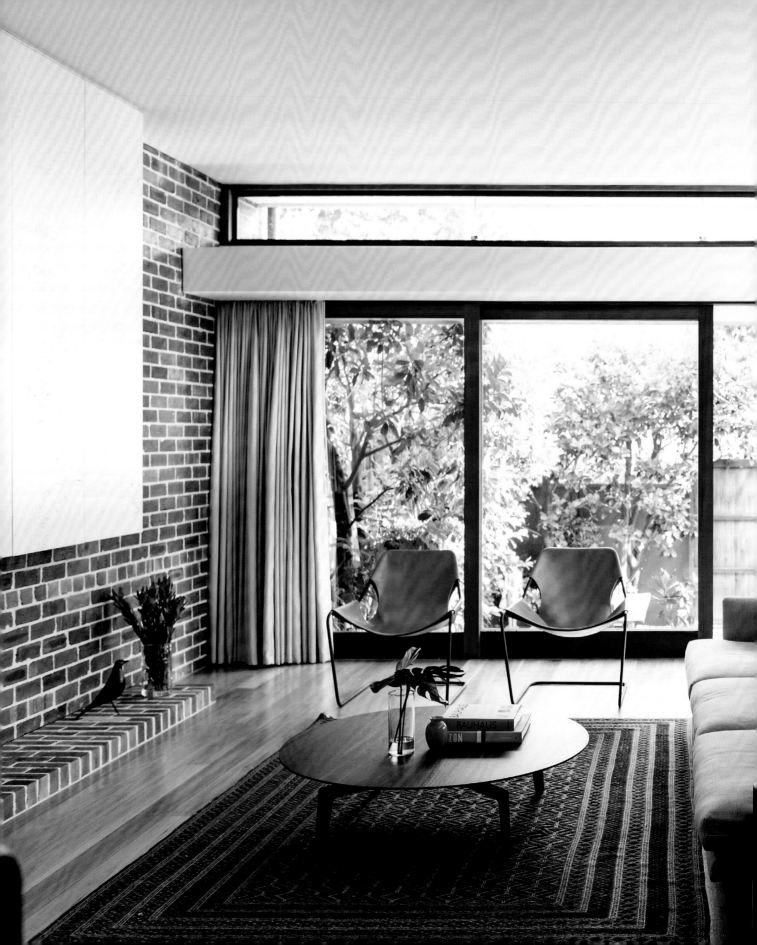

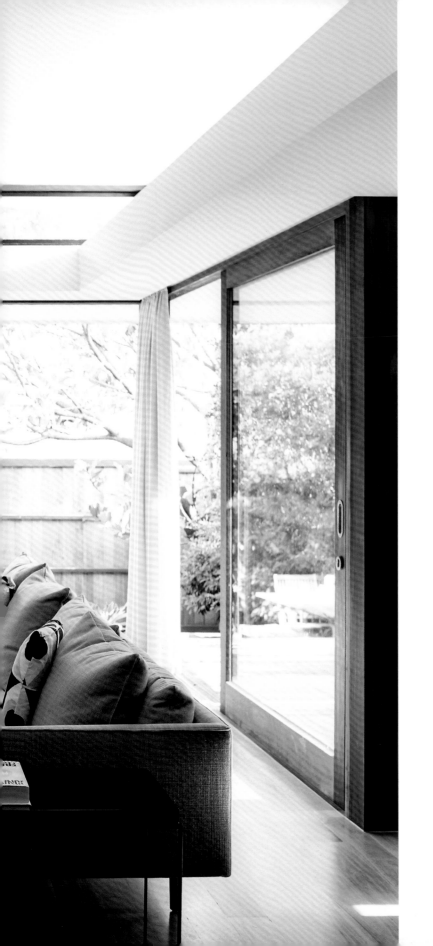

LIVING ROOM

CHAPTER TWO

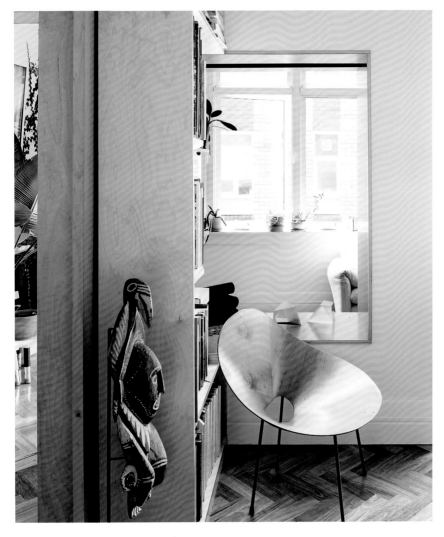

the home. Families go through the need for soft
rugs and Meccano sets, movie gatherings, the
teen years of separation, perhaps a time of fine
wine and dining, the need for a rumpus room, a
guest area and maybe a work and study space.
This is an important room to get right – it will
have a huge impact on the practical functioning
of your life and family.

SPACE

If you are building or renovating and have the
opportunity to locate your living room, then this
is the most vital room to position well; it is often
regarded as the most important room in the
home. It's where you relax and rejuvenate, gather
with family and friends and where you are
entertained through conversation or by the
plethora of different forms of media today.

CHASING THE SUN
Always try to orientate your living room windows
and openings to the sun. The sun is what gives us
life and therefore it makes perfect sense that the
living space should capture a bit of that goodness.
In the southern hemisphere (and the opposite for
the northern hemisphere) try to ensure you
position your living room within 30 degrees of
either side of north.

Most of us are more likely to gather in the living
room in the afternoon and evening so I will usually
orientate a living room window more to the west
of north than to the east, to ensure that sun is
entering the room when people are most likely to
be in there.

Western sun can be very intense and hot in the
Australian summer; however, there are many
design devices that can control that issue. For me,
a favourite design challenge is to capture winter
sun in the afternoon in a living area – this is the
most wonderful uplifting experience during a cold
winter – and avoid it in summer.

If you are renovating, then work hard with your
design to ensure your future living space captures
some sun. Locate north on your plan and then

▲ More than just a corner of
a room, this slice of space is
multi-functional. An internal
window ledge extends the
corner, letting in light and
capturing a view to the
sunroom and windows beyond.
The depth of the ledge is
perfect for resting a cup of tea
as you relax in the chair.

▶ The comfortable sofa makes
this an inviting space, however
it is the quality of light
coming from beyond that
really draws you in.

TODAY'S LIVING ROOM HAS many, many roles
and therefore has to be flexible. In one household
at any time there can be chatterers, movie
watchers, video gamers, sports nuts, book
readers, snoozers and lazy-bones. All these
activities (or non-activities) are expected to occur
mainly in one room: the living room. Not only that,
if the house were to hold an event or party this
space needs to be versatile enough to cater for it.
If all that wasn't pressure enough, this is also
your most 'public' room. This is the room that
practically all your guests expect to see and
spend time in, and they will judge you on this
room and its comfort and character.

The living room changes its role during the
ageing of a family more than any other room in

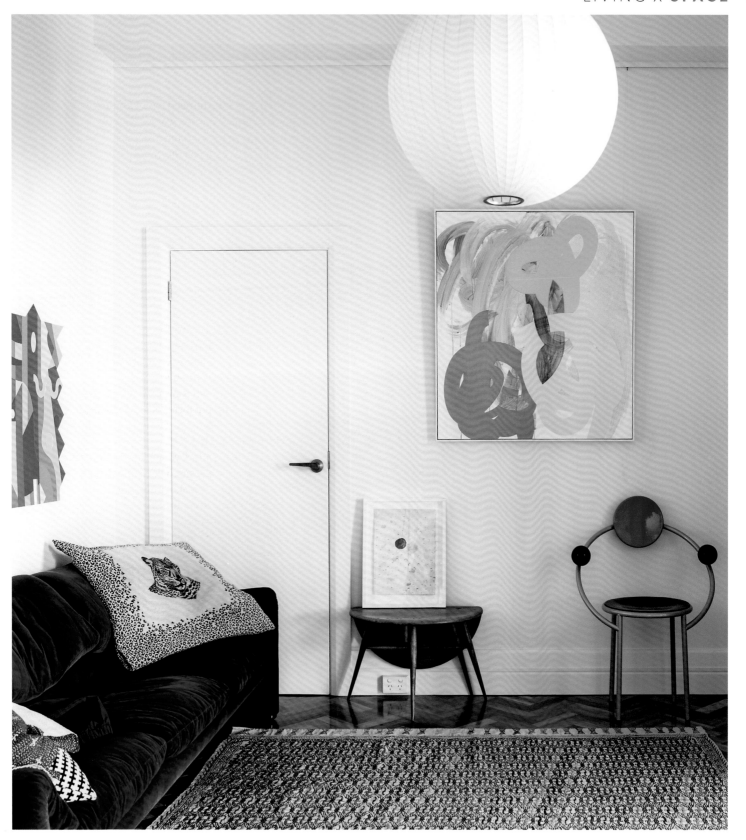

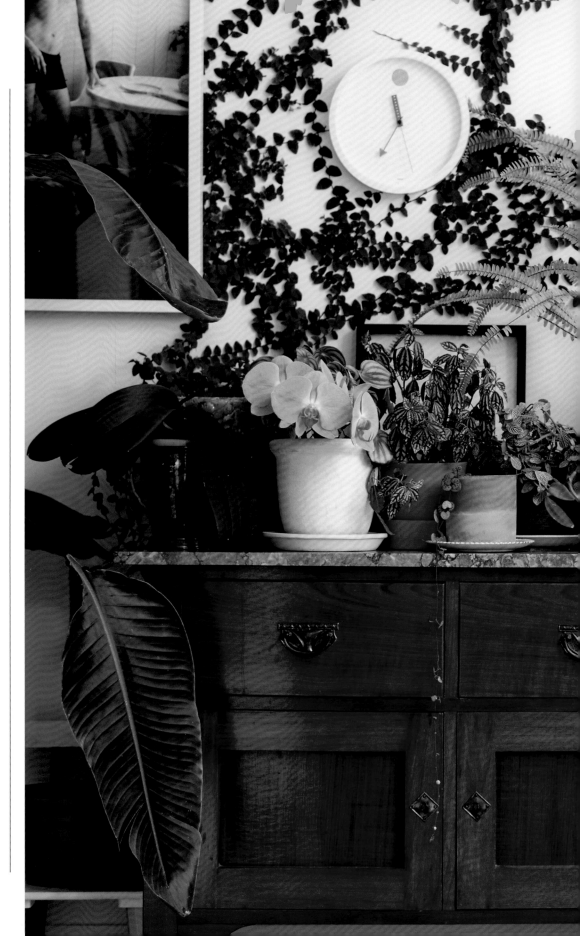

▶ Build your interior gradually.
Collect and keep the things you
love and a narrative will slowly
emerge that is authentic,
which is always going to be
better than the instant styling
of a new space.
Indoor plants always look best,
and most comfortable, in
direct contact with daylight.

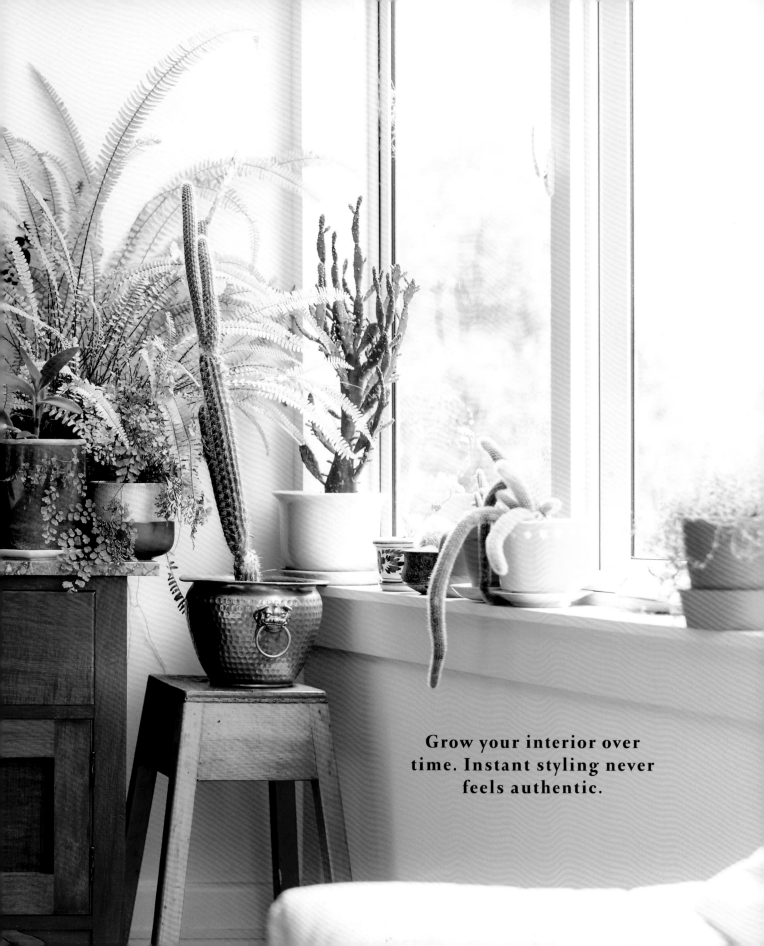

Grow your interior over
time. Instant styling never
feels authentic.

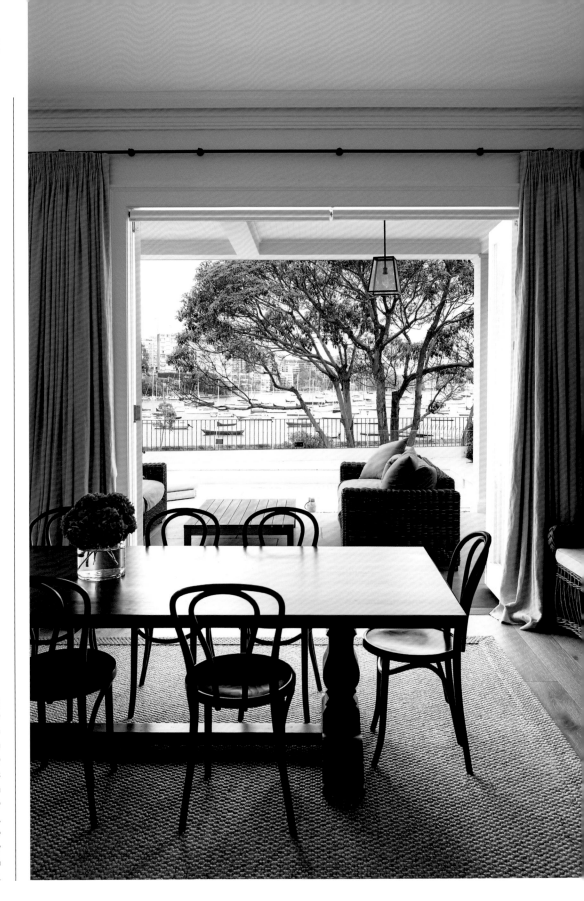

A simple dark timber dining setting is defined in the overall living space by a light-coloured sisal rug on a timber floor. Curtains frame the view and the French doors let in light. Note that from a standing position this eyeline crosses low-level dining, outdoor lounge, pool and the harbour beyond: perfectly designed to be viewed from this kitchen space.

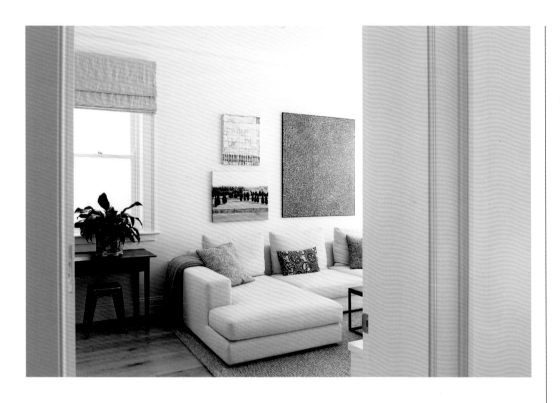

◄ A comfortable sofa makes an inviting space and is given context with the use of console, plant and window and then a series of artworks. The real key here, however, is the sense of light coming from beyond, which truly invites you into the space.

draw two lines, one at 30 degrees to the east of north and one at 30 degrees to the west of north. This is 60 degrees of sun-catchment potential with north right in the middle. You will quickly see opportunities to capture morning and/or afternoon sun in your primary hangout and relaxation space.

Or think more freely and start to look at rooms that already capture the best sun – can that room become a future living space? Consider where you like to sit and have a cup of tea. Do you find yourself not in the living room but in a patch of sun off the kitchen instead? Or always at the forgotten table in the hall? There have been many times where we have designed a renovation around the most comfortable spot in the home – and it often didn't start off as the intended living space. I always enjoy watching where builders take their breaks on a building site – the building site is unfinished and there is no indication yet which room is which – but if you find they naturally are having their morning tea in the future breakfast area and their afternoon tea in the proposed living area, then you know you are onto a winner. If, however, you find them always

gravitating to the proposed position of the garage, you should have a rethink.

Consider also if you have the opportunity to create more than one living space – depending on the orientation of your home and windows, you could consider a morning room and an afternoon room. You will probably find you use one more than the other in the middle of the day, depending on the season.

If you can't relocate the room and it does not have a good orientation then consider other methods of getting some sun in, such as skylights. In my home state of New South Wales you are legislated to receive two hours of sunlight a day.

EXTENDED LIVING

For many families the preference is for the kitchen, dining and living room to be together as part of the same larger space. When you see this working well and in action it is very conducive to conversation and keeping a family together and happy. So, as an architect, I tend to think of a living room as a room with as few walls as possible. To make a great living room I often borrow from the spaces/rooms beside it.

NOTE TO SELF

IN YOUR HOME, TRY TO MAKE THE ROOM THAT CAPTURES THE BEST SUN YOUR LIVING SPACE.

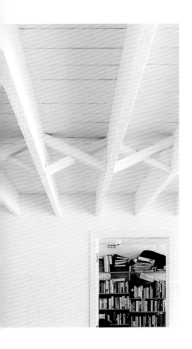

Removing the ceiling and exposing these herringbone struts and the floorboards above gave this room a wonderful new lease of life, as well as increasing the sense of space. The white paint makes the room feel fresher and also bigger. Just be aware that there can be acoustic issues with noise from the floor above; however, if that is a problem you could add acoustic panels.

For example, create some big doors and windows to the garden, so that the living room feels as if it extends into the outdoors. Or design the hall so that it is partly in and partly out of the living room, so the living room has a connection to the rest of the home.

It makes sense to me to combine the uses of different areas into one large room – you get a larger room and therefore a better sense of a bigger and more valuable space for your money. For me, it's better to have one large multi-functional space than a series of pokey little rooms; it always feels better to walk into a bigger room than a little room.

Many centuries ago in our homes we all lived, slept and ate in the same space. It was highly efficient to have everything in one room. It was only with the development of social hierarchies that our homes changed: the upper classes had servants and separate discretionary spaces that could be serviced by the extra help. Dining rooms, drawing rooms, libraries, studies and embroidery, writing and smoking rooms were all made possible by an elite who could afford extra help in their abodes. Of course, these extra rooms became associated with status and the trend filtered down through society. By the twentieth century, many middle-class households aspired to a separate dining room, despite the fact that it added so much cost and maintenance time to a household. I remember when I was growing up my mother always refused to live in a house with a separate dining room: it made her feel like a servant. She insisted on being part of the conversation, not stuck in a separate kitchen, so she demanded that the kitchen and dining area be part of the larger living space. It seems perfectly natural now, but it was a pertinent issue back then. Today the baggage of these separate rooms is slowly disappearing and we are going back to where we started: one major room for the functions of preparing meals, dining and hanging out. In the homes I am asked to design now, we try to create ancillary spaces to that major living space to allow for other activities, such as a train set, study nook, or just a space to get away from the family and return to the main room later on.

Ideally, you should be able to hear and partake in the conversation at the dining table when you are in the kitchen. That way you'll avoid those awkward dinner parties where everyone ends up standing around the kitchen sink because the scale and proximity of kitchen to dining room is not correct and everyone has drifted away from the table.

TOGETHER APART?

Having said all that, I sometimes get very detailed and considered briefs from families who insist on more separation of their spaces. This often becomes more prevalent as the kids grow into teenagers and there are different activities and needs going on under the same roof. It is important to drill down in these situations to find out exactly why the separation is needed.

It might mean something as simple as moving the television out of the major gathering space into its own room so that the one TV viewer doesn't dominate the experience of the other family members.

What separation is required? Is it acoustic or visual privacy? Flexible screens can make a big impact on visual privacy, while acoustic privacy is more difficult – unless the solution is headphones. In bigger houses separation is not an issue because there are just more rooms that can be dedicated to different uses, and you will still have a bigger space to gather in. However, in smaller homes it is difficult to create permanent separation without also reducing the opportunity to gather. In my opinion the best sense of gathering is around meal time, so as long as the space supports that you can afford to have more separation in the rest of the home.

SCREENS AND SEPARATION

While there are many advantages to open-plan living, you sometimes do just need some separation from other people. Consider moveable flexible screens that separate an area. There are many great built-in options, such as sliding walls and doors, with different levels of opacity and acoustic separation. Also available are bifold screens that can be bought at your local furniture store and joined together to become larger. Often we design a room that is an extension of a major living space and has doors hidden in, or against, a wall. Quickly you can draw the doors across, turn

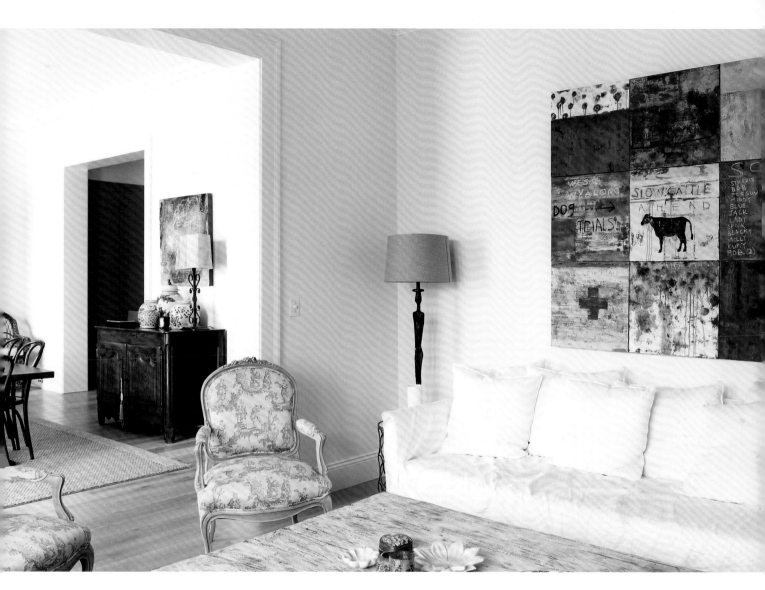

the sofa into a bed and suddenly you have a guest bedroom. The beauty is that this temporary bedroom makes your living room bigger every day that it isn't being used as a bedroom.

LEVEL CHANGE

In a large open-plan living area you need to define zones, whether through placement of furniture, change of materials, level changes in the floor or ceiling, or through screening. Without clever zoning, it will end up as one big bland space.

One of the most important tools of an architect is the level change; this can mean changing the floor level up or down, or doing the same with the ceiling. You can make a space feel special by raising it up and putting it 'on a pedestal' – this is often done with a dining area, to separate and lift it above the main living space. You can also sink

an area down to make it more cosy and special. A sunken lounge is an opulent area, especially if you include a fireplace in it. By raising and lowering a ceiling, you can clearly define different areas in an overall space – drop the ceiling down over a dining area or raise it up to make a living area feel bigger, particularly if it lifts to let in light.

ONE RULE...

There really is one rule to rule them all and that is that the ceiling must be white. White lifts the ceiling away from you, ensuring that the room feels as big as possible. Unless you are intending your space to feel like a cave, paint the ceiling white. And I recommend using a low-sheen paint finish; this gives a soft patina that will recede even further, letting your room's walls, floors and objects become the defining features.

▲ Consider punching a hole in a wall, rather than removing it altogether. In this room the part wall gives definition between living and dining areas, despite the fact that they are essentially in the same space. It allows for an architrave to support the overall styling of the room, as well as providing corners for dedicated seating and lighting.

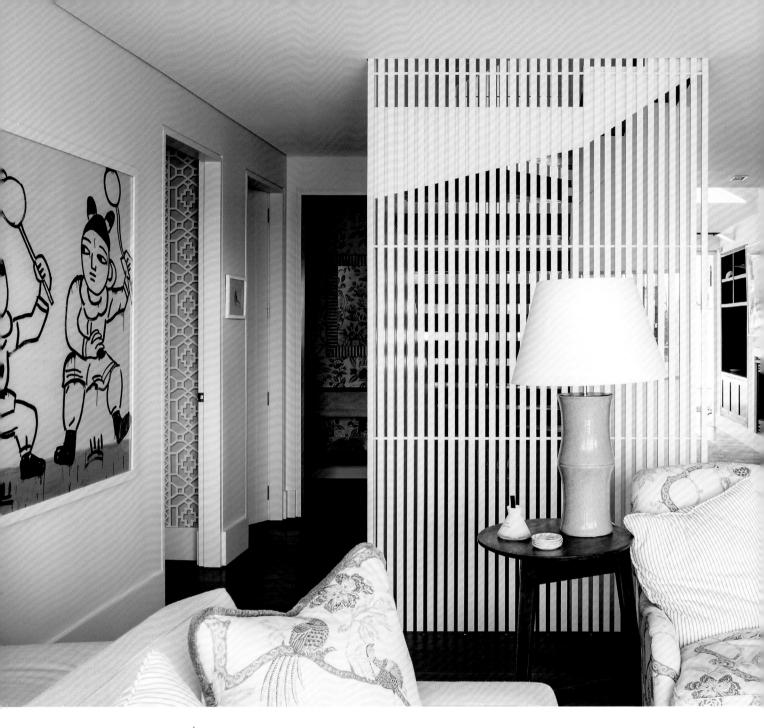

The vertical timber slats are a focal point, not only of this room but of the whole house, signalling vertical movement and allowing the transfer of light and some vision of the stairs. Views extend on one side to the bedrooms and on the other to living space and kitchen.

GO WITH THE FLOW

Where to put your furniture? Make it natural. Moving naturally through a space feels much better than having to negotiate a space. In too many homes I find myself doing a slalom through the living room furniture to get out through the back door into the garden. Or doing a sideways crab walk to get through a too small space. On a plan, map out the foot flow through your house. Draw a line along a pathway that you imagine using. Then keep drawing over the same pathway if you feel your family is going to use that route a lot. So, if it will be used twenty times a day, you'll have twenty lines. Or maybe you think it will only be used twice a day? Very soon you will have some pathways with heaps of lines and others with hardly any. This is your flow map. Now you can feel confident to work on the busy pathways of the home, making sure you have natural lines of sight and natural walkways so that you feel comfortable

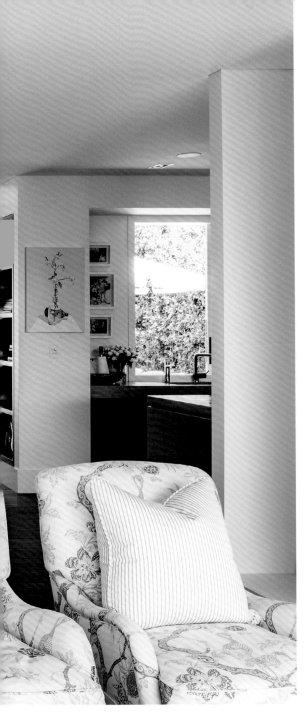

attention to them; and the fact that these pieces fit comfortably in the space diverts the mind from the size of the space. However, put too many small pieces in a room and it quickly feels cluttered and seems small. Choose wisely.

SPACE TO BREATHE

The most opulent rooms always have a sense of space. The easiest way to achieve this is by thinking about the space between things. Filling the whole room with furniture, cheek by jowl, will never feel opulent, no matter how valuable the individual pieces are. Choose furniture pieces that do not dominate the room entirely.

Never put furniture directly against the wall. Allow around 10–20 cm (about 6 inches) between a piece of furniture and the wall to give a sense of space. When we walk into a room we register immediately if furniture is pushed up against the wall, whether we think we've noticed it or not! It gives a feeling of claustrophobia, if not desperation, and makes us uncomfortable. (And, subconsciously, if there is a gap between the sofa and the wall, I always feel that the home is cleaner. That gap seems to signify freshness – allowing air to flow, allowing access to clean.)

THE FOCAL POINT

Once you have captured sunlight in your living space, there are two main things to consider: what activities will take place there, and how many people will usually be in the room. The most common activities are conversation, watching television, reading and listening to music. Decide early on what is to be the focal point of the living space. For many families it is a television, which, unfortunately, when it is switched off, becomes a big black negative space in the room. If you can't conceal the TV behind joinery, at least try to add another focal point to the room to distract from it. That could be a fireplace, a fantastic artwork, a view to the outside, or even a coffee table with a selection of books. Once you have that focal point, you can design your furniture around it.

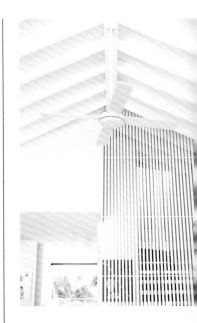

▲ The vertical white timber slats reach up to the exposed rafters in the living space, drawing your eye upwards and making the area feel bigger. All in white, the room feels fresh and even more so with a lazily circulating fan. By exposing the rafters and extending the ceiling upwards the fan has a defined space to exist in and do its job, away from the human habitation.

in your movement. With the right room for flow, your space will feel less cluttered and cramped.

GENEROUS IS BETTER

Be generous with each piece of furniture in your living space; the trick is to only have a few pieces. Whether your room is big or small, my tip is to always furnish a space using a few relatively large pieces, rather than lots of smaller pieces. If you choose three or four great pieces, you draw

SMART HOME

TECHNOLOGY WILL ALLOW A FAMILY TO MONITOR ITS ENERGY USAGE AND MAKE CHANGES TO SAVE MONEY ON POWER BILLS. THE SMART HOME WILL ALSO BE ABLE TO IDENTIFY WHO IN THE HOUSEHOLD IS THE MOST ENERGY EFFICIENT AND WHO IS THE LEAST. IN MY FAMILY AWARDS WILL BE GIVEN OUT AND CHORES WILL BE ADMINISTERED, AND IT WILL CHANGE BEHAVIOUR.

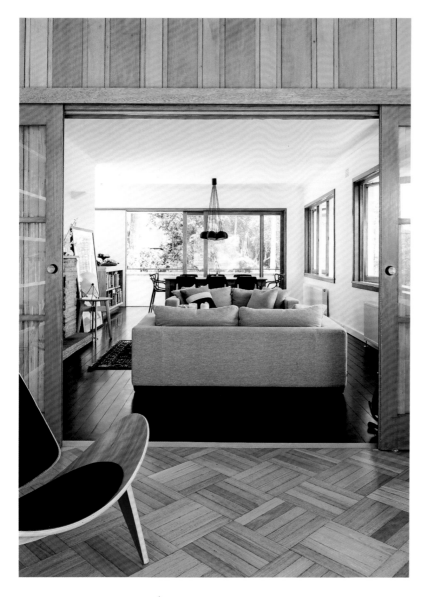

This pair of sliding doors offers a natural sense of symmetry and is a flexible way to divide or join the spaces. The doors are glazed and offer visual connection even when closed. Note the room in the foreground has timber floor, panels and doors; in the room beyond, the floor is dark and the walls are white plasterboard. Although the spaces are connected they are defined by these changes.

Living rooms are an exhibition of who you are and how you want to represent yourself. Family photos, heirlooms, art and special objects are often displayed in the living room so you can involve them in your daily life, as a talking point and to tell a story for whoever joins you there. Traditionally, a mantelpiece over the fireplace was a prominent spot – and if you don't have a fireplace you might still want a mantelpiece. Perhaps a long joinery shelf – some parts behind glass, others not? You only get a short time on earth, so why not bring your story into your main living space?

AN AUTHENTIC STORY

When a space tells a story it has a much bigger impact on you. Just as an artwork with a story is more powerful, the same is true for a home. That is why heritage spaces are so appreciated – much of their beauty comes from the story they bring and what it tells of the time when they were created. Many people can't articulate why they don't like some 'new buildings', but I think it is because we are not able to read a story into the space. Any well-designed modern space will always have a great sense of story and narrative as you move through it, making the space much more valuable.

SYMMETRY, PROPORTION AND BALANCE

Symmetry plays a major role in our make up; it is so deeply part of our own biology that it has a huge effect on how we appreciate space. When you walk into a space and it feels 'right', one of the reasons is probably symmetry. Simple examples are placing the fireplace in the middle of the lounge area (and that doesn't have to be in the middle of the overall room). If the fireplace is the major focus, and the sofas and coffee table are all arranged to honour it, then the fireplace needs to be central. If it is a bit off to the side then things will start to feel odd, without you necessarily realising why.

Proportion is important in design: it is basically how shapes respond to each other in your eye and is all about size and scale. If you walk into a living space and there is an artwork that is half a car hanging off the wall, and it is too big for the space and feels as if it is going to fall on you, then you could say that that artwork is out of proportion with the room.

Good proportions make us feel comfortable; bad proportions make us feel uncomfortable. A common example of bad proportions is when a home has a lovely generous sofa and armchair setting, with a very small rug sitting in amongst them. The rug doesn't fit the scale and proportion of the other pieces and feels out of place – it needed to be bigger and disappear underneath the sofa to make the space work.

Balance is made up of both symmetry and proportion and is about making the room hang

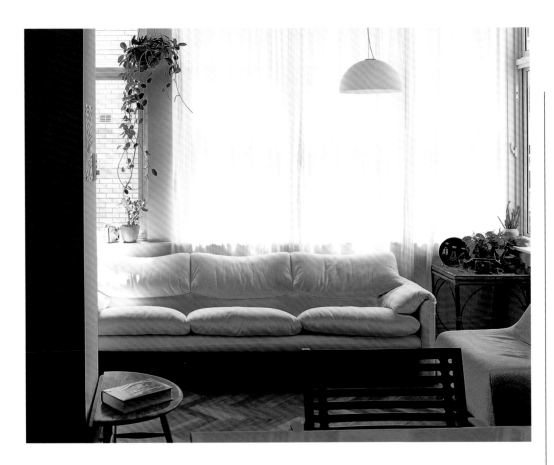

together well. If you are going to put a rich dark brown leather sofa in a room, then you need to anchor it somehow so the room doesn't feel off balance. Perhaps placing it against a navy blue wall will anchor it and make it feel 'right'. Or perhaps a rug or another piece of furniture will anchor it in the room.

HOW TO SEAT HUMANS

Seating arrangements are important. A rule of thumb is to form an informal circle, which makes everyone feel included and involved. Everyone knows the sensation of getting the dud seat at the party, so I try to design that dud seat out early. (I'm not only thinking of you; I've found myself caught in that seat all too often!) If you have guests, seat them with their backs to something solid, such as a wall or window – this will make them most comfortable in a new space – while you take the more exposed seating. This is just natural human emotion: we prefer to have security at our back and a good view from the front so that we can survey the room.

Also make sure that the gap between two sofas or chairs is not the major pathway through the living space. Put the thoroughfare outside the lounge area so that you create a sanctuary that isn't constantly interrupted by people moving between the kitchen and garden, for example.

The basic rule is that whatever lounge room furniture you have, it must at the very least cater for the people who live in that home. It's not very encouraging to gather the family together and find that not everyone has a seat! Once you have the core family catered for, you can start to consider space to seat extended family and friends. Humans are complex creatures and there are many ways we interact, depending on how well we know each other. If you are creating conversation then it's difficult to have an intimate talk across a room. Allow opportunities for people to sit relatively close to each other so that they can have a private chat, while at the same time allowing for people to spread out and not be on top of each other. If you have friends over they will feel more comfortable having their own space. You will notice that talking volumes will change depending on the situation.

You need comfortable chairs, side tables for drinks and coffee tables for books to fill out your living spaces. Depending on your lighting choices you should consider tables for lamps as well.

SOFAS AND ARMCHAIRS

Always consider what job the furniture is doing. Choosing a comfortable couch is a personal choice, but also consider: is this piece of furniture to encourage sitting up and talking, or lying back and watching a movie? It is rather lovely to be able to do both of these on the one sofa: that is one of the reasons larger sofas have become so popular. With some strategically placed cushions for sitting up straighter, they can be all-purpose. If your living space is intended only as a place for conversation or book reading, choose furniture that offers good back support and encourages a more upright position.

I am 190 cm (6 ft 4 in) tall and the sofa in my home suits me – my 170 cm (5 ft 6 in) mate sits on it and his legs stick straight out in front of him. Ensure the primary occupants of the home are catered for, but also make sure you have a variety of furniture that suits various body sizes; you want to make sure people feel comfortable.

When I'm designing seating for a living room, I work with the following basic sizes as guides.

▶ Depending on your personal style, joinery does not have to be expensive or highly sophisticated. Instead, it can be seen as a support to your things, the belongings that tell a story about you, not only to your visitors, but also as a narrative for you as you move around your home.

▼ Good comfortable dining chairs will let people stay at the table longer and take the heat off your sofa.

Sofas (all 90 cm/35 inches deep):
180 cm/70 in (2-seater)
190 cm/75 in (2.5-seater)
215 cm/84 in (3-seater)
260 cm/102 in (4-seater)

But do consider that a 3-seater will often not actually properly cater for three people. Maybe in a family situation with dad and two kids curled up on the lounge, or maybe mum and dad and the dog. Certainly three of my mates would not feel comfortable all sitting shoulder to shoulder on a 3-seater sofa: it would feel awkward.

Corner sofas:
220 cm/86 in square (2-seater with corner)
310 x 210 cm/122 x 82 in (3-seater with chaise)

Arm chairs:
95 cm (37 in) deep x 85 cm (33 in) wide

Coffee tables:
100 x 60 cm (39 x 23 in)
120 x 80 cm (47 x 31 in)

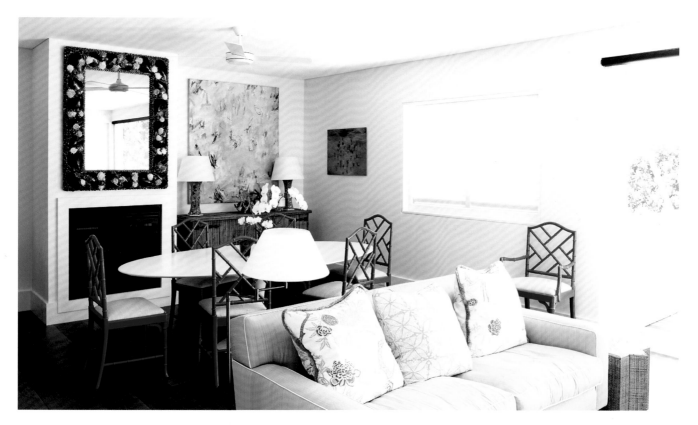

Coffee tables and side tables come in so many different sizes that I work out what will fit the space and then search for a corresponding size. Unless it is a favourite heirloom I try not to design a living space around a side table.

DEFINING THE FLOOR SPACE

Rugs can work beautifully to define a space. Whether on hard floors or carpet they can bind furniture together and make the living area a cohesive 'place', especially if it is part of a larger room. Rugs fail when they are not connected to anything else; they can end up looking like an unwelcoming island in a space. Choose a larger rug that can run under sofas and disappear under an armchair to 'ground' the room.

A safe decorating option is to have a light white room, with a good-quality floor in a neutral tone, whether that is timber, carpet or tile. The floor can be light or dark. Once you have this neutral floor background, you can go wild with the rug. Make it psychedelic, if you want – or jet black, or bright red – it is easily replaceable, so take a risk.

Standard rug sizes:
160 x 230 cm (63 x 90 in)
200 x 290 cm (79 x 114 in)
250 x 350 cm (98 x 138 in)

THE BLACK HOLE

A fact of life for most families is that a TV screen will be in the living room. This is great for catching the news, watching the Olympics or enjoying a movie; however, the rest of the time the TV becomes a dead black hole that dominates the room. And those black holes are getting so much bigger!

It is good to give that black hole some context, some framework, so that it is considered and cared for. I often create custom joinery to hide the TV behind sliding screens or drop down doors. This can be quite an expensive option, so if it isn't possible then we encourage the use of a good-quality entertainment unit; the best ones give the TV a setting in the room. Because a TV is so black I usually choose black or white entertainment units. However, colour can be a great foil and a long timber unit will look fantastic.

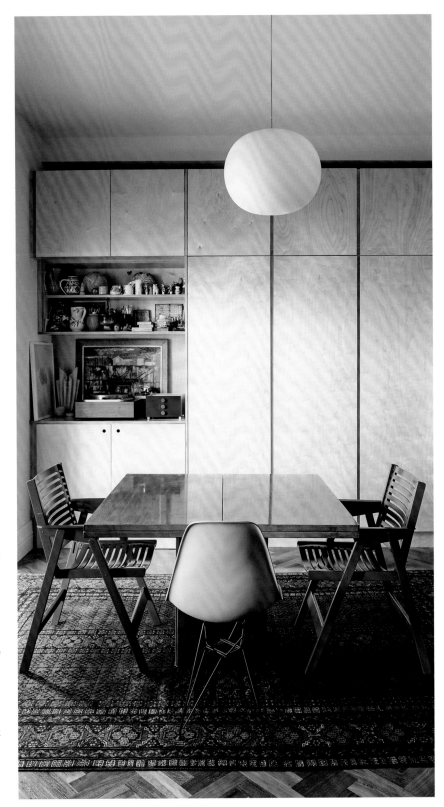

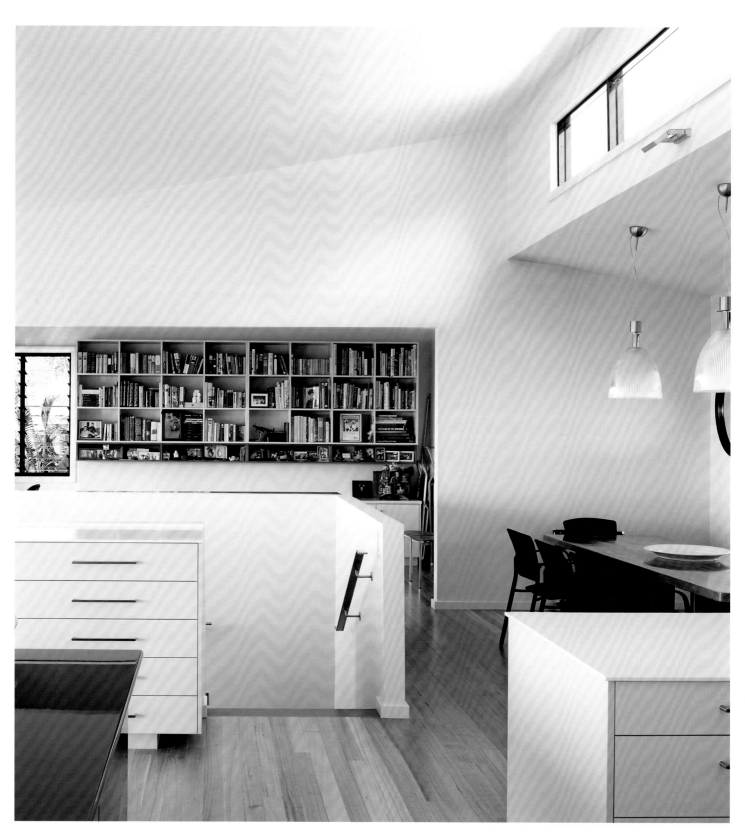

SOPHISTICATION THROUGH CONCENTRATED CLUTTER

Another option is to merge your TV cabinet with a library of books or artwork. I often treat a whole wall as an entertainment unit – I call it the 'service wall'. This can feature the TV, audio equipment, books, games, artwork, ornaments... Everything. This becomes your go-to wall for things to do. It gives the TV context so that it isn't left looking lonely (and, yes, a TV can look lonely). Also, concentrating all these items onto one wall will allow your other walls to breathe and be uncluttered. You will find this gives a sense of space and is more relaxing than having stuff spread over all the walls. Concentrating these items together makes them stronger aesthetically and more organised – you can keep the other walls bare, or perhaps feature a large singular piece of artwork.

DINING IN THE OPEN-PLAN LIVING ROOM

So, these days the open-plan kitchen/living room also often incorporates dining facilities. Increasingly the dining table has many more roles than just a place to eat – it is a workplace, a conversation place, a place for homework, a place to build the latest Lego set. A dining table that doesn't look as if it belongs can throw the rhythm of the whole living space. The size of the table needs to be perfectly suited to the size of space it is allowed in the room, or it will very quickly feel cumbersome and clumsy, or small and mean. Get the size right by careful planning and then choose a solid piece that looks as if it means to be there. Then everything around it can be lighter and more transient.

◁ The raking ceiling up to the clerestory windows not only lets in light but also makes the room feel a lot bigger. Note the pendants over the dining table to define the space.

▽ By adding an unexpected upper window, the space of this room has totally changed. The lower ceiling under the upper window distinguishes the dining from the kitchen and living, while the horizontal bulkhead connects the living and kitchen at each end of the overall room. The window of the dining area was designed to be enjoyed at sitting height.

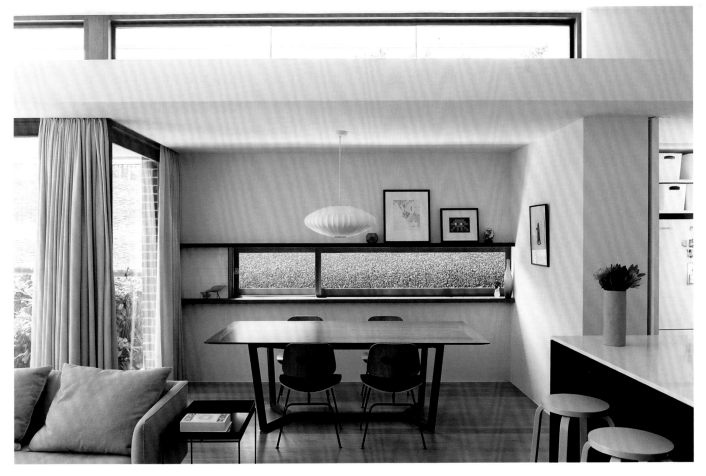

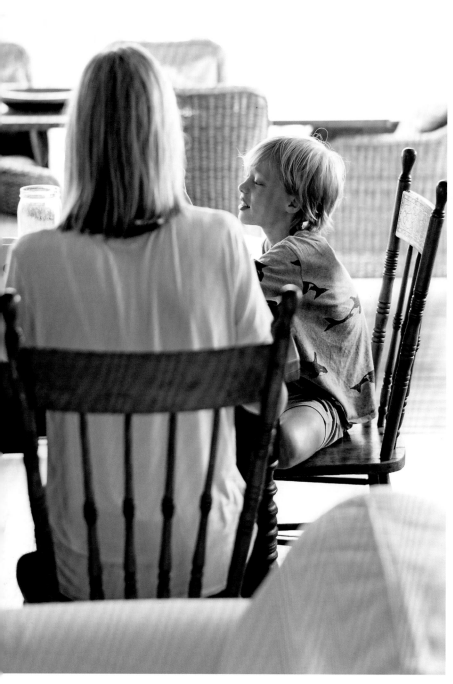

DINING COMFORT

The seating you choose for your dining table can take the heat off the living room furniture. If you choose good comfortable dining chairs then the diners at your table may never feel inclined to move to the sofa or armchairs. If the dining chairs allow people to sit in a relaxed way for a long period of time, then suddenly you can seat eight at the table and your sofa will only need to be large enough for immediate family. In a lot of ways, the dining table is more important than the sofa as it promotes conversation. In our house, the sofa is often only used if we want to watch a movie together – and that is easily fixed by a few floor cushions. In the best restaurants the chairs are almost lounge chairs – they are comfortable enough to keep you at that table for hours.

THE 20 POSSESSIONS RULE

Less is more. I believe you will have a much happier life with less stuff in your space. This doesn't mean nothing; it just means having the things you care about around you and getting rid of the rest. How good does it feel to walk into a room that you have just cleaned? Well, imagine having that feeling every day – the way to achieve it is by having fewer things, with each thing having its own spot. If you can tidy up a room in 5 minutes by only having 20 items to put away instead of 200, and then doing a quick vacuum, you are in control of your space.

CONTRAST IN DECOR

Contrast is a key factor of design. Used well, it can make a space; used badly, it can break it. The rule of thumb is that dark colours recede and light colours come towards you. It is difficult to rely on this rule, as it is broken surprisingly often. In general, the lighter and brighter a room, the bigger it will feel. If you fill a room with dark colours, it will feel smaller. If you have timber floors, then choose furniture that is lighter coloured than the timber and the space will feel bigger.

When it comes to artwork on walls, hang them at eye level; on average, around 150 cm (59 in) above floor height. This ensures the perspective of the room is defined at average human height. If you hang artworks higher or lower it can make the room feel awkward or top-heavy.

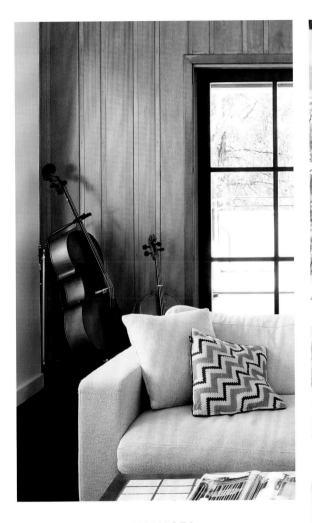

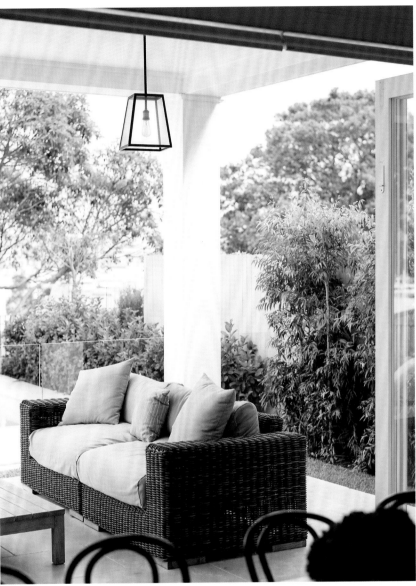

SEASONAL CHANGES

In your living space, think about seasons. When you want to be warm and cosy you can't beat a fireplace. When you want to be cool in summer it's good to be able to open up your space and let in the sun and air. In our house we have a summer rug and a winter rug. We change the cushions over to darker, more comfy cushions in winter. Some friends even have spring and autumn cushions – they use the same cushion and just change the covers. We hang warm blankets over the back of the sofa for people to snuggle up with when watching the telly or reading a book. When the weather warms up and spring arrives, we enjoy changing the rug and cushions and putting away the blankets so that suddenly the room becomes fresher and lovelier. This is a cost-effective way to change your space quite radically.

CHANGE YOUR TONE

Just by introducing black into your space, you can formalise it very quickly. For an executive and sophisticated look, just add a black carpet or rug and black furniture and see how much the space changes. White and colour and fun artworks will create a more relaxed space.

◀◀ Sitting 'up' at the dining table is always conducive to conversation because you are physically more engaged.

◀ Less clutter is better and this empty corner has been given a reason for being with two instruments — no more.

▲ Changing the cushions on this sofa moves the look from summer to winter, or bright to neutral, as shown here.

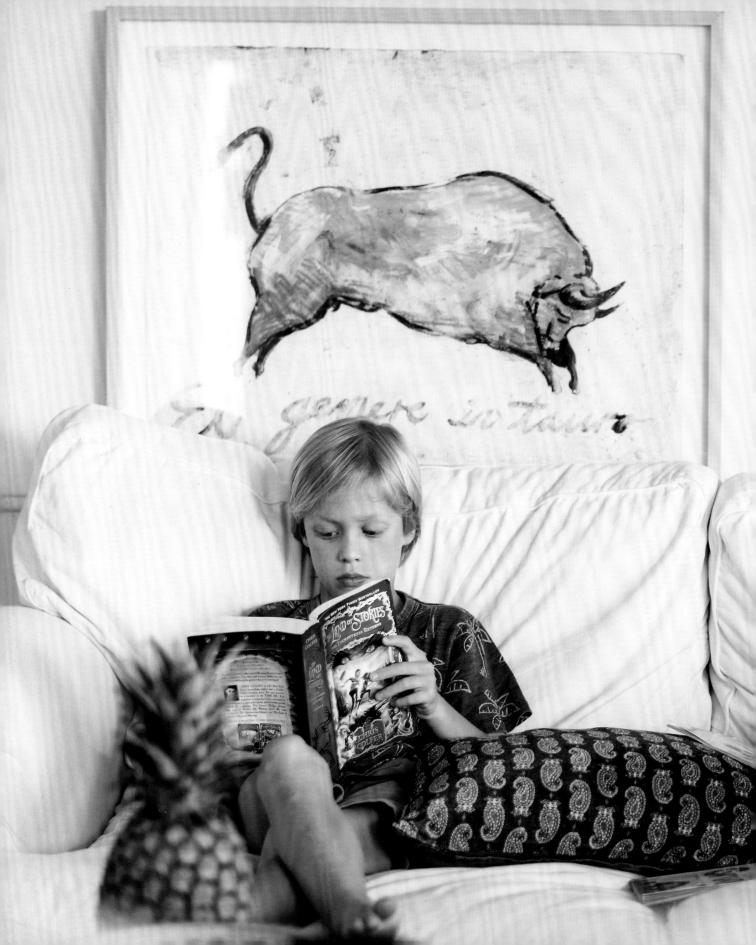

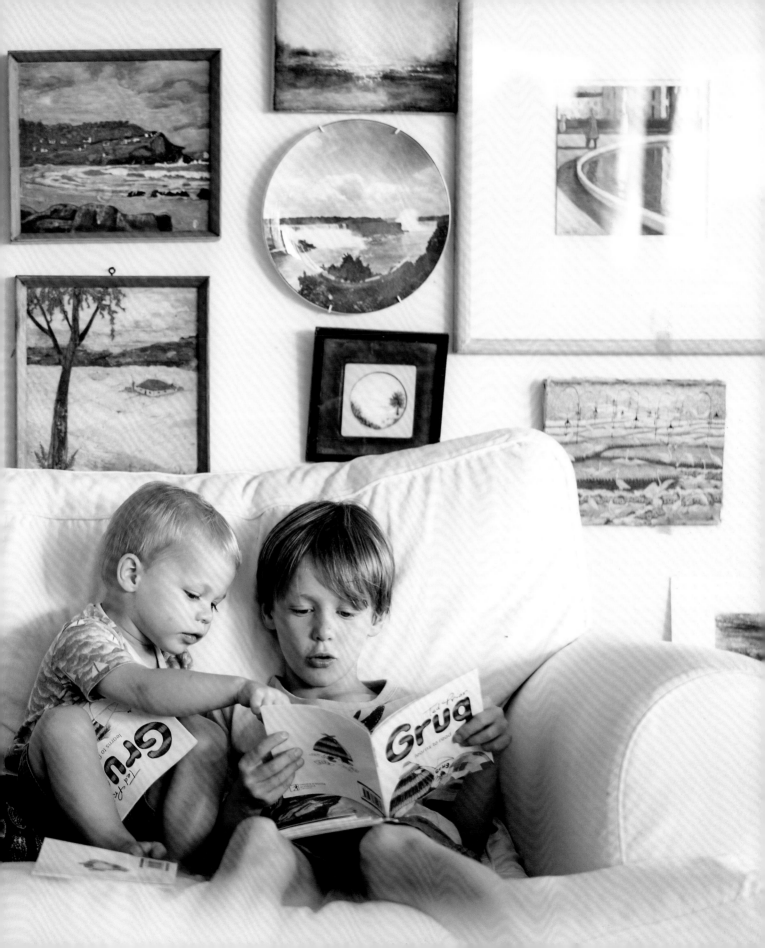

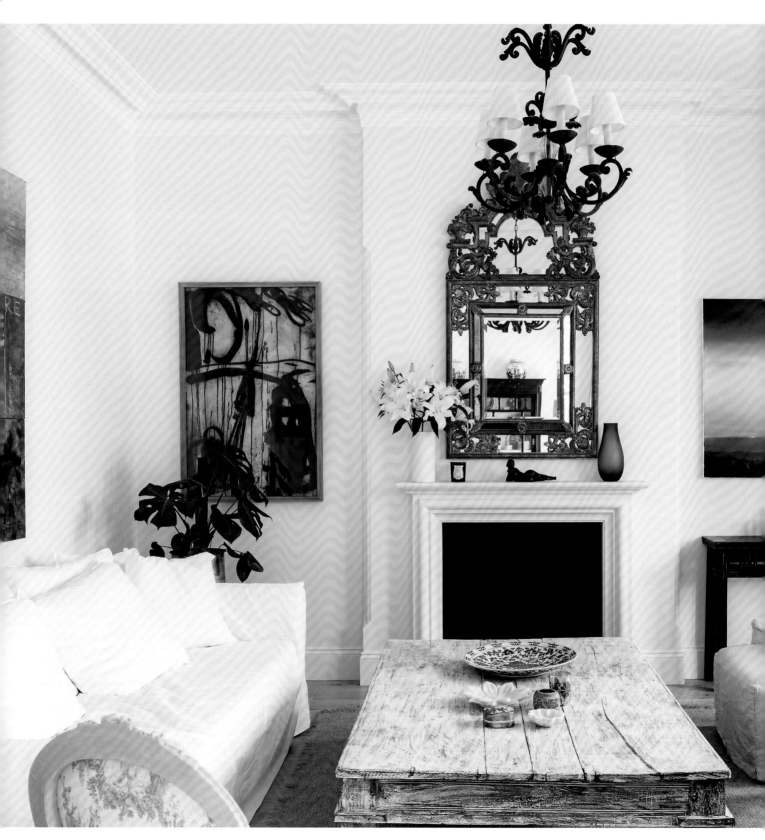

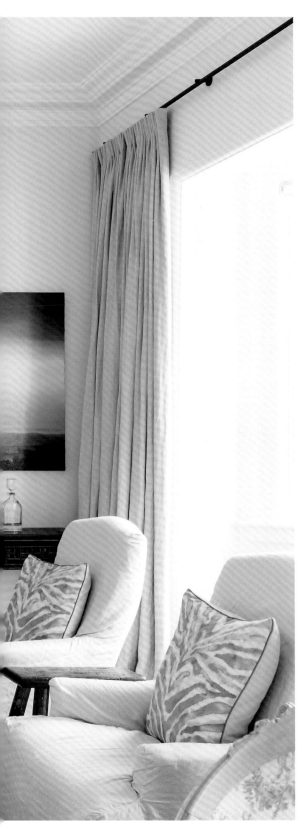

LIGHT

Many different activities take place in the living room – from conversation and watching movies, to relaxing and dancing. Light therefore has to be flexible. Light can emphasise the best qualities of your room. It can make it feel bigger, deeper, longer, higher, or cosier... And all this can be achieved with the same fittings.

A living room without natural light is not really a 'living room'. In fact, it is against the law in Australia to design a living room that does not get a minimum of two hours of sun a day. First, you need to orientate your design to ensure windows face north (in the southern hemisphere; south in the northern hemisphere). This will allow sun to come into the room for at least some part of the day.

An easy change that can make a huge difference to an existing home is to work out where sunlight falls in relation to the house. For example, if there is a part of the home that gets morning sun then that is where I would put the breakfast table. If there is a part of the home that gets afternoon sun, then that is where I would be putting the living room, especially in winter so that the family can enjoy the warmth of the afternoon sun.

SKYLIGHTS AND SUN TUNNELS

Natural light does not have to be direct. Skylights are a very useful way to get soft southern light into a space without being glary. The skylights can be placed on a roof pitch so that they don't get direct sun but let in constant good-quality light throughout the day. I often use skylights to channel direct sun into dark areas as well, and the top brands now have blinds that can be pulled down to stop harsh sun. These can now be up in the ceiling, well out of reach, as they are electronically controlled – they even have rain sensors and automatically close if they are open and sense a downpour.

Sun tunnels can bring light from a completely different area into a space that is dark. They are essentially a tube connecting two small

◀ Grounded with a timber floor and a dark rug, this room makes the most of the light from the bay window. The selection of light-coloured furniture, coffee table and curtains enhances the feeling of brightness.

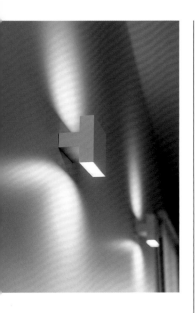

▲ The ambient light provided by these fittings is a perfect combination of uplights onto the white ceiling, with wall washers casting a diffuse light down the walls.

▶ This pendant light fulfils the dual role of task lighting the dining table, while also defining the dining space within the greater living space. Notice how perfectly the light from the dining window illuminates the dining table.

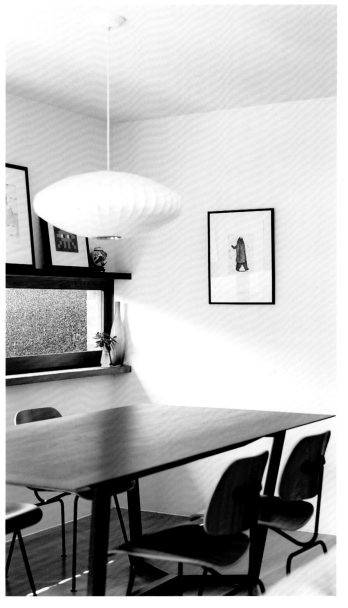

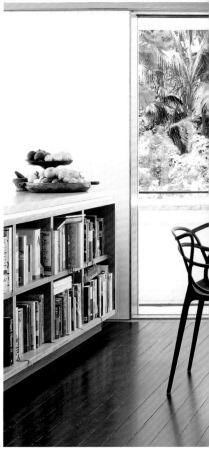

penetrations in the roof and ceiling and can be a cost-effective lifesaver when renovating old dark houses with deep roofs. A skylight is more expensive in a deep roof as you need to create a shaft in the ceiling to fit it – more beautiful but more expensive.

You don't have to be going through a renovation to fit sun tunnels or skylights – just like an air-conditioner, they can be fitted by tradespeople as an individual project.

DOWNLIGHT DOWNER

For me, the great scourge of the average home is the downlight. I find few aspects of my work more depressing than walking into an otherwise well-designed home and seeing a grid of downlights over the living area. Downlights are designed to be task lights, which means they emit strong light in a very directional way. So, in a grid you experience a room that is light, dark, light, dark, light, dark. It is glary and uncomfortable for anyone in the room. You might have even had the experience of feeling uncomfortable and realising there is a downlight directly above you. (In some houses with low ceilings I can feel the heat of the halogen downlights on my head!) It is never pleasant to have a directional light trained on your forehead, and I find it impossible to relax and be comfortable under a spotlight.

You should never be walking into a shopping

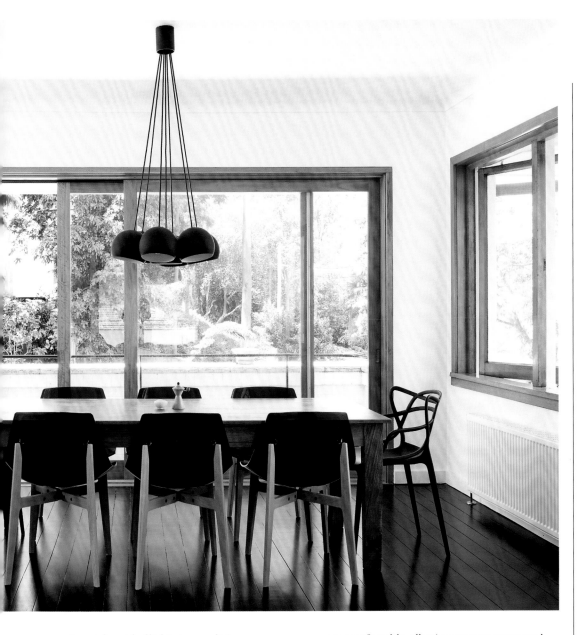

◀ Close to the kitchen bench, this dining table has also become a light-filled spot to sit and chat with whoever is in the kitchen. It is the lively hub of the home and the styling is warm and practical with the dark floor, chairs and statement light in contrast to the white walls and timbers.

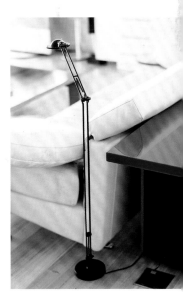

▲ I like to introduce floor and table lamps in the living area. Floor lamps can come up and over your shoulder to light the page you are reading.

centre-style grid of lights in your living room; use downlights purely for tasks such as reading a book or to spotlight an artwork.

AMBIENT LIGHT

For ambient lighting I like to use non-directional light, such as uplights that illuminate the ceiling (always white) and/or wall washers that light the walls. This sort of light that bounces off surfaces is more diffuse and far softer in a room. It is much more sophisticated.

A perfect living room should have gentle ambient hidden light sources that light ceilings and wash down walls. This light defines the boundaries of the room, which makes us feel more comfortable, allowing us to move around and survey the space easily. The light level can be quite low – you would be surprised how low it can be and still be comfortable. The ambient light in your living room need only be enough to show you the extent of the room so you know where you are in relation to it and have enough light to navigate the space.

A basic rule is that you should have dimmers on lights in spaces where you spend time, such as the living room. (It is much cheaper to fix dimmers when the lights are being put in.) Dimmers give you control over your space and how much light is in it. You can have the lights up if you are performing a task or right down if you are relaxing or watching a movie. All light sources, except the most specific, such as a task light for reading or working, should be dimmable. A dinner party in the living room could have the lights dimmed when dessert is over and the wine starts to flow.

MUST DON'T

NEVER PUT A GRID OF DOWNLIGHTS IN YOUR LIVING ROOM. INSTEAD, USE A VARIETY OF LIGHT SOURCES, SUCH AS LAMPS AND WALL LIGHTS, TO GIVE YOU DESIGN CONTROL.

WARM OR COOL?

Warm lighting includes warmer tones of white, yellow and orange. Cool lighting includes cooler tones of white, blue and green. A living room, generally speaking, should have soft warm lighting – it is much more calming. You could introduce cooler lights in a localised and directional way – for example, focus a cool light to bring out the correct colours in a painting. Or have a cooler task light to aid your concentration if you are reading a report in your armchair. In the living room, I use the philosophy of less is more.

ACCENT AND TASK LIGHTS

The living room should have a few different light sources, and I don't mean downlights. Introduce lighting of different kinds at different levels: wall washers, uplighters, floor lamps, table lamps, feature highlights and candlelight. Once the ambient lighting is fitted, I love to introduce floor and table lamps. Floor lamps can come up and over your shoulder to light the page you are reading, and table lamps will light nooks in the room and tell the story of the home by highlighting a family photo, any heirlooms, art, a grandfather clock or an antique chair.

LIGHT SPILL

In these days of open-plan living, spaces merge in many ways, including lighting. Remember, you will get light spill from one part of a room to another. Consider switching the lights off in the living room area, leaving on the accent lights in the kitchen, dining area or hallway. This may give you enough background light to relax in the living space and enjoy the evening news or a movie.

And, of course, during the day, placement of windows is key to allowing light into the room. I always consider it a win the later it is that I need to turn the lights on.

MIRROR, MIRROR

A clever way to bring a sense of light into a living room is through the use of mirrors. By carefully

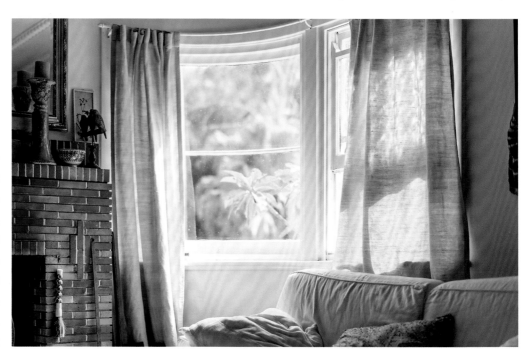

▶ Give yourself options to control natural light. Sometimes this sunny window is too dazzling, and that is when the translucent curtains come into their own.

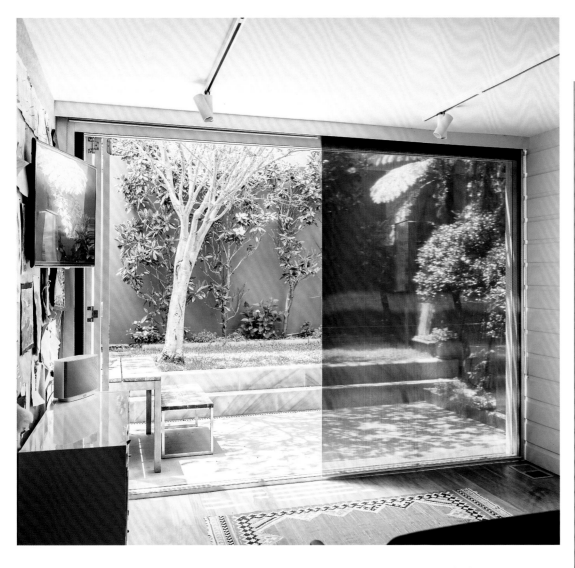

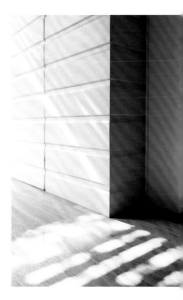

◄ Large bifold doors completely open this living area to the garden. If the sun gets too intense, then sheer blinds can be dropped to stop the glare and reduce heat, while still ensuring a view and a sense of the garden beyond.

▲ Dappled light is not only beautiful to behold, but also brings out the character of the materials that it falls upon.

placing a mirror you can catch light and bounce it into other parts of the room. A classic example is to place a mirror on the wall perpendicular to a window, but you can also think vertically and consider placing a mirror on the wall underneath a skylight. The shaft of light coming down will bounce off the mirror – if you get a reflection of blue sky, that is a bonus!

WARMING THE SOUL

In the days before artificial light we used firelight for vision after dark, whether through fireplaces or candles and lamps. Firelight is an absorbing and relaxing sight (our ancestors have been staring deeply into it for thousands of years). It has also been fundamental to our development and survival. It is not an accident that restaurants introduce candlelight to tables for dinner; the light, the dance and flicker of the flame is an ancient accompaniment to the human evening and encourages conversation and a feeling of comfort. And so candlelight is a welcome addition to a living room – dim the lights and add a few candles and you will greatly enhance the atmosphere for a relaxing evening.

A fireplace brings a presence that produces warmth and security. It has the power to captivate a room and when in use it draws people around it as a gathering point. One of the amazing things about a fireplace is that it allows for a pause in conversation. It is not at all awkward to not talk for a while and to just stare into the flames. Contemplate how the light from a fire warms the room, the body and the soul.

▷ This white room, grounded by a dark floor and with excellent light penetration, allows for an eclectic mix of furniture to show off the personal style of this home owner. The vertical wall of white timber slats bookends the living space, reflecting light from the glazed doors and defining the space.

Once you have the design fundamentals of a room right, it gives you the freedom to explore your personal style with decoration.

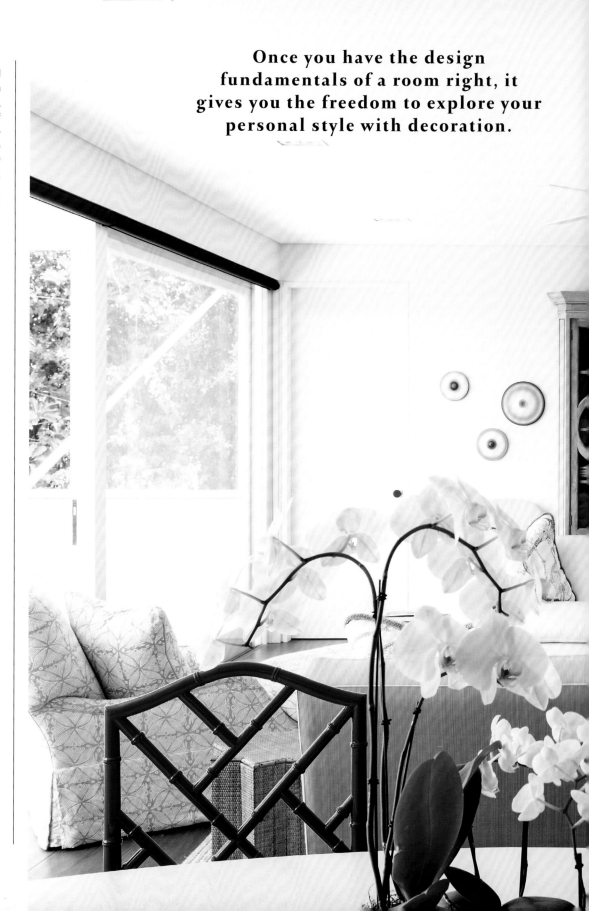

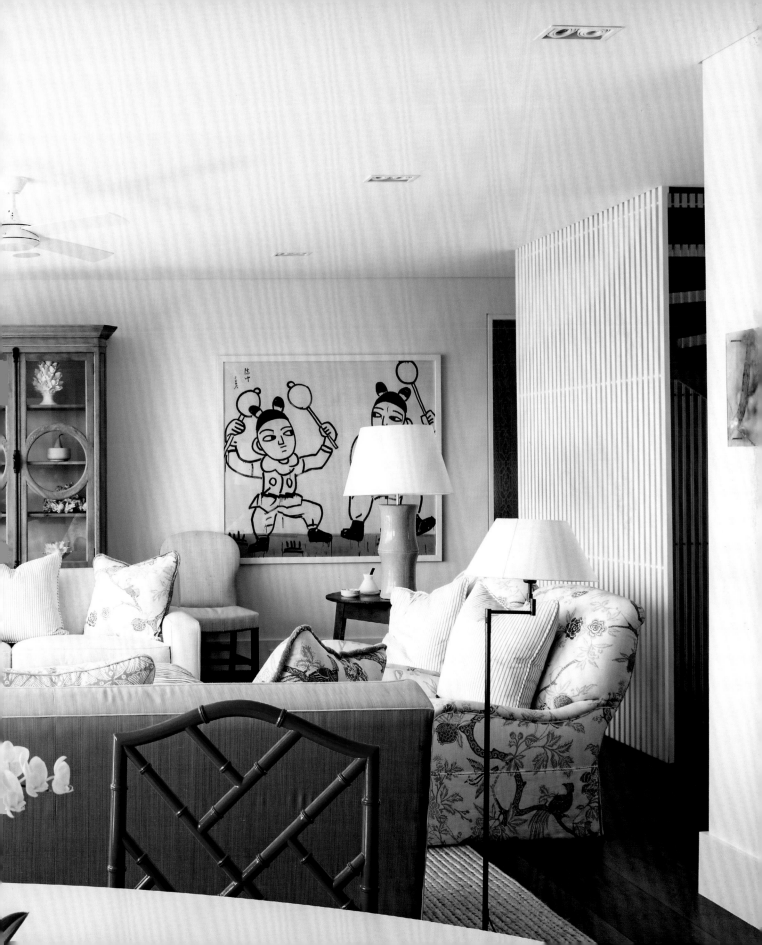

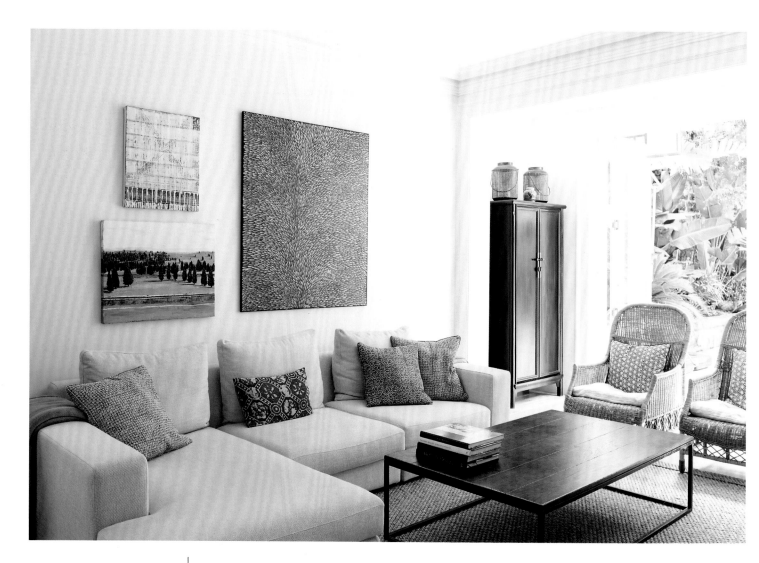

▲ This sofa sits between two openings on either side of the house, ensuring that cross-ventilation passes over the people who are seated. If it gets too cold, closing one of the openings will reduce airflow.

AIR

Once you have positioned your living space with the correct aspect, and taken some time to work out the wind directions that affect your home, you can design your living room to maximise that air flow. If you know there is going to be a cooling breeze just when you need it in the hot summer months, make it work for you. Your living room should hopefully be getting some sunlight, so make sure you put some easily opened doors or windows on the side of the house that faces the cooling summer breeze. Then locate openings to the outdoors on the other side of your house. Once you open both sides, if there is a breeze, and you don't need much, you will instantly feel the air begin to flow. And the air moving across your body is naturally cooling. My dad always placed furniture in the best spots to take advantage of this summer breeze, and I have strong memories of sitting on a couch at a beach house with a door open on one side of the house and a window on the other. I could feel the breeze moving over my legs and arms as I sat and read *Tintin*. It was something that, once I understood, I always marvelled over; it was so glaringly hot outside, but inside, with correctly designed cross-ventilation, we felt cool and comfortable.

MANUFACTURED BREEZE

If there is no breeze, never fear: that is why man invented the fan. The best way to get the air moving is a ceiling-mounted fan. A ceiling fan can also work *with* your air-conditioner to cool your space: add a chill factor with a fan and it takes the pressure off your air-conditioner so you don't have to turn it to such a low temperature. Buy a great-looking fan that suits the aesthetic of your home, but, even more importantly, ensure it is quiet. There are few things more annoying than a repetitive squeak in your living room.

There are so many fantastic options on the market, but please oh please don't combine a fan and a light. I know they seem like a great deal – two for the price of one – but they are so inelegant. I have never seen a good-looking fan-light – and please send me a picture of one if you feel I am wrong – but I really don't think they exist. There tends to be a slight shake you get in the light when the fan is rotating.

EASY OPENINGS

To capture that breeze, make sure you fit practical and manageable openings, such as sliding doors and windows or banks of louvre windows. Louvres are my favourite – they not only provide the breeze but they also *look* as if

they do. An open wall of louvres instantly gives an impression of cooling, even if you haven't yet felt the airflow. If you are worried about insects, such as mosquitoes, you can fit flyscreens for louvres and even for bi-fold doors. There are elegant systems now that can span 6 metres (18 feet), using vertical rollers at each end that meet in the middle and connect with magnets.

CROSS-VENTILATION IN APARTMENTS

Because apartments are often a box with only one face to the outside, it can be difficult to achieve airflow. In these circumstances ceiling fans and/or air-conditioners are mandatory. If you are looking for an apartment keep your eye out for one that is a through-building apartment – so it has window openings at both front and back. This will allow through airflow to keep it cool and fresh.

TEMPERATURE CONTROL

Openings in your roof are key to controlling the temperature in your house. By designing clerestories into your house with windows you allow hot air to escape and then also draw cool air in.

MUST DON'T

PLEASE DON'T EVER FIT A COMBINED CEILING FAN-LIGHT. THEY DON'T LOOK GOOD, AND THEY INEVITABLY END UP DEVELOPING A RATTLING SHAKE, WHICH IN TURN LEADS TO A SHAKY LIGHT FLICKERING AROUND YOUR LIVING ROOM.

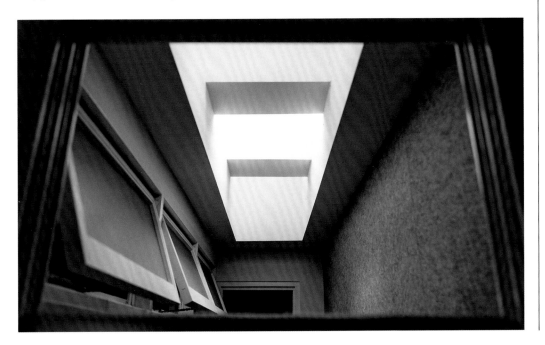

◀ An air and light chimney in a terraced house offers a lot of opportunity to enliven a home. Creating a two-storey void from the ground floor living room up to electric-opening skylights allows air and light to travel through the house. The family bathroom, ensuite and a bedroom all have windows opening into this space, allowing airflow and light into these otherwise landlocked rooms. In summer hot air gathers at the top of the void and can be released through the openable skylights, which in turn draw cooler air through the house.

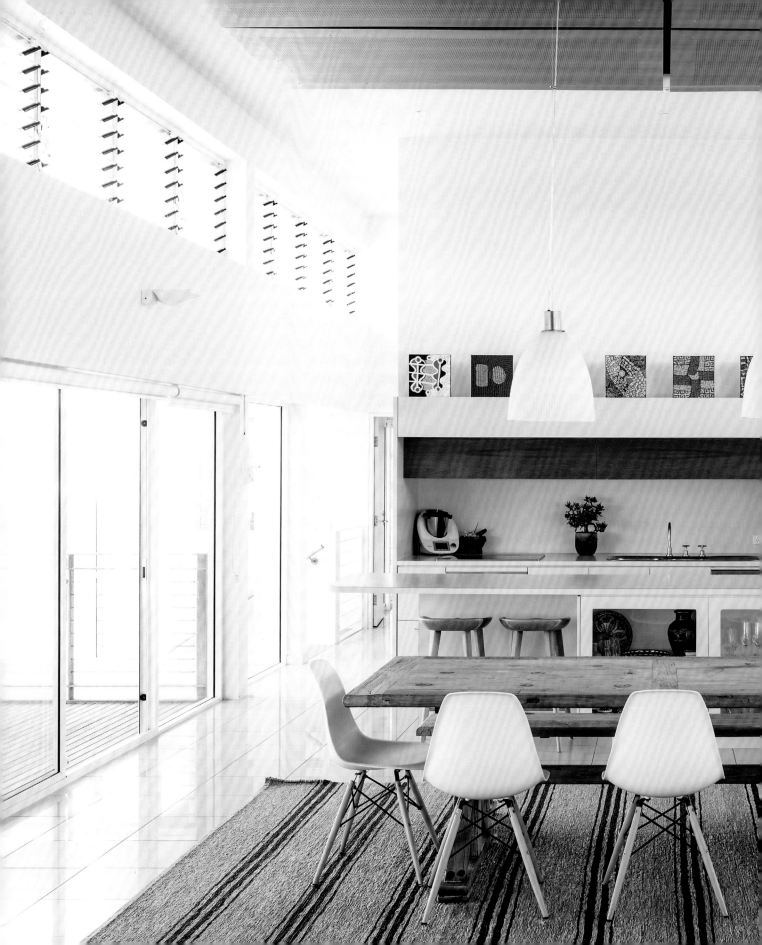

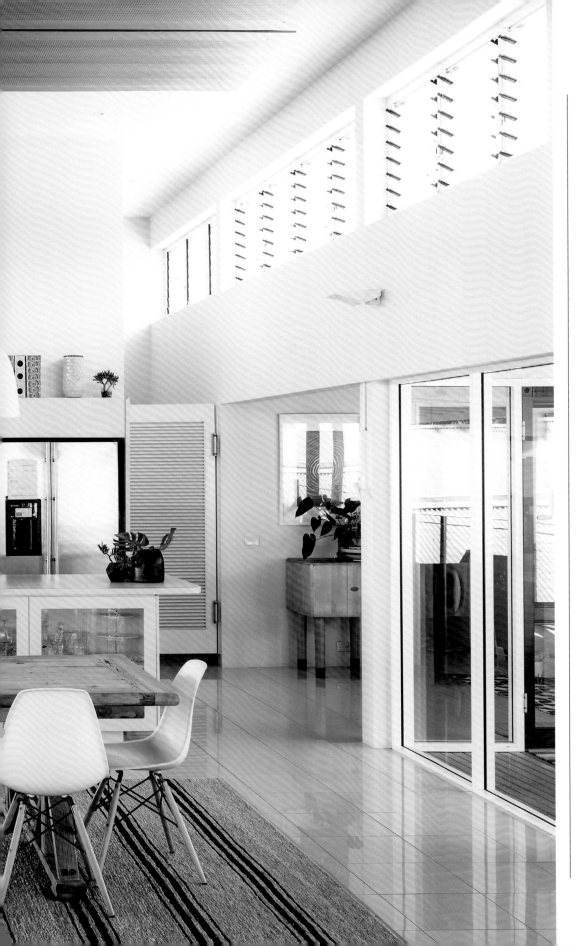

◀ A magnificent room of light and air. The clerestory windows not only let in light but also allow heat to escape on hot days. The tall space is capped with timber acoustic panels that dampen echo and add a warm aesthetic. Wall up-lights illuminate the acoustic panels and ceiling at night, creating a soft diffuse ambience, while the pendants provide focused light on the dining table.

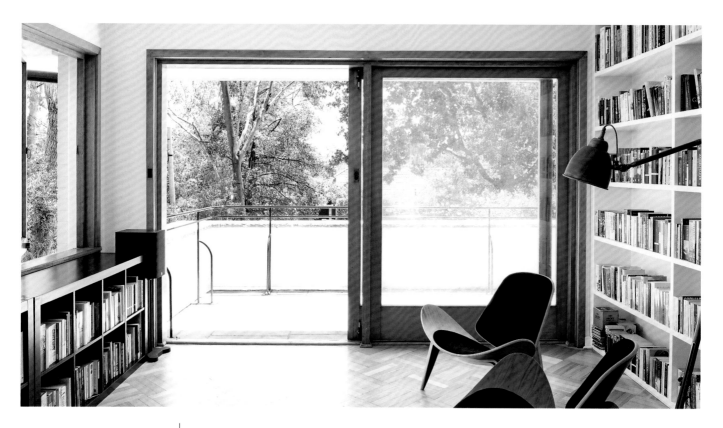

Give yourself options for letting air in. In this room you can either open the door, open the window, or open both for cross-ventilation. It depends on the day and the breeze.

Openable skylights do the same job and there are many electric varieties on the market now that open at the touch of a button and let hot air out. In winter, warm air from your heating system rises and gathers in roof and ceiling spaces. Keep clerestory windows and skylights closed and introduce a ceiling fan on slow reverse to push the warm air back down and make your heating more efficient.

A COOL TRICK

If you create shaded gardens full of plants on the cool side of your house and put in plenty of windows on that side, you will have a bank of cool air to draw on in the summer months. They also rid the air of carbon monoxide and add oxygen, making a healthier environment – if the plants are where you want to draw in the cool air, you will be bringing fresh oxygenated air into your home at the same time as cooling it.

THERMAL MASS

You can control the temperature of the air in your home by using thermal mass – the absorption of heat, either man-made or from the sun, into solid materials such as stone, concrete or earth. These elements take a long time to transfer temperature and so can become great insulators. If you let the sun hit a concrete floor, after the sun has gone you will feel the heat emanating from the floor, keeping you warm through the evening.

Good insulation in walls and ceiling is imperative for controlling temperature. In summer it insulates your home from searing heat; in winter it keeps warm air inside and prevents it escaping.

DOUBLE-GLAZING

One of the biggest problems I find in Australian housing is that we have not invested in double-glazing in our windows. Single-glazed windows transfer temperature freely, so, even if a home has well-insulated walls and roof, it might then allow heat or cold to enter through the windows. And I won't even get started on the gaps around doors and windows. Many houses are extremely poorly sealed, which is very energy inefficient and bad for the environment.

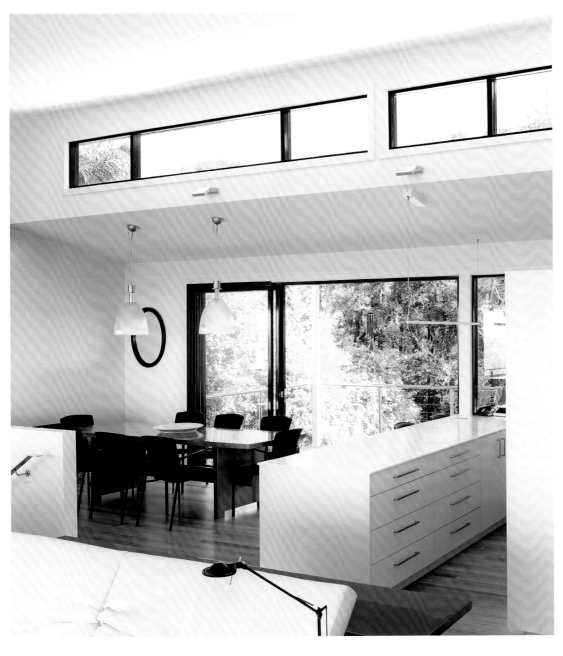

◁ During the day the clerestory windows and glazed wall of sliding doors allow airflow and light into the kitchen, dining and living spaces. Note that no downlights are used in this room. Uplights under the clerestory windows direct their beam at the ceiling to bounce ambient light back down into the space. Two pendants hang over the dining table and a linear pendant hangs over the kitchen bench to provide suitable task lighting. And in the foreground a floor lamp is perfectly poised for anyone reading on the sofa.

We need to learn a lesson from Europe and spend a bit more upfront during building to get substantial cost-saving benefits down the track, including using less energy to artificially heat and cool our homes.

The correct use of shutters and blinds over windows will help to stop the sun at its harshest. Or you can shade windows from the outside with hoods or eaves, or maybe even plant a tree. It is a lovely idea to consider a deciduous tree that provides cool shade in summer and then sheds its leaves to let in the precious winter sun.

Of course, one particularly mind-blowing form of temperature control is to put on a jumper. Fancy that! Unfortunately, many of us would rather turn up the heating and burn the earth's resources, so that we can sit around in our shorts in the middle of winter. Ridiculous.

▶ Designed with sliding doors, this living space is alive with air and light. In winter you can close up, keep the cold air out, but still feel aware of the passing day.

▼ Form and function: the brickwork in this hearth supports and frames the fireplace. And the brickwork will also absorb heat from the fire and give off latent warmth, even after the fire has gone out.

AIR-CONDITIONING AND HEATING

In Sydney, where I live, we can get away for most of the year without air-conditioning, by using natural (and cheap) systems of cooling. And that is good for the soul. Air-con has a poor reputation in the design world as being bad for the environment and often unnecessary. It is true that air-conditioning is often required, but that is because the building itself has been poorly designed and doesn't take advantage of the environment it is in. Or the occupants of the home are not aware that by opening and closing a few windows they could create a cooling breeze. You often don't need air-conditioning if you get the fundamentals right – house orientation, site position and openings to catch cool airflow.

However, there are always days that are stiflingly hot with no breeze. As a purist, I would fix this with ceiling fans and an attitude of embracing the weather wherever I live, but air-conditioning can be an absolute life-saver for the elderly or very young. Its efficiency has improved enormously over the past 10 years, so be sure to research which type best suits your home. Be aware that air-conditioning comes in many forms, from ducted to split system. Ask a number of consultants and suppliers what is best for you and make sure what is being recommended is right for your needs, rather than just being right for the installer/supplier.

Reverse-cycle air-conditioning can be used for both heating and cooling; however, don't forget that heating from split-system air-conditioning (these have a cassette in your home that is connected to an outside unit housing the condenser) is not always the most efficient, as the hot air has to be pushed down from a height. Any heating you have is better created at a low level so that the house is heated as the air rises. A ducted system through the floor is always a pleasure.

Take care when working out where the compressors and evaporators will go – they are often noisy and certainly aren't pretty. Try to put them somewhere on the exterior of the house that isn't obtrusive – please consider your neighbours.

OTHER HEATING

An electric portable heater on wheels can heat a small room quite efficiently if the room is well insulated, but as soon as you move to larger spaces, such as living rooms, it starts to struggle. A gas heater can be a great option in a living room (but do note that they create emissions so are not for bedrooms or anywhere you intend to sleep). It is best to have some ventilation in the living room when using one – although current gas heaters

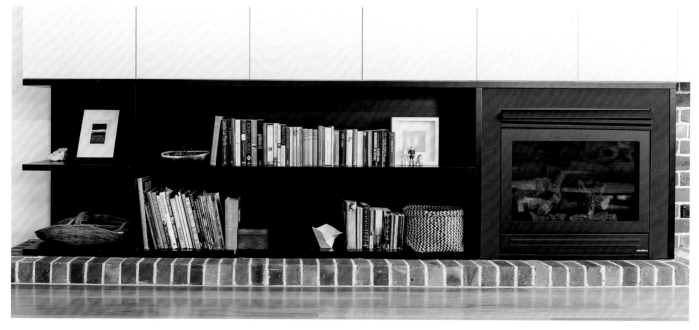

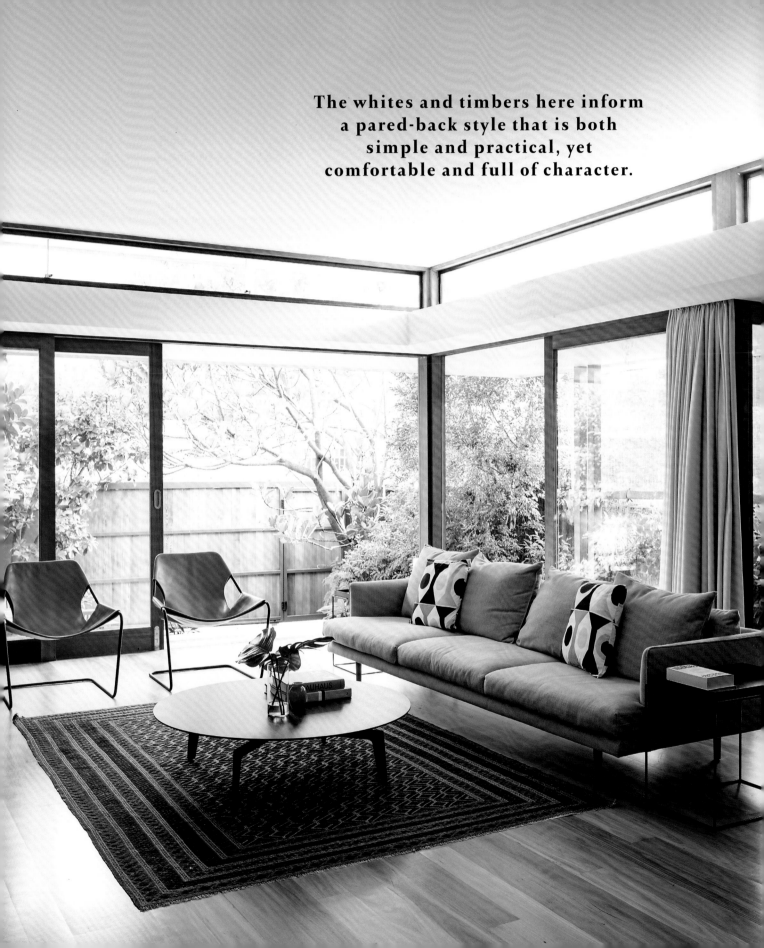

The whites and timbers here inform
a pared-back style that is both
simple and practical, yet
comfortable and full of character.

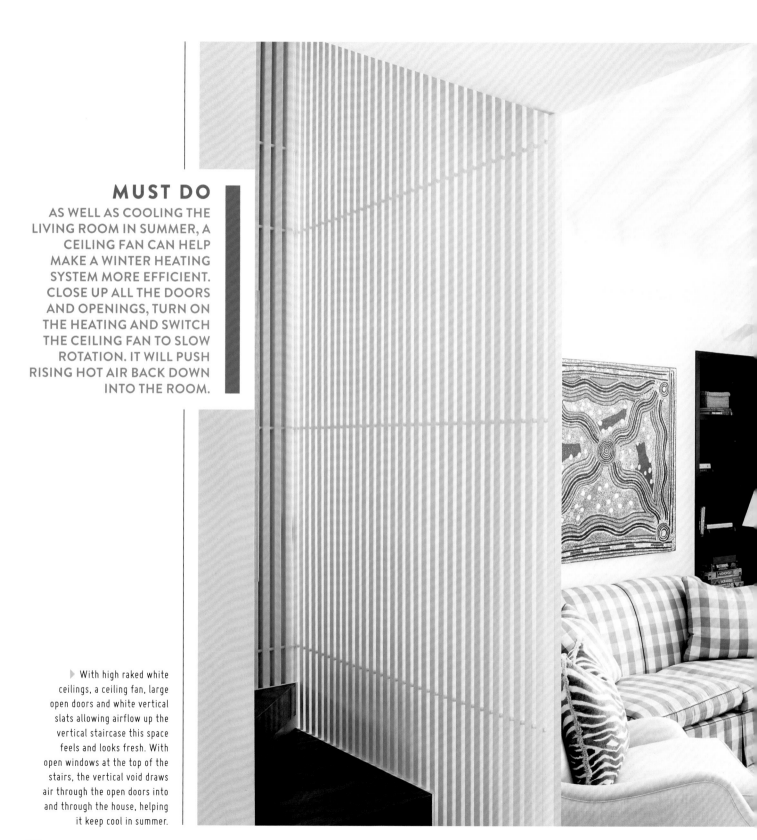

MUST DO

AS WELL AS COOLING THE
LIVING ROOM IN SUMMER, A
CEILING FAN CAN HELP
MAKE A WINTER HEATING
SYSTEM MORE EFFICIENT.
CLOSE UP ALL THE DOORS
AND OPENINGS, TURN ON
THE HEATING AND SWITCH
THE CEILING FAN TO SLOW
ROTATION. IT WILL PUSH
RISING HOT AIR BACK DOWN
INTO THE ROOM.

▶ With high raked white
ceilings, a ceiling fan, large
open doors and white vertical
slats allowing airflow up the
vertical staircase this space
feels and looks fresh. With
open windows at the top of the
stairs, the vertical void draws
air through the open doors into
and through the house, helping
it keep cool in summer.

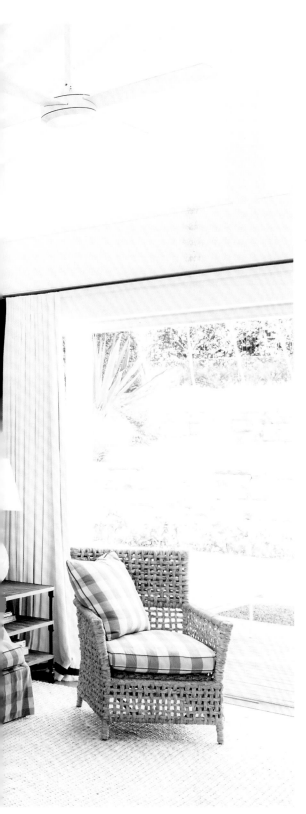

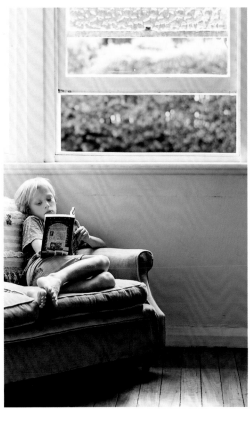

◀ Asger enjoying a book
and some excellent
cross-ventilation!

have clever technology that switches them off if it detects lower than usual oxygen levels.

Another way to heat your home is to warm the floor itself with hydronic heating – this system puts tubes under tiles or carpet, or in a concrete floor, and then runs hot water through them. It can be an efficient mode of heating, particularly if your water is gas- or solar-heated. However, it can become very inefficient if left on for too long throughout the year. The technology has improved a lot, though, and while it was once used only in bathrooms it is now becoming more popular throughout the home.

Central heating with radiators is very popular in colder parts of the world, such as Europe and North America. It is not used much here in Australia but is slowly increasing and can be an efficient way of heating your home, particularly when the water that passes through the radiators is gas- or solar-heated. It does mean having radiators through your home, but I have never minded this – I see them as functional objects that are performing a role.

SOUND

The sophistication of a home is often determined by its qualities of sound. Restaurateurs have been on to this for years; they understand that if they get the sound quality wrong in their dining room, then patrons will not enjoy the experience and won't come back.

If you visit a house where all you can hear is people clip-clopping around, then you are given the subconscious impression that the house isn't well made – it sounds cheap. Too much echo is also unsophisticated.

▼ The sisal rug not only defines this living space by generously embracing the furniture, but it also absorbs sound in the room, reducing echo and absorbing the noise of footsteps.

THAT SHOUTY FAMILY...

It is important that when you are having a conversation you are able to hear reasonably well; if you are having an important conversation, then you don't want to have to shout. In fact, some families are the product of their environment; that loud and shouty family you know might, in fact, come from an acoustically poor house that bounces noise around so much that everyone is shouting to be heard above the din. If that same house had been better designed in terms of noise, then the need to shout would be less, the house would be quieter and the family perhaps feel calmer. We all find ourselves shouting in a restaurant if the background noise is too much, and the situation is no different at home. Having a

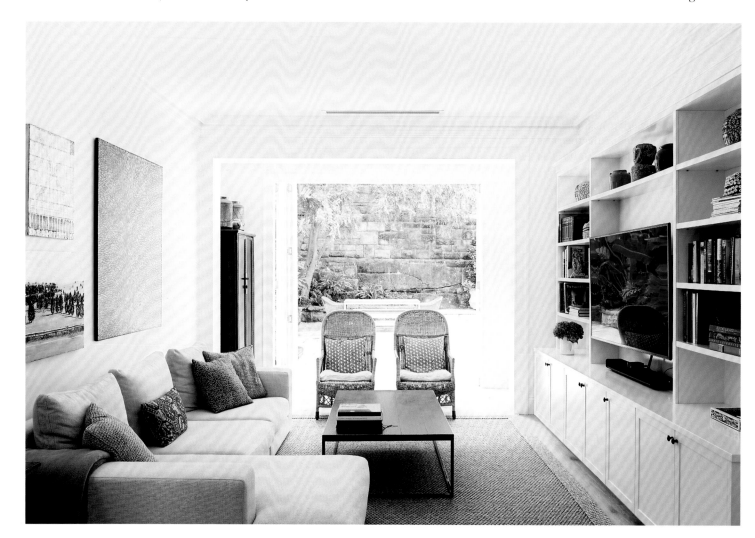

home that is too noisy is just not good manners: it is forcing your family and guests to be hyper-aware of each other at all times, which is not pleasant. Sound privacy is a large part of feeling comfortable in the home.

FLOOR ACOUSTICS

The sound in your living room can be radically changed by the introduction of an acoustic material. More echo makes a room seem bigger, while a muffled space sounds smaller. The trick is to reduce echo, but not to completely deaden the sound so much that you create a sense of claustrophobia. Soft furnishings can make a huge difference. Just adding sofas and chairs to an otherwise hard-surface room will completely change the dynamic. By contrast, if you added hard furnishings to a hard room the sound will bounce around and be uncomfortable. Rugs and cushions absorb sound and soften the acoustics. A deeper, thicker rug adds more acoustic absorption than a thinner rug, and will feel more luxurious. Of course, you can also introduce carpet to a living room. If you feel it is too much to carpet everywhere, either because of expense or worries about cleanliness, then just carpet an area that defines the living space. That way you alight from the thoroughfare onto the living room carpet area and know it's time to relax.

CEILING ACOUSTICS

Adding an acoustic ceiling panel can reduce echo and dampen sound. There are many types on the market now: from all white with tiny perforations (that you can paint to any colour) to timber and felt materials. I often use a ceiling panel not only for acoustic reasons, but also as an aesthetic definition of space. For example, I position a set of acoustic timber panels directly over the dining table in an open-plan setting. This gives an acoustic device right where it is needed – over a chatty table – as well as defining the dining area with a ceiling of warm timber. The panels are perforated with tiny holes that disrupt sound waves as they hit, preventing them bouncing back cleanly to create echo. Any sound that does get through the perforations hits an absorbent material behind. The panels should be set off the wall, leaving an insulating air barrier between.

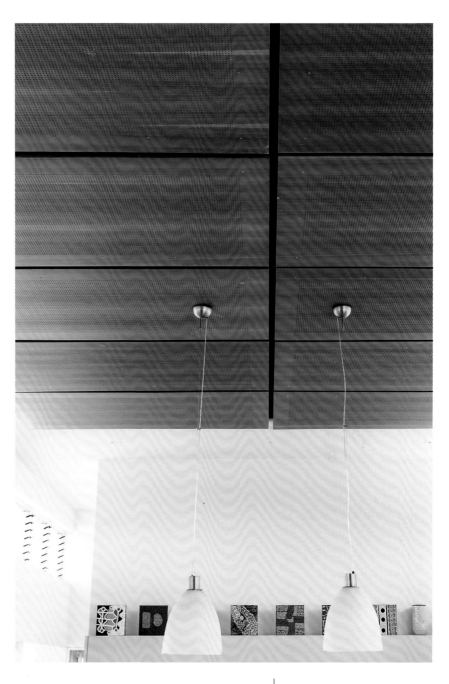

I have covered whole walls with soft acoustic panels – this also acts as a giant pinboard for artwork and kids' paintings as well as being aesthetically beautiful. Any piece of design in your home should attempt to have more than one function: if you can get a functional device to be a lovely addition to the overall look and feel of your space then you are on to a winner.

These timber ceiling panels are lovely to look at, define the living and dining areas below them, and ensure the dining table has comfortable and sophisticated sound levels by reducing any jarring echoes.

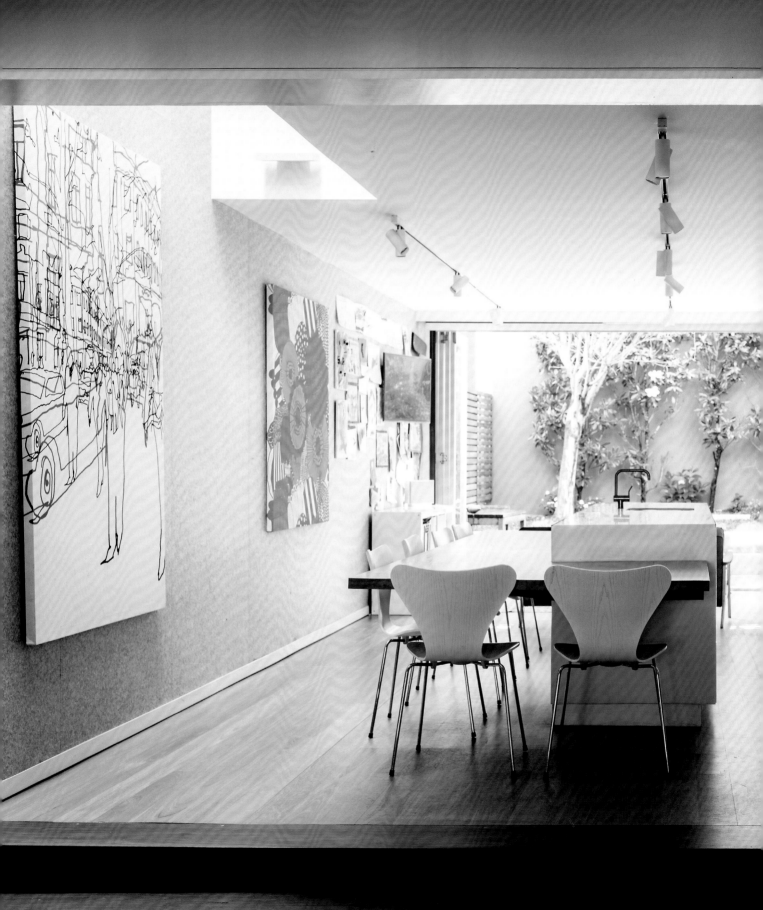

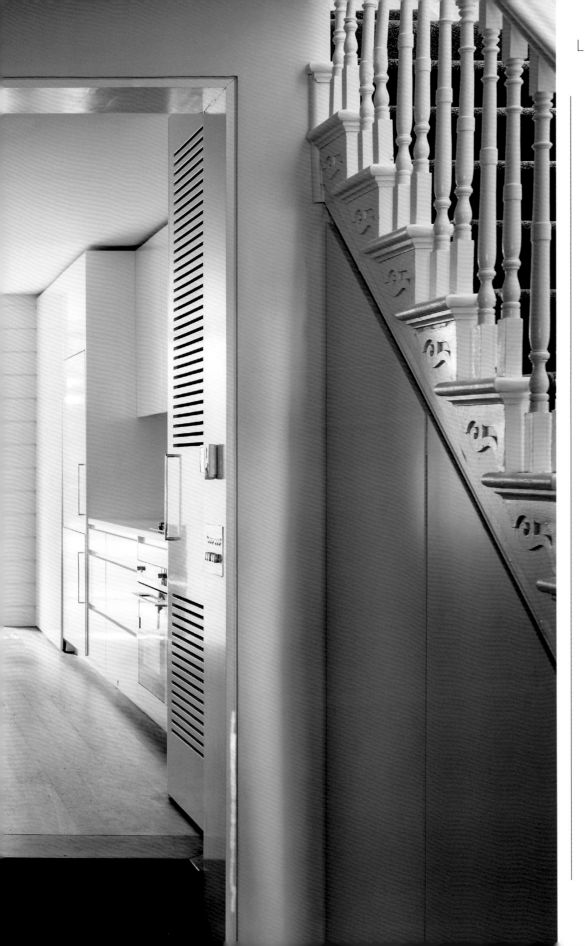

◀ Terraced houses are notorious for being echoey spaces, as many renovations knock out all the downstairs walls and leave one large open-plan room of hard surfaces, such as timber floors and plasterboard. In this home, a whole wall has been covered in soft grey sound-absorbent panels. Traditionally used as office pinboard material, this product, with acoustic properties, has been turned into a holistic wall covering that even reaches up into the void between upstairs and downstairs. The effect on the space is remarkable; it is much more acoustically comfortable with dramatically reduced echo. Aesthetically beautiful and acoustically sound, the soft wall has the added bonus of providing a giant pinboard for family artworks.

NOTE TO SELF

NO ONE ENJOYS
SOLITARY
CONFINEMENT. OPEN
UP THE HOUSE TO
HEAR THE WORLD.

▼ A well-stocked bookcase acts perfectly as an acoustic baffle. The varied, uneven surfaces of the books and their soft paper and board disrupt and absorb sound waves. So, not only does a bookcase make your room look more sophisticated, it makes it sound more sophisticated too.

ABSORBING BOOKS

One forgotten technique to reduce echo in a space is to have a well-stocked library. Not only is a collection of books lovely to look at and have in a living space, but it is also an excellent acoustic device. The broken surface of different sized books and their soft paper and board disrupt the sound waves bouncing around the room, stopping echo as well as absorbing noise. If you think about visiting older houses with walls covered with books, they often have a serenity; part of that is simply down to the effect a library has on the sound in the room. It is also part of the reason libraries are quiet, although designers and architects also bring in other devices such as acoustic panels and baffles and carpets to further enhance the sense of concentration.

SHHHHH

It is important to provide good separation in a house between the living and sleeping areas. This enables multiple people to occupy the same space, rather than everyone having to change to suit one person's sleeping or living patterns. And that can be a big issue as those kids of yours turn into teenagers.

The best place to deal with this, of course, is in your early planning. If you have the room, make sure you design a natural separation between the noisier living areas of the home and the quieter sleeping areas. Distance helps, but so do doors. I often design cavity sliding doors that disappear into walls when a sense of openness is required. It is nice to make a door disappear when you are not using it, particularly when it is a space divider: when you want a space to feel 'open', seeing a door, even if it's open, speaks of closure. However, when someone is trying to get some sleep and others are up and chatting, then the door can be closed and acoustic separation improved. Closing this door is also an excellent signal to others that there is a need to be quiet – there is someone trying to sleep in the bedrooms beyond. I love this kind of quiet telepathic communication that a house can provide. You can design a house to truly speak to you.

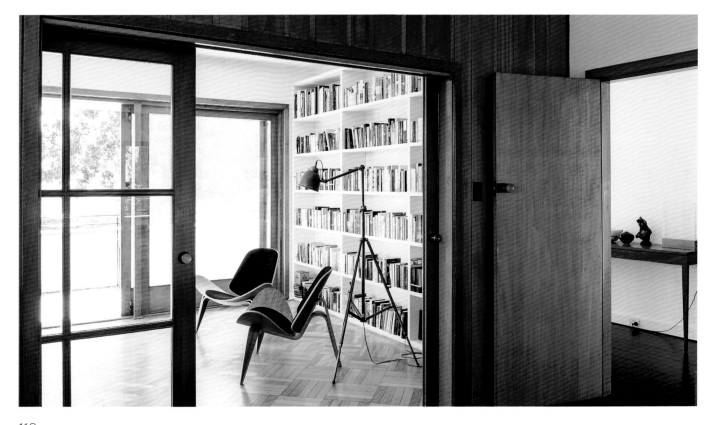

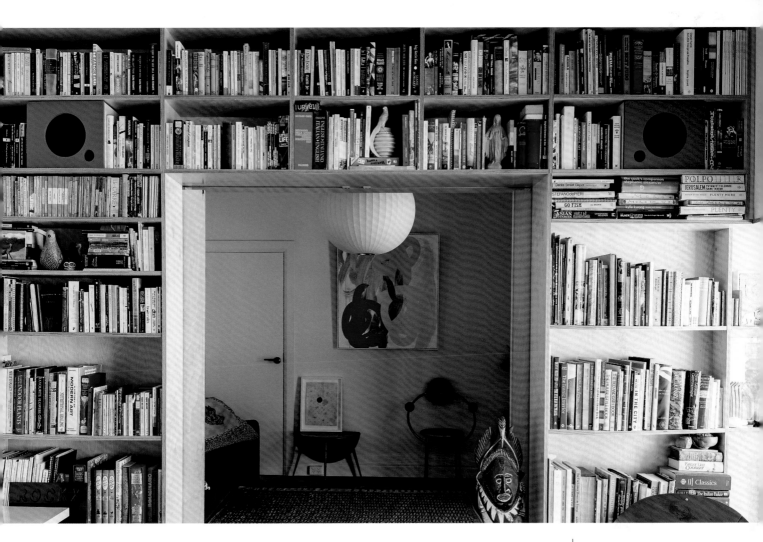

In smaller homes, where doors from bedrooms must open directly onto living spaces, it is important to use good-quality solid-core doors with a density that stops sound. Hollow-core doors are just lighter and less sound proof. The door must be well fitted with no large gaps and then seals can be placed around the door to further insulate it. Both these techniques also reduce the transfer of temperature; any device that does two jobs at once is always a bonus.

SOUND-PROOF, OR WORLD-PROOF?

Sound-proofing is about keeping out unwanted noise from the outside; for example, traffic noise. However, some of the most disappointing homes I have visited are those that are so self-focused that they have become sensory bunkers. No one likes navel gazers and the same goes for our homes. Don't make your house so 'separated' that you create a stale, stark and sterile environment.

A desensitised environment is an unhappy environment – think solitary confinement – and no amount of styling can fix it.

It is important to know the sound of where you live. It will be something you become familiar with. When you go away and come back, the familiarity of your home is often due to the sound of place. Sound also has a lot to do with security; odd sounds are sometimes the way that humans realise there is a potential security issue.

If you shut yourself off from all the sounds of the outside world then you become isolated and oblivious to your surroundings. The natural sound of your home can be an auditory joy – don't delete that. Birds herald the beginning and end of the day. Church bells, the town clock, school pick-up time, ice-cream van music, the last train or bus of the day, a late storm spattering on the roof – all form a patina to life that makes your home more of a home and forms its strong connection to the outside world.

▲ Now this is what I call an acoustic wall! The library of books frames the entry, disrupting and absorbing the sound so the room has less of an echo. Notice the speakers, placed among the books — this wall not only absorbs unwanted noise, but is also a source of chosen sound.

▶ When designing your living space, think of all the facets of life in your family. Make it a flexible space — in this room the chairs can be pulled back to allow for dancing.

▼ Large open doors not only let in light and air, but also sound. It is great to be connected to the voices of family on an outside deck while you are indoors. And, if they are too noisy, you can always close the door!

A QUICK MUSICAL FIX

A technique that shops and restaurants use is to play music. The music has to be at the right volume to not dominate the space, but enough to cover the standard uncomfortable noises of people moving around and chairs scraping on the floor or the sound of a cash register. The same technique can be used in the home, where some quiet music can be just enough to take the edge off an otherwise not great sounding space.

MUSIC FOR LIVING

Music is such a part of human mood and consciousness that I believe access to it should have the fewest barriers possible. Today's technology means there is no excuse for not ensuring you can access music anywhere in your house. It could be the hand-held; it could be the built-in system. Either way you should be pursuing surround sound like never before, because it is so much more accessible today. I enjoy retro-installed speakers that function on the home's wifi system.

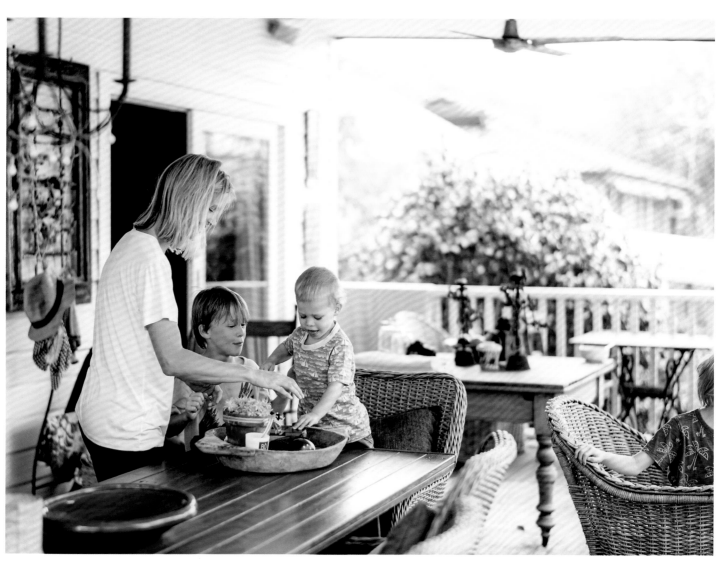

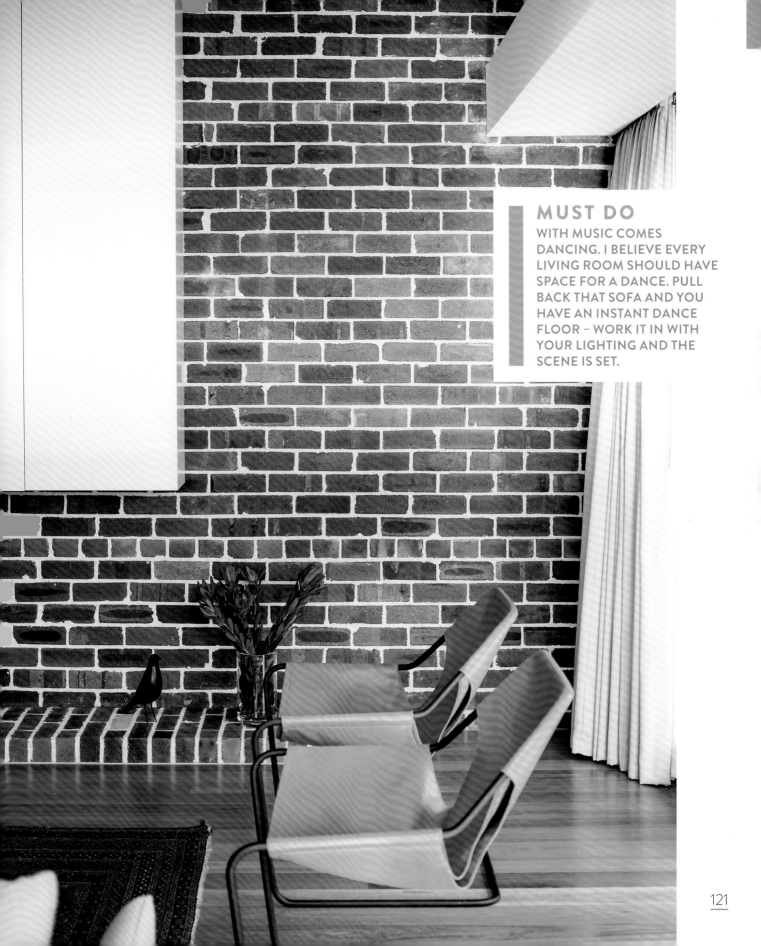

MUST DO

WITH MUSIC COMES DANCING. I BELIEVE EVERY LIVING ROOM SHOULD HAVE SPACE FOR A DANCE. PULL BACK THAT SOFA AND YOU HAVE AN INSTANT DANCE FLOOR – WORK IT IN WITH YOUR LIGHTING AND THE SCENE IS SET.

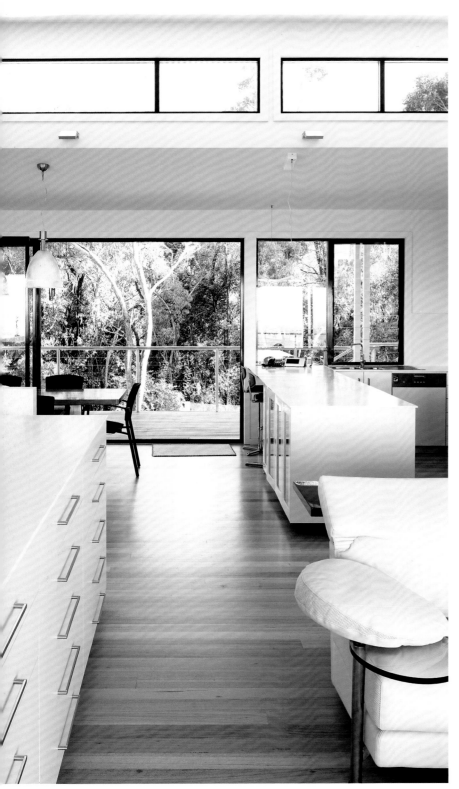

VIEW

Looking out over water, city or paddocks is a wonderful plus for a home; however, not many of us can afford a million-dollar view. What we don't realise, though, is that we can create our own views *within* the home to optimise our feelings of spaciousness and ownership.

When I design a house I am always thinking about views. Not only to the outside, but also on the inside. As I design the home I think about where people are and what view they will have. As they move around what will they see? Will it be a pleasant view or a nothing, banal view? There is so much that comes out of getting this right: not only a pleasant outlook for your life and your home, but a sense of ownership – a sense of ownership over your domain, your place, your nest; a place that you have nurtured to uplift you and your family every day to create a better life. Ensuring that the views are right in your home will give you a sense of pride, as well as a sense of safety and refuge. It is imperative that you create the best space possible for you and your family.

BRING THE OUTSIDE IN

Bring the outdoors into your living room through windows, glass doors and skylights. If you are sitting reading a book on your sofa, it is good to have a sense of the weather and light outside, so you keep a connection with your environment, the time of day and so on. Having this connection with the outdoors will also make your room feel bigger and less closed in, and with good doors you will have a sense of being able to spread your living space outwards.

A living space simply must have an outside aspect. You need to be able to see into an outside space of some kind, whether that is a deck, a courtyard or a garden. When we as a society decide to punish someone, one of our worst penalties is to put them into solitary confinement where they are desensitised from the outside world and from human contact. This is an inhumane punishment – yet, amazingly, I have been into people's homes and their living room is

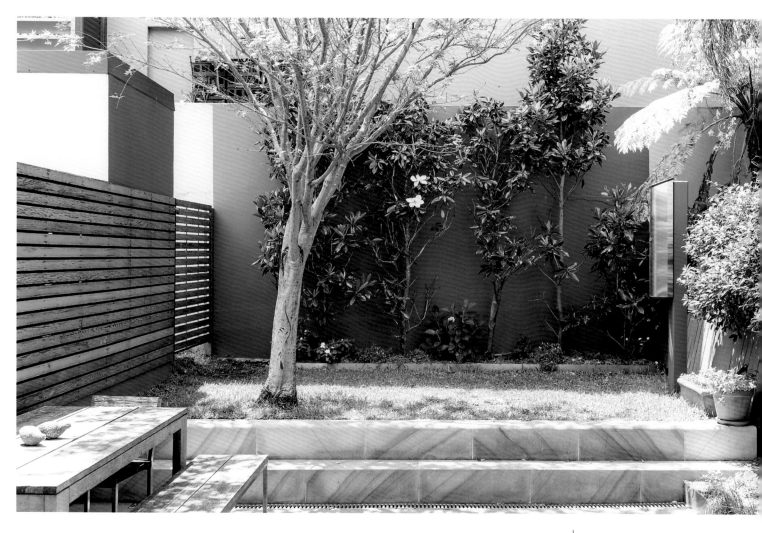

not far off such an experience! It is not surprising that the space you inhabit can have an enormous impact on you and the relationships around you.

FRAMING AND CROPPING

One of the best ways to make a home feel bigger, more spacious and more valuable is to consider its views. Views go hand in glove with window shape, size and position. Give the spaces where you sit and spend time the best and longest views possible. Think about what you want to see from those spaces. The view to the outside does not have to be a million dollars but it does need to be considered. If you have a view outside that is not great then think about how to improve it. Is it possible to frame the best bit and exclude the worst? For example, design a perfectly square

window that captures a vine growing on the wall, but crops out the ugly air-conditioning unit on the neighbour's house.

Can the French doors perfectly frame a pathway leading to a favourite part of the garden? You might not walk that pathway today, but because of the placement of the French doors your mind does, every time you look up. It is all about focus. Your view could be as simple as some dappled light on a wall. Views can be defined by a single window, or by a series of windows. It is imperative to know from where you will be seeing the view. It is surprising to me that people will buy a house for a view without realising that the only time they see that view is if they are standing at the window purposefully looking at it – something that they might do a couple of times a year!

◄ Thoroughfares not only allow for movement through a house, but can also frame a long view.

▲ This small garden is framed by bifold doors that fully retract to the side. The back wall is painted a dark recessive colour that gives the illusion of extending, and forms a background for the green foliage and tree. The garden is divided into two levels and the solid sandstone steps become furniture as well as creating a layered view from the kitchen and living spaces.

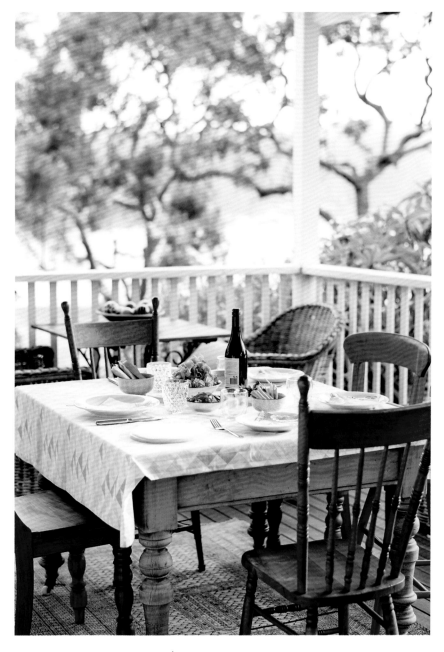

the tree in the distance perfectly framed in a window. As an architect, I work hard to make the most of any view that might be available. I've designed window seats to raise you up enough to see over rooftops, and have not been averse to using a ladder to get people up to the right height.

TAKING THE LONG VIEW

The view is all about where you are seeing it from. Are you sitting on the sofa? At the dining table? Then your eye height is definitely lower than when standing. When standing, the average adult eye height is 150 cm (59 in) off the floor. Once you are aware of this you can start to design for that viewpoint. You can ensure that when you are washing vegetables at the sink you can glance up and see into the garden – I plan specifically for moments like that. And when I plot the location of the dining table, I ensure there is a view to the outdoors and the sky beyond – it might be a long view, from the dining chair over the table, over the sofa and out over a deck. We have to ensure that the sofa and any other objects do not impede the view. Don't take the short view – always try to create the longest views possible.

Remember that window style, and how they are decorated, can also influence the feeling of view. Looking out into a green garden feels different if the view is bordered by a black aluminium minimalist window frame or a white timber heritage-style frame. The way that garden is perceived from inside will be vastly different.

Remember that a kitchen benchtop stands at a height of 90 cm (35 in). So, if your kitchen is between your living area and garden, when you are sitting on the sofa you will not have a view into the garden; you will only be able to look over the top of the kitchen bench and see a sky view. Conversely, when you are in the kitchen you are generally standing, so you have that added height and are able to look over the relatively low living room sofa area and still see the view. It is up to you to think about whether a view from your living space or kitchen space works best for you.

MIRROR, MIRROR

Not every spot in your home is going to be able to take advantage of whatever view you have, or have created, but you can use secondary design

▲ The view from this table is lovely, but, even more importantly, the view from inside the house to this table and view is even better. Invest in decent outdoor furniture; it often ends up in your most frequently seen view.

Remember that in a real estate viewing you are not doing natural everyday things like having breakfast, sitting on the sofa or at the dining table, or cooking dinner – so you don't consider the view from these aspects.

Have you got a favourite tree in the distance? If you have, you can try to design the space so that when you are sitting in your armchair reading a book, you can look up from that book and admire ideas to make the best of these. For example, your armchair has a perfect view of your favourite tree outside, but now the sofa has no view? Consider mounting a mirror on the wall in the perfect position to reflect that same tree through that same window right into view from the sofa. This can be done in a big house or a small apartment; it is about reviewing the space you have and the aspects it has to enhance every moment you spend in your living space.

Clever placing of wall mirrors can also appear to extend the rooms of a house by giving a sense of depth that is otherwise inconceivable. I often use the two walls on either side of a fireplace as an opportunity for a mirror. They can be relatively small and awkward spaces and the mirror can give them a lift and make them feel more spacious, not to mention giving the impression that the room continues beyond. It is also a nice unexpected variation to putting a mirror above the fireplace – I often reserve that space for a favourite piece of art.

STREET VIEW

A view to the street is important to give you a sense of safety and an overview of what is happening in the neighbourhood. Being able to view the street does not mean that you are on view yourself – you can design the aspect so that you can see the street, but you can't be seen *from* the street. This is something very important to me – it forms the basis of community and neighbourhood watch. I don't like to see houses being built that turn their back on the street, or the street becomes an unwatched void that we don't feel comfortable to let our kids play in. As an architect, I often introduce screening up to shoulder height to the front of a house so that the occupant can see out when standing or moving inside. But if you were looking in from the street, all you see is the occasional head moving around.

If your living space is at the front of the house on the road, sometimes the view is just not great when looking straight out. In that case I would use screening to block out the unsightly aspect and introduce higher windows and skylights to capture the sky and bring it into the home. A changing sky is very attractive and can make a lovely feature in a living room.

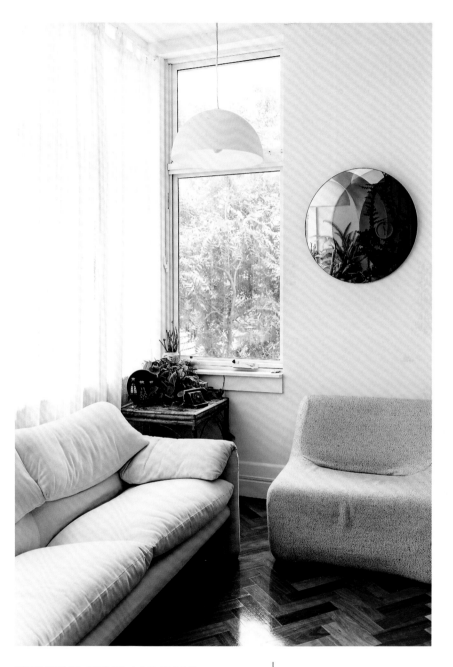

THE WINDOW BLACK HOLE

Many people spend big bucks on a property with a great view, perhaps over the sea; however, they don't realise that at night that view becomes a pitch-black hole. The only thing they see out of the window at night is a reflection of themselves and their space. In these cases it is possible to create a night view across the living room to the outside space.

▲ A window that frames the view of an attractive tree is left unadorned, while translucent curtains obstruct nearby buildings that are visible from the other windows. The round mirror adds to the overall view by reflecting greenery from the opposite side of the room.

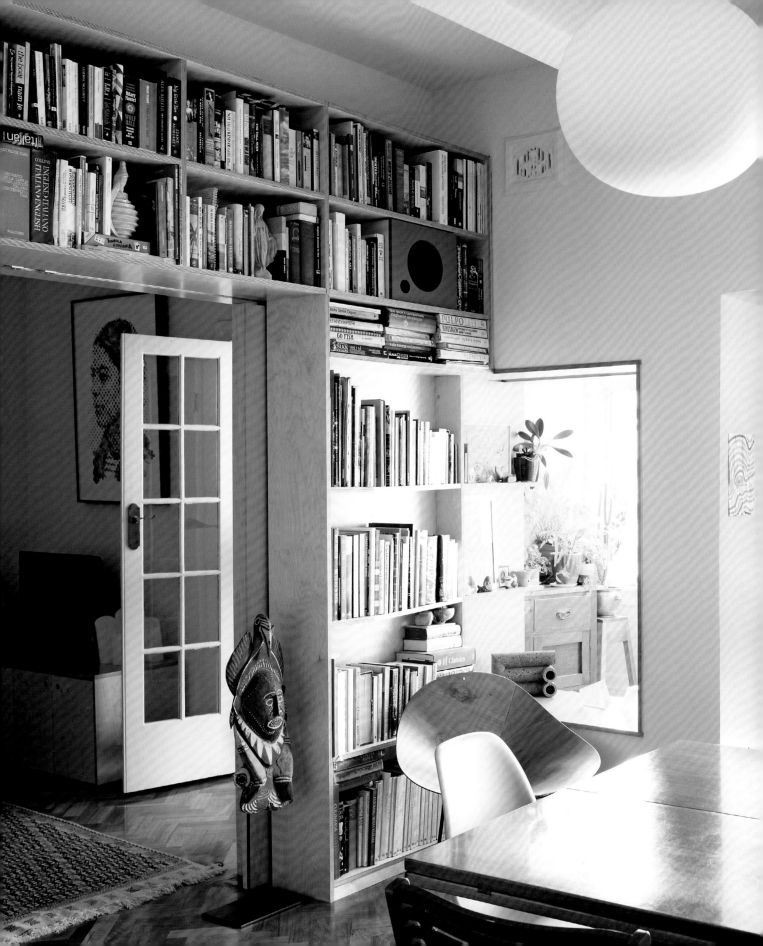

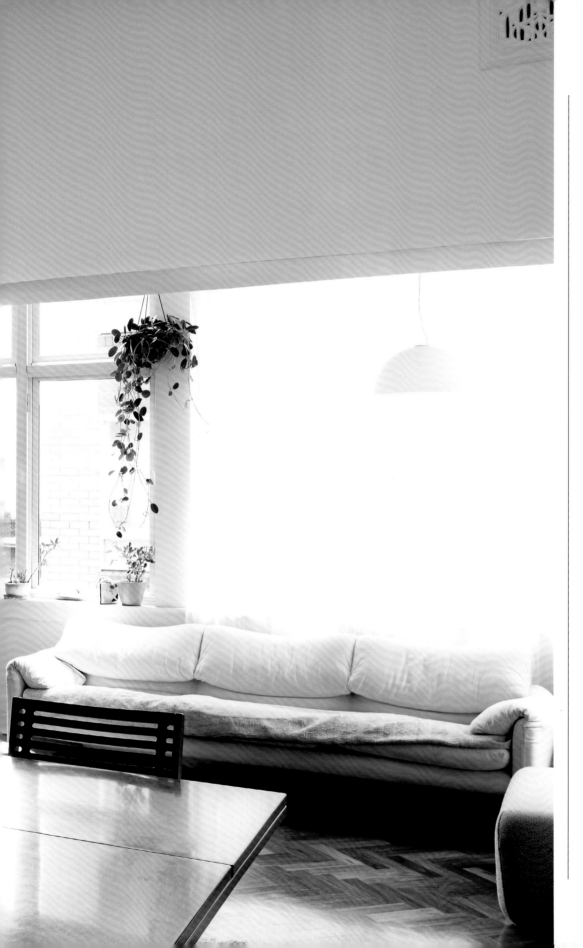

◀ A plethora of interior views
have been created in this
apartment using depth,
layering, character and story.
No million-dollar outside
views required.

You could create a body of water – such as a pool, plunge pool, reflection pool or even a pond – and then light it from within. As the sun goes down and the sea view darkens and disappears, the light of the pool rises and it becomes the focus and view from the living room.

Another technique is to simply light your garden. Introduce garden lights to define areas, spotlight a beautiful sculpture or plant, and create depth by uplighting trees at the rear of your garden. This will provide you with a beautiful and interesting view after dark.

BEWARE THE DECK

It sounds counter-intuitive, but be careful not to ruin your view with a deck. You are in your newly designed house, standing in your living room, looking out over a wonderful deck to the beautiful sand, sea and waves beyond. You have made it! Well done! Tired of standing, you take a seat in your armchair and suddenly you can't see the sand, the sea and the waves; all you can see is some bulky outdoor furniture on a deck. You realise you have built a deck right across the front of your house, facing the view, and now the only time you can see the view is when you are standing up!

This is one of the most common mistakes I see. It is also something that's often missed by people buying a home or beach house – they conduct the viewing standing up – they never sit down and so will never realise that the view disappears immediately. In a new home or renovation, the design solution I use is to create a part-deck, part-conservatory. We bring the inside space as close to the view as possible and then have the deck to the side. That way an inside space and a deck both have the view; if the inside space can be opened up, you have the best of both worlds.

IF THERE IS NO VIEW

If there is absolutely no view to be captured, then don't waste valuable wall space with windows that reveal something unsightly – instead, create storage and artwork opportunities on your walls and then install high windows to capture treetops or sky while also letting in sunlight. I have even taken this same idea and installed low-level windows to create a view out onto a specially planted garden bed. This works wonderfully on side passages where a normal window would just reveal a view of a fence or neighbour's wall. Instead you have a low-level window with a view to a green garden bed, and then perhaps a wall unit for books or storage or art above it that appears to be floating as the light from the low window pours in.

You can also create powerful internal views, or views of interest, by using voids, atriums, contrasting timber rafters, views across courtyards, bridges, interesting balustrades or level changes. Remember that internal views are something you can control, but they do need to be planned in a fundamental design sense.

AND IF ALL ELSE FAILS

One architectural device I have used for a house is what we call periscopes. These use mirrors to capture a view the house doesn't actually have. This particular house had no view of the sea from the ground floor – however, the rooftop did have a sea view, so I designed and installed pop-up sections of roof with glass fronts facing the sea.

▶ Invest in oversized indoor plants to create fantastic and unexpected interior views if the external outlook is not the best.

▼ Large sliding doors are designed to disappear behind the drawn back curtains so the separation between inside and outdoors is minimal. The continuation of the exposed rafters between both areas further enhances this.

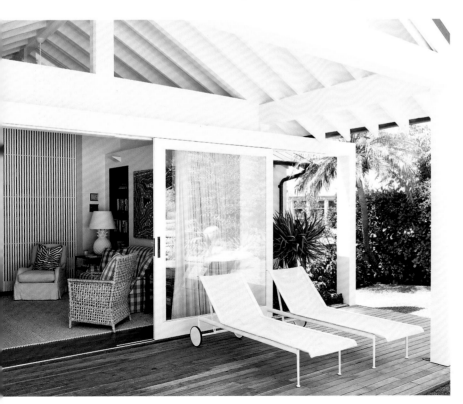

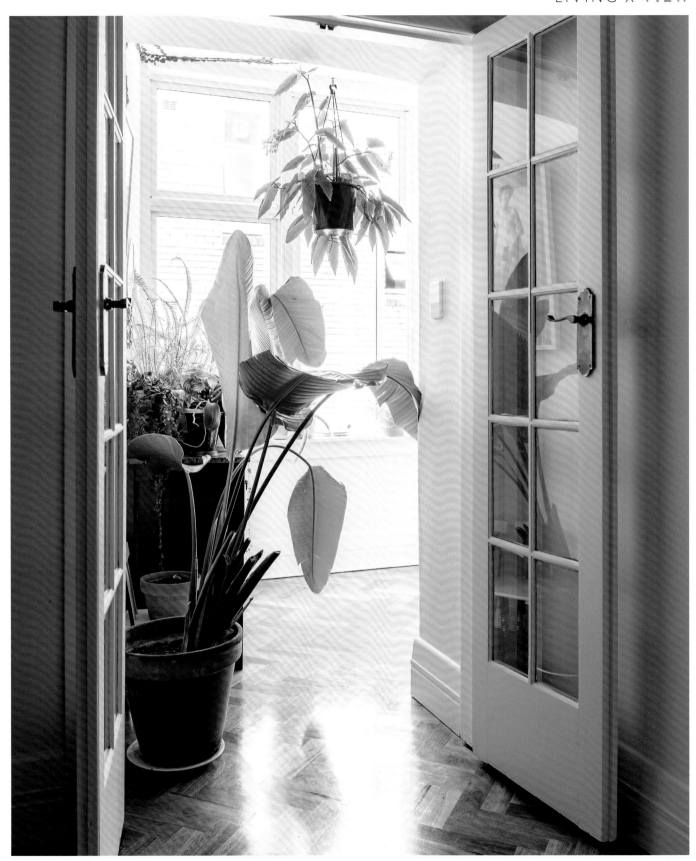

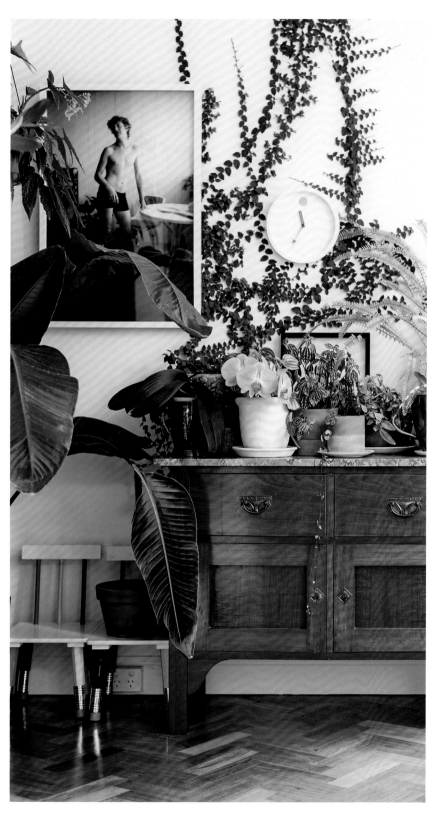

On the sloping inner side of the pop-up sections we installed mirror. The mirror was designed at the perfect angle to capture a view of the sea when you looked up at the skylight from the lounge. The added bonus was that the pop-ups also let in light and air with motorised clear glass louvres. Importantly the pop-up was designed so that sun did not directly hit the mirror and send unwanted harsh light into the living room, only the view.

THE SLOW REVEAL

Once you are confident at understanding and designing views into your home, you can become more sophisticated with ways to use them. I work hard to control the view so that everything isn't revealed at once. I often try to design a sequence of spaces that hold back the view and only reveal it when I want the full impact. I think this is a sign of good design, and I can always feel when moving through a well-designed house the hand of the architect guiding me and challenging and surprising my perception. Sometimes there is nothing more disappointing than the obvious. Like a piece of music, a space should be a journey with a few surprises along the way. Make your home a progression of experiences with sliding doors and walls, revealing part and then whole rooms and new and unexpected views. Use curtains to partially hide or reveal a room or view.

WINDOW SEAT

I think everyone should have access to a window seat in their home. Take the living space and identify a wall to carve out a nook. Most commonly, you would push part of the wall outwards to create space, but you can also simply build a ledge under a window that is big enough to furnish. Once you have created the defined space, add seating with soft materials. Give the window seat a reason for being, a purpose: is it a place for reading, an IT nook, for catching a view or basking in the sun? A purpose is absolutely key for a window seat, otherwise it will just start to fill up with stuff that people leave there. If it is for reading, make sure it is comfortable and has good natural light and perhaps a reading light for when the sun goes down. If it's to catch a particular view, arrange extra cushioning at the right end

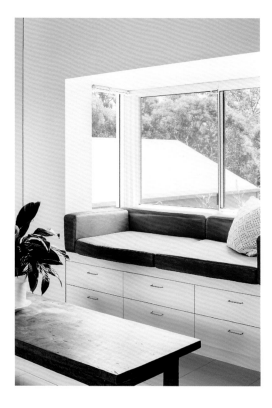

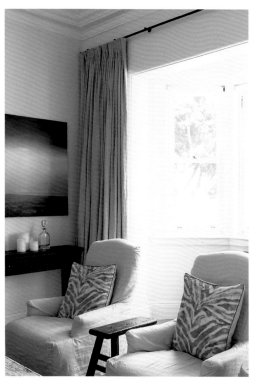

◀◀◀ It is not often you see a vine on an inside wall. It creates a captivating and interesting internal view and I love how it seems to have grown up and around the clock.

◀◀ A window seat offers the opportunity for a new experience and perspective, different even from the room it is in. Every home should try to have a window seat.

◀ Depth of view comes not only from the windows, but also from the painting with its deep view across an ocean.

for sitting. For an IT nook, consider a window desk; build the desk as an extension of the window sill and create a dedicated space wrapped around the view. This will feel like an escape from the main living space even though it is still connected. A window seat becomes a major feature in a room and can become such a character filled and friendly addition, so make sure it looks good with great materials and a splash of colour.

ART AS VIEW

Consider placing art or photographs so they can be appreciated from a certain vantage point, such as when sitting at the dining table or the breakfast bar. If the artwork has an element of depth then that is a bonus – it will have a sense of extending the view.

CURTAINS AND BLINDS

Be aware of orientation. If a window is on the western side of the house then it will get strong sun in the Australian summer. You will want to protect yourself from harsh sunlight with shutters or blinds, which means, in turn, you lose

your view. Slim-line louvre blinds can be used, but your views will be filtered at best. So try to understand the orientation of your views and don't put all your eggs in one basket. Try to create options, such as capturing a particular view at breakfast and another one in the afternoon. Only architecture can do this for you. No amount of interior design or decoration can make these changes and take full advantage of these opportunities.

And be careful with heavy curtains in a living space as they can be oppressive. Having said that, they can have great thermal properties for keeping rooms warm or cool. The trick to curtains is to use light colours and to ensure that they are designed to be well out of the way when not in use. I have always loved thick navy blue curtains for their luxurious feel; but I would only use them in a very large space; in a small room they would be oppressive.

MUST DO
EVERY HOME SHOULD HAVE A WINDOW SEAT. NOT ONLY ARE THEY LOVELY TO LOOK AT BUT A WINDOW SEAT ALLOWS YOU TO CLIMB RIGHT INTO THE VIEW.

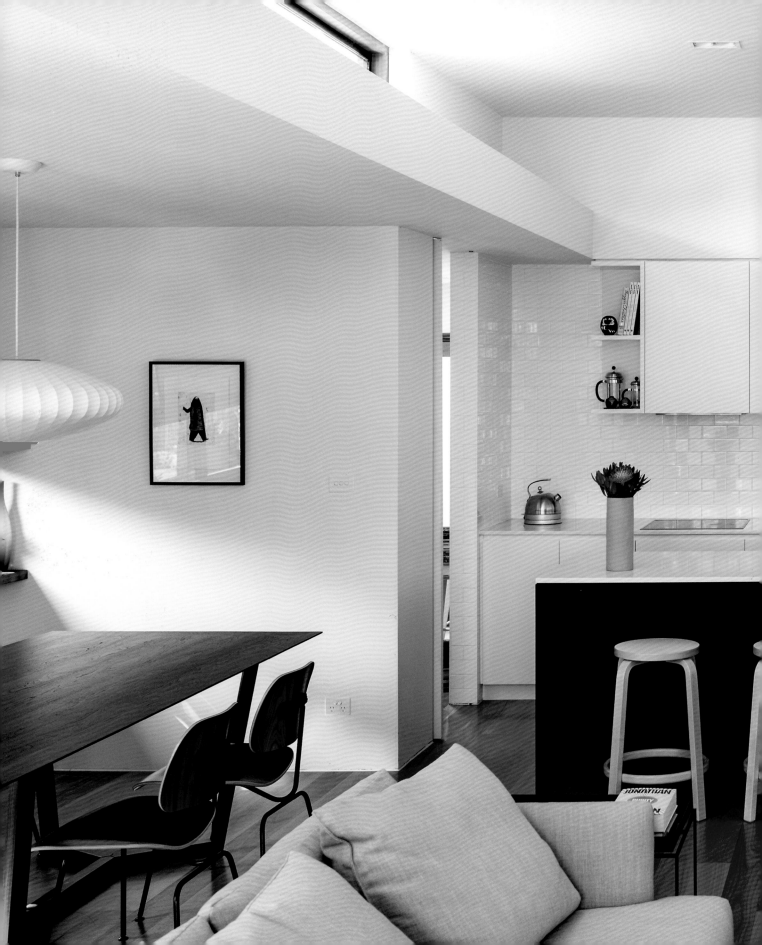

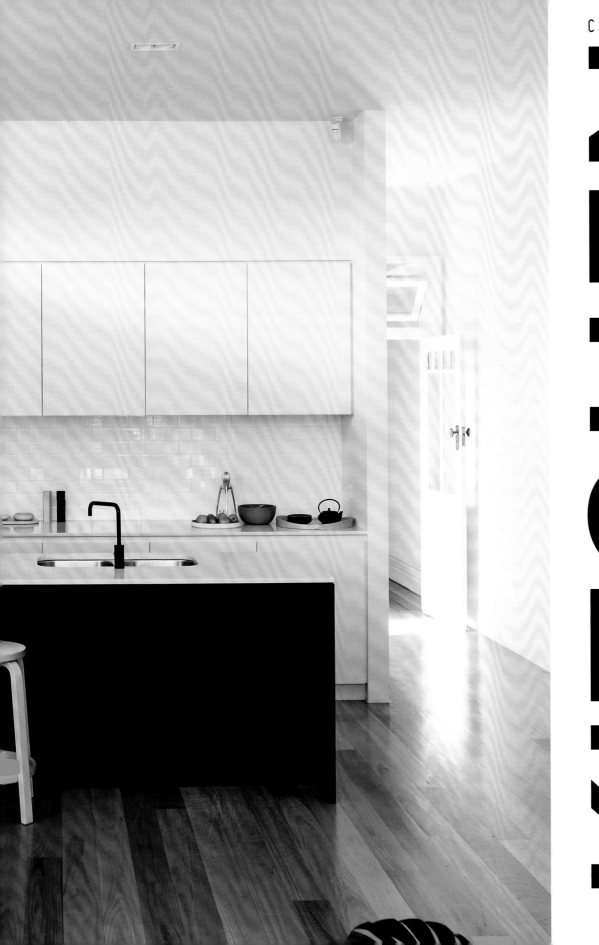

CHAPTER THREE

KITCHEN

▷ This kitchen is located to be the perfect vantage point for overseeing the rest of the house, even the outdoor areas.

▽ Creating the family meal is a great chance to spend time together while contributing to a common goal.

THE KITCHEN IS THE MODERN-DAY HEART and hearth of the home. In our busy lives it is the place where we are watered and nourished, and where there is a wonderful opportunity for the family to spend time together and find out what is happening in each other's lives while food is prepared and eaten. It is the touchstone of the home. But the kitchen is foremost about cooking and food preparation, so the space needs to be practical and provide storage for ingredients, appliances and equipment.

Never underestimate the power of a chat while preparing the evening meal. Sometimes the best time to broach a sensitive subject or difficult topic is while sharing a practical task. Make the kitchen a place where you can be approached by your kids and be available for a quality conversation while you chop and cook. Sometimes while you are concentrating on an activity, yet with open ears, is the least confronting time to have important discussions as children grow up. The kitchen is one of the best daily opportunities for that, making it the true heart of the modern home.

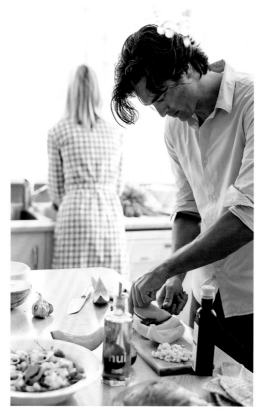

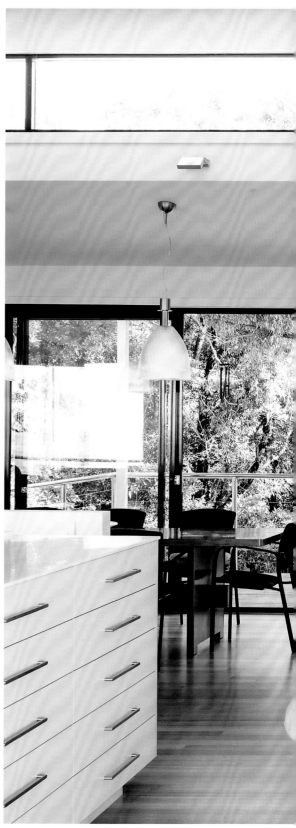

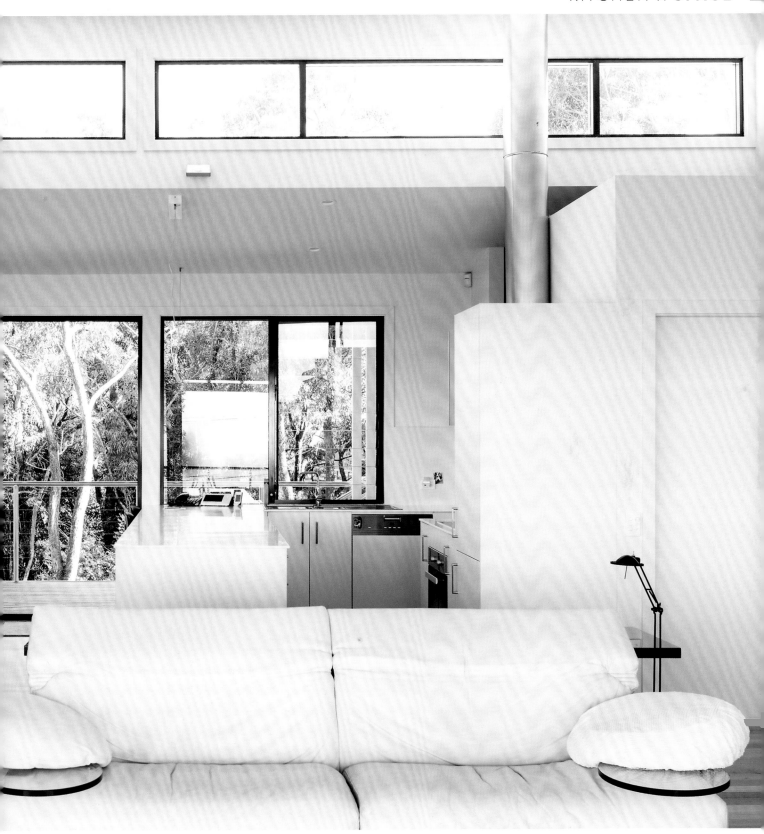

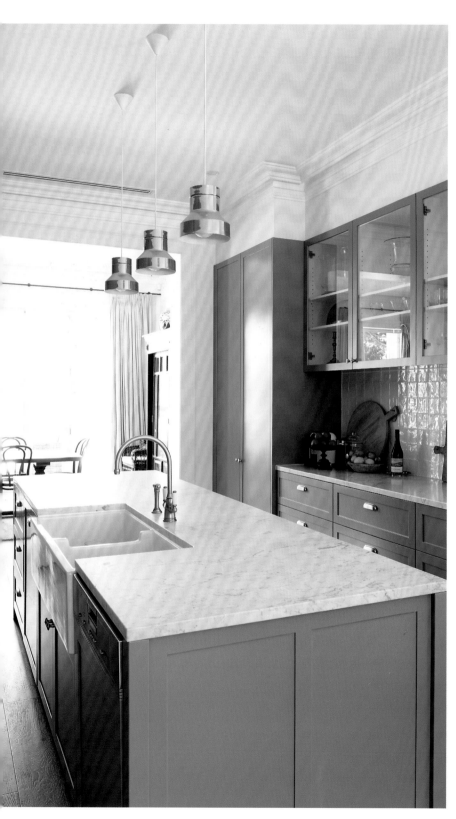

SPACE

Increasingly in the modern home the kitchen is part of a much bigger space, including living and dining, and not in its own separate room. This change has occurred for many reasons: firstly, because most of us no longer have servants in the home! In the old days, the host and hostess of the house entertained while staff prepared the meal in another room called the kitchen. Nowadays the host and hostess want to be with their family and entertain at the same time as preparing the meal: hence the combining of rooms makes sense. The last century of technology has also allowed the kitchen to come into our living spaces: we used to cook on open fires, which were hot, polluting, smelly and hazardous, so keeping the kitchen removed from other areas of the house – usually out the back – was a safety precaution. Today, we don't see the modern kitchen as a safety risk and smells can be better filtered out of the space.

SPLENDID ISOLATION

Very rarely these days do I receive a brief to design a kitchen in an altogether separate room. However, occasionally someone will request a kitchen that is able to be separated or is not located completely in an open living space. This is usually for one of two very different reasons. Perhaps my client is a mad keen cook and sees their time in the kitchen as an opportunity for 'me' time, and in this case a sense of separation from everyone else is not a bad thing. When talking about it, they almost seem to regard the kitchen as akin to a study. In that case, I try to design a way of separating the kitchen using flexible doors, so that at other times it is part of the greater room for the rest of the family to enjoy.

The other reason is kitchen smells. Some people absolutely abhor the idea of cooking or food smells in their main living space. And when they describe the strength of their feeling, you certainly don't want to argue – even the best air exhaust won't completely eliminate all cooking smells. In this instance, I do design a completely separate space for the kitchen that can be sealed from the rest of the house.

As with all aspects of home design, you should do what suits you and how you want to live. The only point to make is that if you might be selling in the not too distant future, then a kitchen combined with the major living space is what most buyers would choose.

RELOCATING THE KITCHEN

If you move into a home with a separate kitchen, there is a real opportunity to add value by bringing it into the major space. Moving a kitchen is generally something you should try to avoid for cost reasons: look for opportunities to make a connection without moving the major plumbing services. Moving a wall can open up the kitchen, but so too can punching a hole through a wall.

However, if the best option is to relocate it to a different space, then try to place it where some plumbing already exists, such as a previous or adjoining bathroom.

CONNECTION TO LIVING SPACES

We have to recognise that the kitchen in a modern family home is about a lot more than just cooking: it is about family connection. The cooking experience should be part of the communication experience amongst the family – it is about healthy eating and healthy chatting. The key is to get the fundamentals of the kitchen right – the practical basics – so that it functions as a well-oiled food preparation machine, and then work out how to integrate it with the other activities of the household. The first area I place and design in the home is always the kitchen.

In terms of planning the space, the relationship between the kitchen, dining and living areas is key. Generally speaking, the dining table needs to be within easy reach of the kitchen, for carrying food and crockery from kitchen to table and vice versa. And both in terms of living and dining, proximity is important so that conversation can carry on between these three focal areas of the

◀ The key feature of this kitchen is a central island bench with wall joinery on two sides. This creates a huge amount of prep space as well as storage, and allows for plenty of people to be together in the area, helping out.

▼ The kitchen does not end this space, rather there is a sense of being able to continue beyond, with the glimmer of light and the reflection in the splashback all working to create a three-dimensional space. Note the connection of the blue in the dining chairs and the artwork.

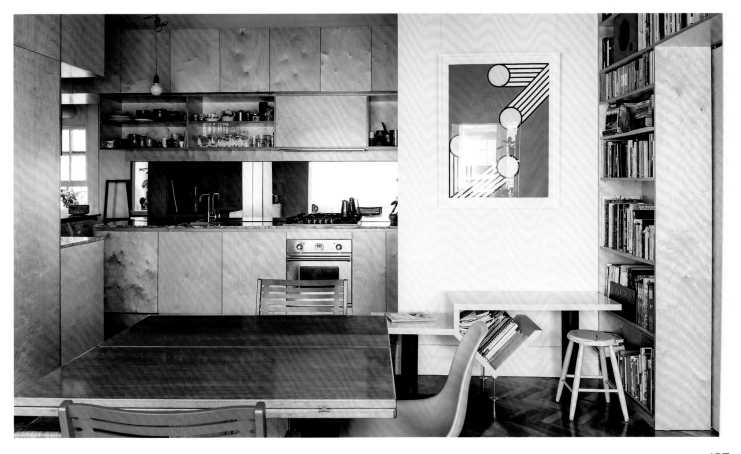

▶ A window into the kitchen brings light and air and can also act as a servery to an outdoor eating area — a great way to get the pancakes out, quick and hot!

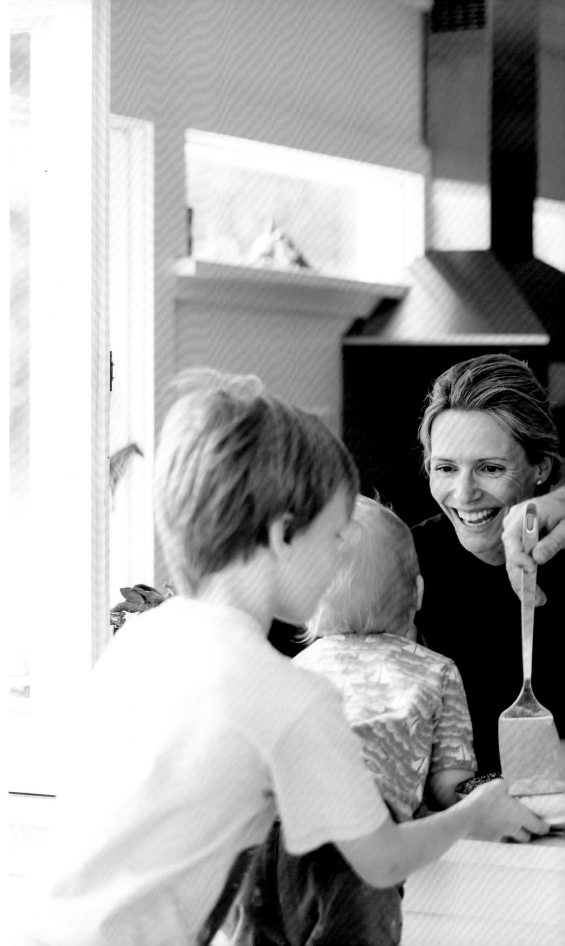

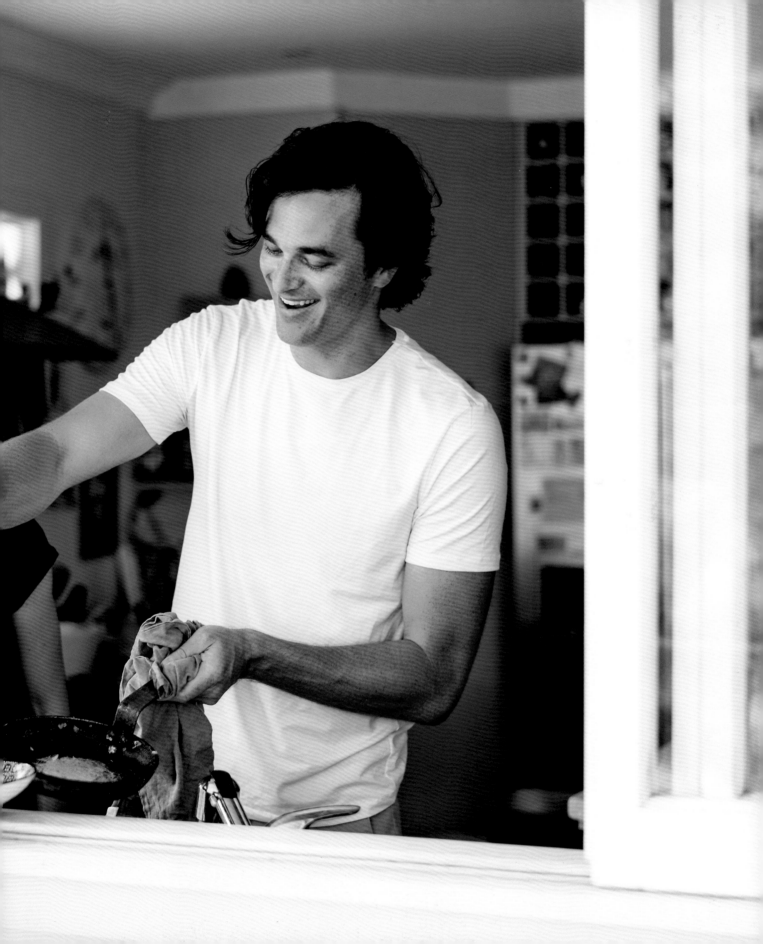

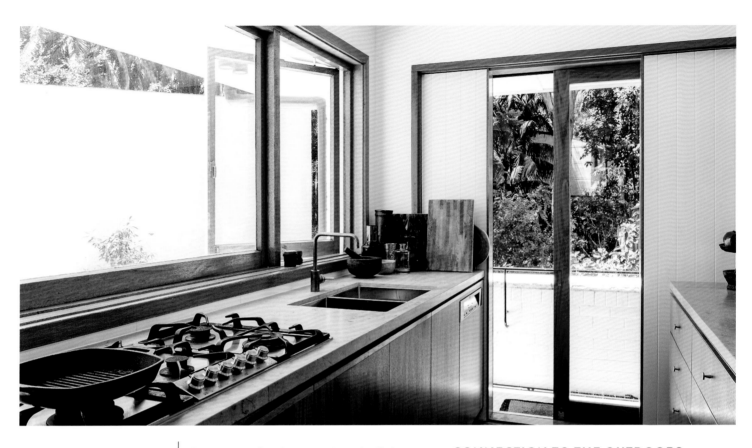

▲ This relatively small kitchen feels much bigger due to the backdrop of opening windows and the door to the outside, which also allows great serving access for the outdoor area.

house. A good cooking experience is all about communication. No one wants to be stuck in the kitchen feeling that they are slaving away while everyone else is off having a great time in another room. And, anyway, preparing a meal can be theatre, so why not show it off and include everyone in the show?

Another common request from clients these days is that the living room television be visible and audible from the kitchen, so that the person preparing the meal can watch the nightly news at the same time. This is also a great way to chat about the news as family members can be spread throughout the living, dining and kitchen areas and still be part of the conversation.

(Although I do tend to avoid a separate TV for the kitchen – I am a firm believer in the telly being off during meal time so that proper communication can occur.)

SMART HOME

THE SMART FRIDGE WILL MONITOR THE AGE OF PERISHABLE FOODS AND RECOMMEND RECIPES TO USE THEM UP. RUBBISH BINS WILL NOTE EMPTY PACKAGES THROWN AWAY AND AUTOMATICALLY PUT IN THE ORDER TO RESTOCK.

CONNECTION TO THE OUTDOORS

The kitchen can be a great way to merge a house with the outdoors. I have designed many kitchens that extend into the garden, where the kitchen service area extends into a barbecue and an outdoor sink. We have also designed a house so that no barbecue was required: instead we positioned the kitchen so that in good weather all the doors opened and slid back completely, the kitchen suddenly became an outdoor area and we included teppanyaki hotplates instead of a barbecue.

KITCHEN LAUNDRY

Many kitchens, particularly in apartments and smaller terraced houses, have to include other aspects of the household, such as the laundry. The washing machine, dryer and laundry sink can all be completely hidden behind bi-fold or sliding doors. This can also be an efficient way to plan your space, because it is always cheaper to group your plumbing and waste into the same area of the home.

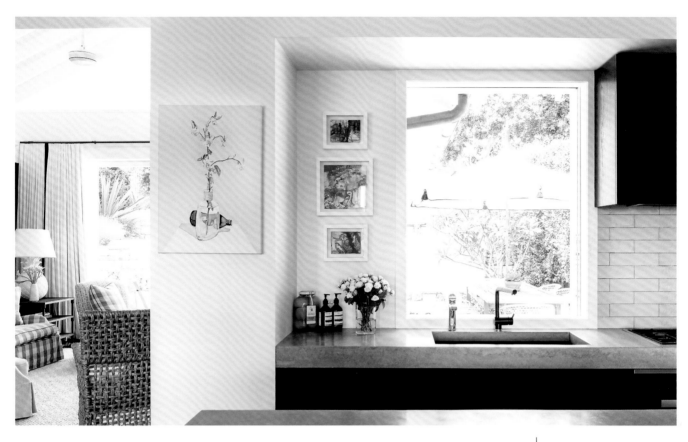

Do consider, however, the noise implications of including the laundry in your open-plan living space. If you can organise the use of washer and dryer to occur when you are at work then that is not an issue, but if you are at home in the living space then it can be tiresome to not be able to shut the door to the laundry as your drying spins away noisily. With any washer and dryer, it is imperative that they have good exhaust and ventilation, so make sure that your cupboard space is as well ventilated as you would expect a laundry room to be. You don't want condensation in your living room.

DEFINING THE KITCHEN

Spatially speaking, if your kitchen is part of a large open-plan living area there is an opportunity to make it a focal point, give it character and make it play a part in the particular style of your home. By its very function, your kitchen will have unique characteristics compared to the other areas in an open-plan design. You can play up some of these characteristics with strong benchtops, colourful splashbacks and potentially interesting industrial aspects such as ovens and range hoods. On the other hand, you might prefer your kitchen to merge into the overall room, so that when not in use it disappears behind joinery cupboards and screens and becomes simply an extension of the living space.

KITCHEN CEILING

You can lower the ceiling over the kitchen to define the cooking area within the overall room, bringing the focus down over your cooking task surface. This can be practical and cost-effective too – it can aid task lighting by bringing it closer to the task surface, and your exhaust system will also be closer to the cooking surface, increasing its effectiveness in sucking up steam and smells. A lowered ceiling also provides the perfect cavity in which to hide the unsightly exhaust machinery, pipes and wires that are always more numerous in a kitchen than in other areas.

▲ Behind the island bench, the rear of the kitchen is also a concrete bench supported by black joinery. This is repeated in the upper cupbards, which are set back to reveal the lovely window onto the garden. Rather than wall-to-wall joinery, space has been left to allow for artworks.

5 X 5
KITCHEN X **SPACE**

▷ This design merges an island
bench and dining table as an
efficient way to deal with an
open-plan kitchen in a narrow
terraced house. The timber
bench wraps around the island
at a lower level, so that more
comfortable standard chairs
can be used for eating, rather
than barstools.

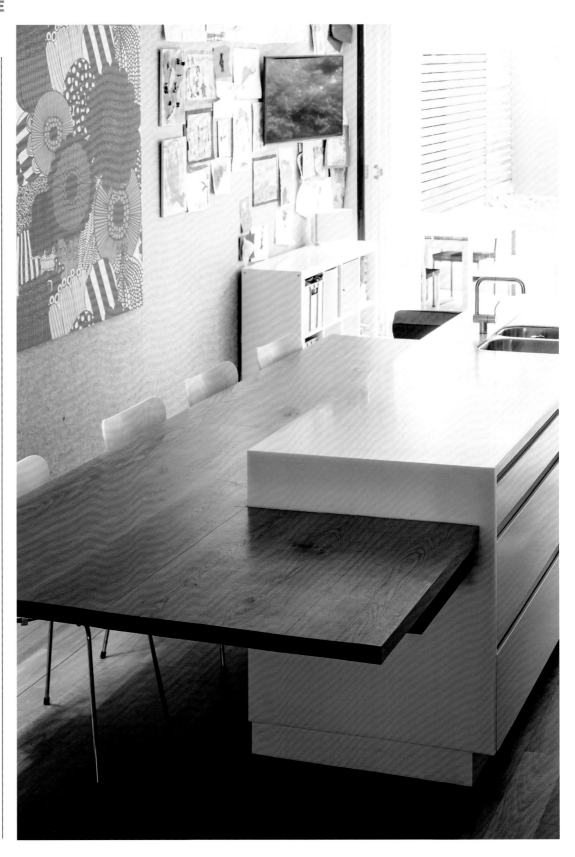

KITCHEN FLOOR

In an open-plan design consider defining your kitchen space with a different floor material. This is practical if the living area is carpet, but even if it is timber a material change into the kitchen can be a good thing. Consider whether you want to go dark or light. Use your kitchen joinery as reference and either blend or contrast the floor depending on which you want to be a standout feature. If you create white kitchen joinery and benchtops and introduce a dark tile floor then the kitchen joinery will appear to float.

Primarily, the kitchen floor needs to be practical; it must be easily washed and cleaned. You should also consider floor traction – it is easy to slip in a kitchen if there is spillage and that can lead to bad accidents if you are carrying a heavy pot or hot pans. A textured non-slip tile or stone floor can be beautiful. Polished concrete is becoming an increasingly popular choice but make sure it is sealed or it will absorb and stain with red wine and oils. You can even put a seal on your concrete that has a bit of extra grip in it for traction.

In Europe I experienced a few kitchens with rugs in them. They were usually farmhouse-style kitchens and often had a decent amount of open space; the rug was never in the major spill zone. These were also quite cold climates and it was cosy to have a rug in the kitchen. In fact, a kitchen fireplace with a hearth rug is something I am going to enjoy designing one day.

CASUAL DINING

Informal dining is now a major feature of the kitchen space in the modern home. For many of us, sitting up to grab a quick snack or meal at the kitchen bench is a big part of our lives. Some of my clients have requested this space as an alternative to sitting at the dining table. I have even designed kitchen benches that merge with dining tables to complete the scenario. As a guest it is the best place to sit; you can be at the kitchen bench, chatting to your friend, watch the meal being prepared and even be helping – all from the 'living room side' of the kitchen bench. If this is how you like to live, you should strive to integrate the cooking experience with casual entertaining.

If you have the space, bring in a farm table for rustic charm. A big farm table is conducive to

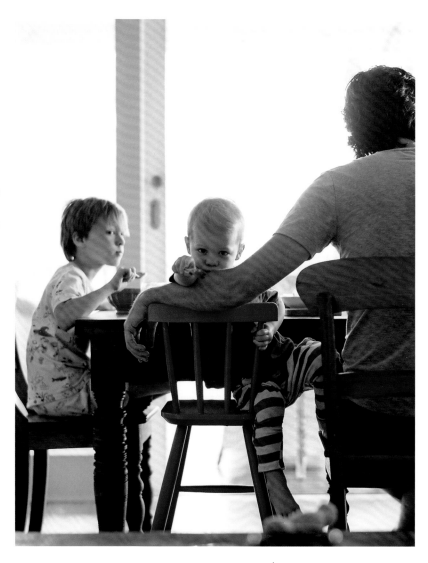

large informal gatherings and can be a stylistic lead for your whole kitchen. There is something homely and friendly about eating in the kitchen (and you are close to any second helpings). I think all those old TV shows where the house staff sit around a kitchen table and have a lot more fun than the posh people upstairs in the stiff dining room definitely had an effect on me.

THE BREAKFAST NOOK

Create a breakfast nook, or maybe just a cushioned nook where you sip a glass of wine while 'helping' in the kitchen. If you have the opportunity build a kitchen window seat or bench under a window; it doesn't have to be much, just

▲ In open-plan living the dining table can be central to the action, letting you keep an eye on things, just like Peter is doing here.

The refrigerator is undoubtedly a large and bulky item and not everyone likes to have it on show. In this kitchen the fridge has been put in the laundry area to the side, allowing a more streamlined kitchen in the open–plan space. This only works when there is easy access from the main living area to the room with the fridge — otherwise everyone visiting the fridge passes through the kitchen and annoys the cook.

enough so that someone can hop in and chat to whoever is preparing the meal. There will be an opportunity to store wine above and below this nook as it is always used seated.

THE ESSENTIAL TRIANGLE

The primary consideration when laying out a kitchen should be circulation during cooking and food preparation. The 'two-step rule' advises that no more than two steps be required when transferring a hot pan from the stove top to the sink or other bench, or vice versa. If you are taking more than two steps, then room for accident increases enormously. Less than two steps and the space will start to feel very tight, especially if there is more than one person in the kitchen – suddenly you will find you are bumping into each other.

The key is the relationship between the fridge, stove top and sink – commonly referred to as the 'kitchen triangle'. The rules are that no side of the triangle should be too short or too long. There are even specific measurements sometimes given out for how many metres these should be, but they span a pretty big range, so don't worry about them too much: they are just a guide. As long as you are aware of the triangle and plan accordingly, it really is just common sense. Anyway these days we are often juggling more priorities than just these three elements, so I often refer to different parts of the kitchen as 'zones' and then ask the home owner to establish their own hierarchy of relationships between the elements. You might include your frequently used appliances in your design, as well as common pantry ingredients such as salt and oil. You might

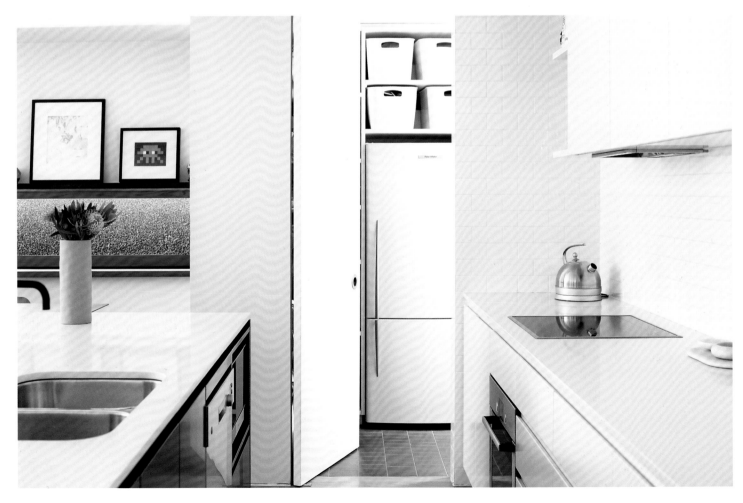

even have a dedicated configuration for baking and then another one for preparing the evening meal. These days there are often multiple people in the kitchen doing different things, so bring that into your zoning hierarchy and circulation.

WHICH SHAPE?

The design of your kitchen has to be led by the demands of the overall building and where the kitchen needs to be located to make it the centre of your home. It should occupy an important location among living, dining and outdoor areas. The main options for kitchen plans are U-shaped, G-shaped, L-shaped, single-wall, galley kitchen and island bench kitchen. Today, the island bench is the most sought after kitchen plan, followed by the U-, G- and L-shapes. Few briefs call for a single-wall or galley kitchen – these are more a product of the past or necessary only because of distinct parameters of the building.

An island bench kitchen is the most liberating design, as it allows the best movement and access to all parts of the kitchen with a minimum of two access points. It is super-efficient for movement, as you do a short spin from the bench to the stove and back again, for example. However, you need quite a large natural space for an island bench to work – in essence you are giving up preparation and storage space for access.

In smaller areas, or where there is a greater demand for bench space and storage, the U-, G- and L-shapes really come into play. These are continuous, and so can wrap around any wall space and configuration, and then also create a forward-facing bench to the rest of the room. The downside is that, unlike the island bench, which has two access points into the kitchen, the U-, G- and L-shaped kitchens have one access point. If that point is not easily wide enough for more than one person it can become a pinch point.

A single-wall kitchen can be an efficient design in smaller houses or apartments. However, it means the cook has their back to the room, shimmying up and down the length of the benchtop as they conduct the different jobs of cooking. Certainly you have no chance of achieving the efficient triangle and in a large kitchen the shimmy up and down would get a bit ridiculous. One solution to the single-wall kitchen

in a small apartment is to create an island bench on wheels that can be pushed away somewhere (such as under the stairs) when it's not in use. Obviously, in that scenario you can't have a sink or power points in the island bench as it won't have plumbing or wiring.

A galley kitchen can be a sophisticated space if it is well designed with room for movement and thoroughfare, as it can become a great connector between other spaces and rooms. However, if it is not big enough then a galley kitchen can feel like a strange combination of kitchen and hallway, leading to uncomfortable congestion.

▼ A mix of open and closed joinery has been used to add interest and display options in this compact kitchen. The joinery is all timber except for the benchtop, which is hard-wearing and practical waterproof stone.

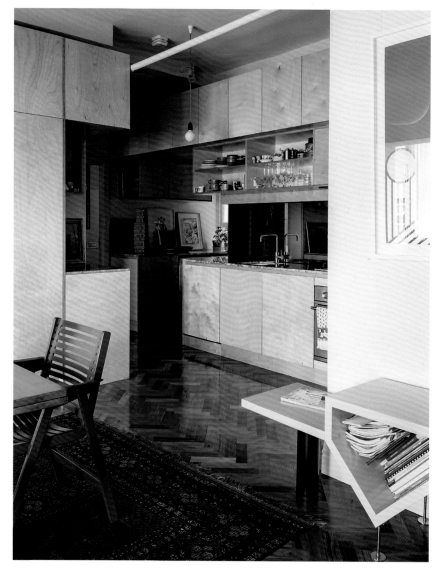

▶ Mirror has been used cleverly here as the face of the island bench, under the concrete benchtop. It lightens the concrete and gives the impression it is floating. Gloss subway tiles are used as a splashback — they catch and reflect the light in a lovely contrast to the dark-stained timber joinery.

WAYS TO BUILD

In terms of updating or building a new kitchen there are two options. One is an off-the-shelf kitchen that is made and delivered and popped into place. The other is a custom-made kitchen that is designed and built to become part of the building, and so takes into account any unusual wall angles, or unique design decisions that have been made. Generally speaking, the latter is more expensive than the former.

There are a multitude of off-the-shelf options these days that they are definitely worth considering: many come with design assistance and a lot of material and finish options. The downside is that if your walls are out of whack you can end up with unsightly gaps – these would be absorbed by a completely custom-made kitchen. A custom-made kitchen will have unique finishes and a more personal design, so if you really want something different this is the way to go.

If you decide to go for an off-the-shelf kitchen, ascertain its exact dimensions, both in plan and height, and then build a cavity for the kitchen to fit into, so that it is built-in. If possible, I try to avoid joinery cupboards finishing in mid-air with no immediate bulkhead or ceiling above them.

MUST DON'T

NEVER PUT THE FRIDGE AT THE BACK OF THE KITCHEN WITHOUT ALTERNATIVE ACCESS – IT IS THE MOST FREQUENTED APPLIANCE FOR THE WHOLE FAMILY AND THERE NEEDS TO BE A CLEAR PATH TO IT.

INTEGRATED KITCHEN

There is no doubt that an integrated kitchen appears more sophisticated; the refrigerator and dishwasher in particular are integrated into the joinery, hidden behind cupboard fronts that match the rest of the kitchen, to create a more seamless look. This makes sense if you are investing in a lovely material, such as a timber veneer, for your kitchen and also if you are avoiding cabinetry handles and the like. The exception to this is to make a statement with your big appliances. Some home owners love to show off industrial or rustic-look stoves that incorporate big hobs and ovens and smack of a serious cooking or farmhouse kitchen. Another example is the resurgence of the colourful retro refrigerator that becomes a feature of the space.

THE MULTI-PERSON KITCHEN

When designing your kitchen, don't make it a one-person dream space. You need to make sure it enables shared tasks – baking with the kids, sharing the chopping of vegies, letting guests find glasses and coffee mugs while you're doing that chopping... Make space for these special shared moments – this is quality time and it's where the best and most relaxed conversations often happen. And consider it not all standing time – as well as the stools on the outer side of the bench, I often introduce a stool on the inner side that tucks away underneath when not in use. Leave an overhang at the end of the bench so you can create a circle around the bench - this is great for not only communicating but also teaching and learning. For families, I find it is always best to provide solid bench stools for the kitchen – the kids will climb all over them and perch on top to see what is going on at the bench. (From their lower vantage point they are always busting to see how the chocolate icing is made!)

For households that love to cook, my advice is get two sinks. It might seem an extravagance, but if your way of being happy and connecting is to be in the kitchen and cooking at the same time, then it's well worth the expense.

Finally, the butler's pantry... Traditionally, this was a room that always contained a sink and was where servants did the dirty work, leaving the main kitchen pristine. In some larger homes today a butler's pantry is introduced to hide dirty dishes and general mess so that they can't be seen by guests. It can also double as a walk-in pantry. A big butler's pantry can be excellent for caterers to use, as all the food preparation can take place out of sight of guests.

THE BUSY FRIDGE

The fridge is the most frequented appliance in the kitchen. In fact, it is also the most frequented appliance by the non-food preparers in the house. In other words, your kids will visit the fridge a great deal in the day without any intention of serving anyone but themselves. Therefore, one of the biggest problems with home design is if the fridge is located at the back of a kitchen. Never do this unless you want a steady stream of grommets under your feet as you try to prepare the meals of

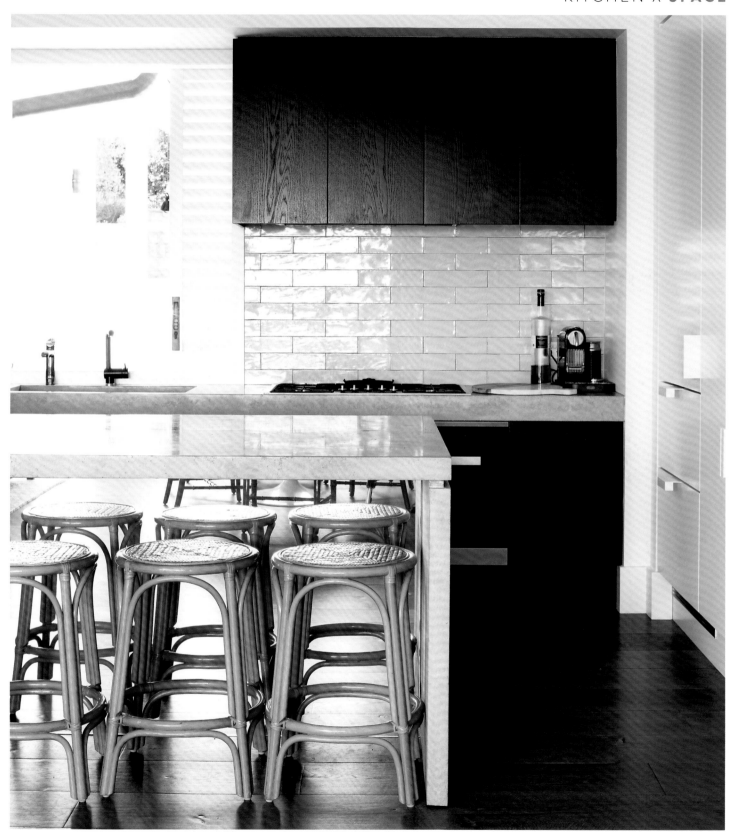

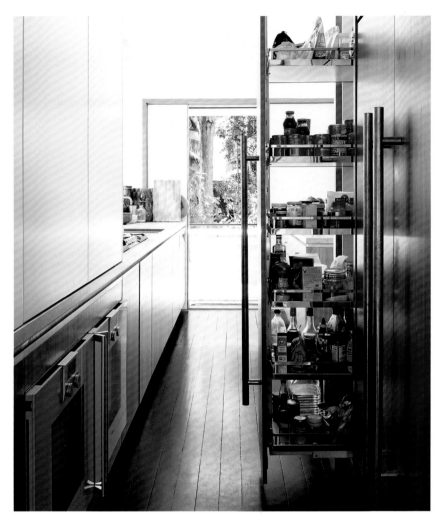

too deep. A pantry with pull-out shelves is a clever way to beat this issue. A full-height pantry is definitely best: it is important not to be constantly bending down or reaching up. Store most-used items in the most easy to reach section, which is at mid-height. I work out a spot on the bench near the stove top for salt, pepper, olive oil and the like – it is an opportunity to have them on show, maybe in earthenware bowls with timber spoons, and add a bit of life to your kitchen. When you walk into a kitchen that has these few things on display it is amazing how much more homely it feels because it represents a space that is being used daily for cooking. For example, a hotel room kitchen would never have these daily condiments on show, as it is not a home. By the same token, a commercial kitchen with all its whiz-bang machinery does not feel like home – it's never that friendly or relaxing to see a whole lot of robots lined up on the kitchen bench.

STOVE TOP

Your stove top is the next key item. Gas or electric is a personal choice, but from my point of view they are quite aesthetically different, so I will sometimes change my kitchen design depending on whether a client has chosen the more slick electric rather than the industrial and bulky gas stove top. The next decision is a 60 cm (24 in) wide stove top or 90 cm (35 in) wide; and I have a rule – no matter which stove top, you must choose the same width range hood. It is jarring to see a large 90 cm stove top with an itty bitty 60 cm range hood over the top. Not only does it not work as efficiently – it looks ridiculous.

There are many types of range hoods. Some hang from the ceiling, which is fine as long as you are aware of them – I have banged my head on many over the years. They need to be set back over the bench, just like overhead cupboards are set back – this allows you to stand at the bench with your head forward, which is a natural position when chopping, for instance.

There are some great new range hoods that are fixed in benchtops and rise up at a touch of a button when you require them. This is a very slick option. However, there is quite a bit of work involved ensuring they are ducted properly though the joinery and/or floor to the outside. In

▲ A pull-out pantry creates super efficient storage that ensures food never gets lost and forgotten at the back of the cupboard.

the day. It is always best to locate the fridge at the main entry point to the kitchen from the living room, so that easy access is available without disturbing the food preparer.

THE ALMOST-AS-BUSY PANTRY

After the fridge the next most frequented store area is the pantry. Spatially, I always try to locate the pantry next to the fridge. If you have the space, it is hard to beat a walk-in pantry. I like to design them with vented doors that allow air flow but prevent light entering. It is good to have varied depth shelves on the walls to provide different storage options – just don't make them too deep or you will lose things and find them again when they are way out of date. A cupboard can work as a pantry as long as the shelves aren't terms of aesthetics, a range hood can be concealed or revealed in your design. If you go down the 'revealed' path then make sure you very clearly understand how the dominating range hood sits in the space with the rest of the design.

OVEN

There are two main considerations here: is it under the stove top or in the wall? This is a personal choice and I have been caught in the middle of many arguments over the years between family partners who have different preferences. My personal preference is a wall oven, simply because of my height – but I can see the planning efficiency of having the stove top and oven combined in a freestanding cooker. A wall oven takes up another 600–900 mm (24–35 in) of your floor plan, as 600–900 mm has already been provided for your hob, so it is more space grabbing. Although, be aware that, when open, a wall oven door usually does not intrude into the space as much as a fully opened stove oven door; and, of course, the associated human takes up a lot more space when opening a stove oven door as they bend over, in comparison to standing up while using a wall oven.

The microwave oven is often a forgotten item – it works best integrated under the bench or, even better, as part of the wall oven column. If it is a stand-alone item it should go in a place where it is not seen, like a walk-in pantry. It's disappointing to walk into a lovely kitchen and find this boxy creature crouching on the table.

THE THEATRE OF THE SINK

The sink for me is the Holy Grail of the kitchen because there is something so alive and so human about running water. It is such a big deal for us not only in terms of drinking for survival, but also for hygiene and cleaning the food that we eat and the utensils and equipment that we eat off. We really are so lucky to have a fountain of fresh water gushing in the centre of our homes at the flick of a tap. We must never take it for granted... but of course we do. With that in mind I tend to celebrate the sink in terms of location. It is always disappointing when the theatre of the sink is stuck on a bench underneath a set of cupboards. It seems to me that the sink and its precious

water source should have some room to move. So, invariably, I bring it out into the open, usually in one of two places... Depending on the brief and the demands of the space, the sink will be in the bench facing the living space (sometimes this is an island bench) and will be the main focal point of the kitchen. The other option is facing the outdoors. There is something lovely about being able to look outdoors to a view while using the sink. Even more exquisite is the idea of sun coming in over the sink and the sparkle of sunlight through the water as you wash your spuds – now that is a slice of heaven. Another element that I like to bring together is herbs and the water source. Edible greenery is a lovely sight and everyone implicitly knows water is part of the health of plants, so it makes sense that the garden comes as close as possible to the sink. Having a living kitchen herb garden, preferably near the sink, is never a bad thing.

In terms of placing a sink in a bench, consider not putting it slap bang in the middle. Position it to one side of the bench to allow a larger, more usable prep area next to the sink.

An undermount sink is one that is mounted underneath the benchtop so that none of the sink

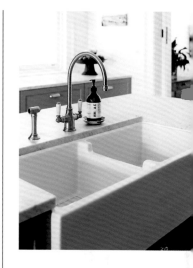

▲ A farmhouse sink has nostalgic charm and this double version offers great depth and usability. The thick benchtop fits well with the solid nature of the sink.

▼ This concealed range hood has been made into a feature with a timber veneer façade. It is the same width as the hob and vented door to the pantry.

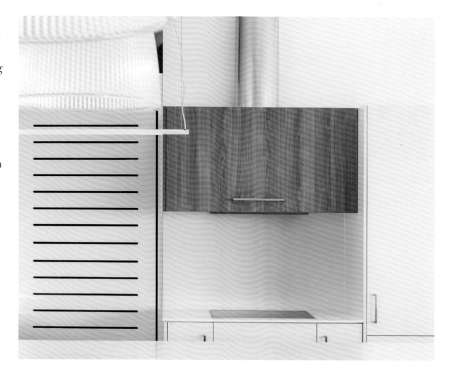

▶▶ Use different textures to create spatial interest. This predominantly white kitchen uses a selection of man-made stone benchtops, polyurethane cabinetry, gloss subway tiles and plasterboard — all in white. The joinery has been seamlessly tucked in under a bulkhead, complimenting the minimalist lack of handles in the joinery. The open display shelf adds character.

▼ The fridge and freezer are entirely hidden in this kitchen — integrated in a wall of sleek white joinery.

is above the bench – instead the edge of the bench is revealed. These were once expensive and not easy to obtain, but now the opposite is true and I would certainly recommend them. If you have a beautiful benchtop and want to show it off then the undermount sink is the way to go – and it is a breeze to clean. The only time I now specify an overmount sink, which is when the benchtop runs underneath the top edges of the sink, is when I am using a cost-effective melamine material for a benchtop that is not waterproof at the edges and therefore requires the protection of the overmount sink.

My favourite type of sink is the moulded sink – but these are a little pricey. They are made out of resin, with the sink and the bench being continuous. You can then mould grooves into the benchtop next to the sink to form a seamless draining board. If you love stainless steel, you can have seamless stainless steel sinks and benchtops too. All are easy to clean, and once you have had the pleasure of using one it is hard to go back.

The sink tap is the vertical centrepiece of most kitchens. It can be a stunning focal point, or it can dominate in the wrong way, so if you are renovating remember to set some budget aside for it. For an easy fix for your kitchen, simply splash out on a new kitchen tap.

BENCHTOP

Your benchtop is an important element in the look and feel of your kitchen. If you choose a benchtop that is 40 mm (1.6 in) or more thick then it will feel quite heavy in the space – even heavier in a dark colour. With that heaviness can come a sense of opulence, especially if you wrap the top down the sides of your bench, often referred to as a waterfall feature. However, do take into account that many people know the 40 mm thickness is often fake and just an attempt to mimic a thicker piece of stone or resin, when in reality it is simply an extra strip of the material added to the edge of the top for effect. Once you know this, it is difficult to be impressed by a thick benchtop that you know is not really thick. Of course, when you see a real thick slab of stone or timber, it is impressive!

Instead, a much finer bench top of 20 mm (0.8 in) or less can be very elegant if you taper it off to a point to make the bench top 'float'. This is much truer to the material and can create a sophisticated look.

Beyond playing with the light and dark of your benchtop, try different finishes. Gloss can give a sparkly reflective look to your kitchen; but also consider a honed look – a more matt finish can bring in some unexpected elegance. Check when buying, because some honed finishes do not clean as easily as the gloss ones.

NOTE TO SELF

KEEP YOUR PANTRY SHELVES RELATIVELY SHALLOW, EVEN THOUGH THEY WON'T HOLD AS MUCH. THAT WAY NOTHING WILL GET LOST DOWN THE BACK AND BE REDISCOVERED IN A FEW YEARS' TIME... YIKES!

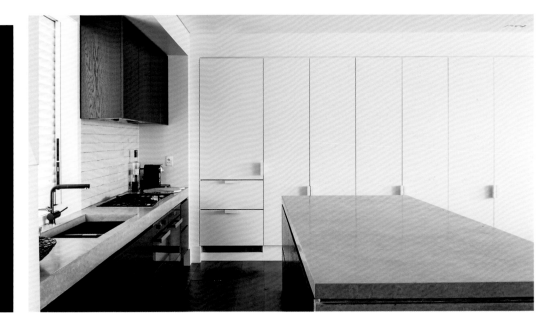

Other benchtop materials to consider are resin, stone, man-made stone, concrete and even tile. Timber bench tops can be lovely; however, they need to be well treated to handle water. A commercial kitchen look of all stainless steel is also an option, but you have to accept that it will scratch, and scratch a lot. For me, that is part of its appeal: it looks used and it is highly practical.

A relatively easy fix to upgrade an existing kitchen is to simply replace your kitchen benchtops. Or, if you have stone benchtops, you can re-hone and polish them to give them a new lease of life.

The standard kitchen bench height is 90 cm (35 in). However, as a tall person, I creep it up to 95 cm (37 in) for my own benches and it makes a huge difference. Another solution I have found for a taller person is to use a big chunky cutting board – you can find some that are extremely thick and they can make a huge difference – good for your muscles to lug around! The key measure is to ensure the bench is between 5 and 10 cm (2–4 in) below your bent elbow height.

If, however, you are stuck with a standard bench height and it doesn't happen to suit you, then using a stool to sit on can make a big difference. Find a stool that ensures you end up at the right height above the bench when seated and it will be far more comfortable than stooping or reaching – of course, you need to be able to get your knees under the bench for this to be practical and comfortable.

Oh, and don't forget the kids. Every family home should allow space for a kitchen stool that children can stand on to join in cooking. A stool is better than finding them sitting on the kitchen bench. The stool is also handy for you if you have high storage – this is something I often design into kitchens, as you might as well use the full ceiling height and it is quite cost-effective to extend joinery that you are already building.

MAKE A SPLASH

The splashback is an important design element for your kitchen space – it enables depth in the middle of what can be quite a dominating façade of kitchen. You can emphasise perspective, contrast or even a burst of colour. I always encourage people to have a bit of fun with the

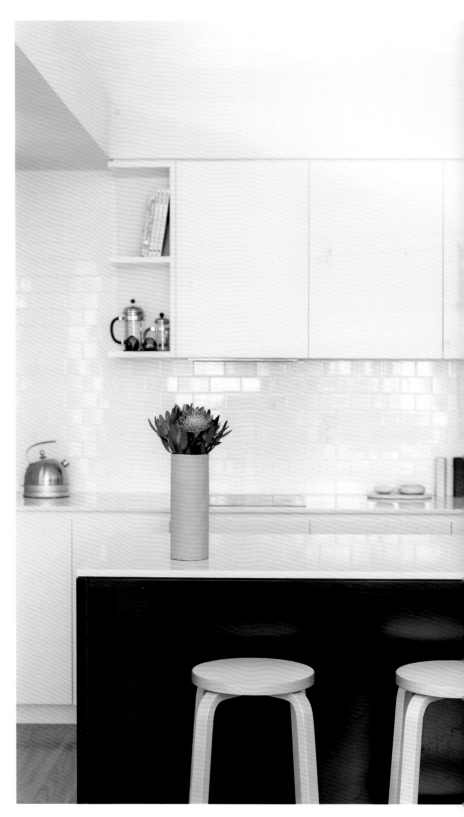

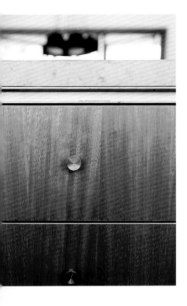

▲ Detail is important and here the coming together of stone, brass and timber is very satisfying.

▶ A semi-integrated dishwasher allows the timber veneer to be the dominant feature, rather than the metal front of the dishwasher.

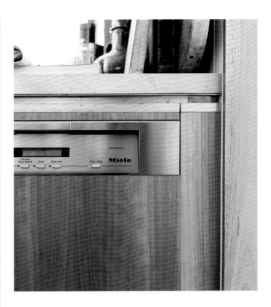

splashback, but that doesn't have to mean bright colours: white subway tiles or silver mirror can both add some spark to an otherwise flat façade.

For a quick style change, replace your splashback. Pressed metal, chalkboard, mirror, tiles or mosaics will all have a big impact.

DISHWASHER AND WASTE

For practical reasons in regard to plumbing, the dishwasher is usually under or next to the sink, which makes double sense as items are often superficially dealt with in the sink before being popped into the dishy. Keep in mind that one of the most backbreaking jobs in the kitchen is emptying the dishwasher, so organise your kitchen so that crockery, glass and pan cupboards are as close as possible to the dishwasher. If you can transport straight from dishwasher to storage without having to stack on the benchtop in between, then you are on to a winner.

The bin and recycling are often also located around this area, if not under the sink then in the cupboard next door. The sink, bin and dishwasher all work together in the clean-up phase, so it makes sense that they are together – you could call them a secondary triangle.

DRAWERS AND CUPBOARDS

Increasingly in the kitchens we design we are utilising large drawers. The technology of drawers with their soft close systems has

improved so much that they are a very practical and dependable part of the kitchen. Drawers are more accessible than cupboards –they bring the rear of the storage right to the front, putting everything within easy reach. You can also create a hierarchy, with heavy, more bulky, items in deep bottom drawers and lighter items higher up in shallower drawers. The top drawer can be the shallowest, with your utensils neatly laid out. I try to avoid designing below-bench cupboards now, except in corners where I use fantastic swing-out corner units (which once again bring the hard-to-reach part of the cupboard to the front).

I design cupboards for above the bench, but make sure they are set back 20 cm (8 in) from the edge of the benchtop below, so that the person working at the bench isn't constantly bumping their head as they lean forwards to work. And I always leave 60 cm (24 in) depth between benchtop and the cupboards above.

For a relatively easy fix, change your old lower-level cupboards into modern soft-close drawers. And then make one of them the go-to drawer for all the miscellaneous stuff that hangs around a kitchen, like batteries and bottle openers and scissors. Let everyone in the family know that is the 'stuff' drawer and that everything must be returned to it. Give it a spring clean every six months to keep it under control and it will become one of your favourite drawers (mainly because this annoying stuff is no longer on the various surfaces in your home).

Drawers and cupboards give you an opportunity to really change the look of your kitchen. Cupboard doors can be any colour, any range of metallic or wood grains, any texture, any finish from gloss to matt. In fact, there are really too many choices. Even more reason to be led by a deeper story of why you are making this kitchen and what home it is in, rather than following the latest fad. For a very easy facelift, just replace your cupboard doors. If you have a white kitchen, change the doors to a contrasting black, or a bright colour such as sky blue.

You could also add glass cabinets to your kitchen. These can provide character and relief in an otherwise opaque expanse of kitchen joinery and are a great opportunity to show off heirloom china, cookbooks – all these add charm and personality. Remember, the kitchen is often the scene of getting to know someone a bit better and there are few better ice breakers than looking through a collection of cookbooks.

HANDLES, OR NO HANDLES?

I love beautiful handles for drawers and cupboards, and they can be a feature of a lovely kitchen. But do watch out that your kitchen doesn't become a mishmash of handles everywhere – some vertical and some horizontal. Many of the kitchens I design don't have traditional handles on the face of the joinery. Rather I use 'shark-nose' pulls on the top of cupboards and doors, and then drop the overhead cupboard doors 20 mm (0.8 in) lower than the cupboard behind, to form a convenient pull so that you can open and close the doors. This creates a very clean look in your kitchen. There is a practical aspect to this as well – with no handles there is nothing to catch on as you move around the kitchen. These days there is often more than one person in the kitchen, so space can be an issue even in a well-designed kitchen. We still often specify handles for the bigger, weightier items, such as the pantry door and an integrated refrigerator, where the finger pulls get difficult – especially for the weak among us.

SMALL APPLIANCES

When planning your kitchen, make a list of all your appliances – it can feel oppressive when a beautiful kitchen is cluttered with a multitude of machines. A toaster and a kettle are fine but seeing every juicer, presser, mixer, plunger and latest 'time-saving' kitchen fad on display can make me feel like I'm in the Terminator's *Rise of the machines*.

In a well-planned kitchen every appliance should have a home, preferably behind a cupboard door or shutter. And make allowances for space for future appliances – a new type of fandangled juicer, perhaps – as they can often be very bulky. In new kitchens I like to design concealable bench space located behind a pull-down shutter, so that the items are easily accessible but can be hidden away. I find that if you store appliances in a low cupboard or on a high shelf, not only are they less likely to be used,

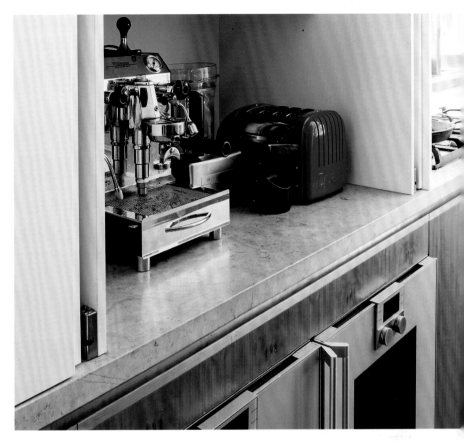

but they are clumsy to move around. Better to have your favourite juicer, coffee machine, mixer, blender and so on all lined up at a usable height on the benchtop behind a screen, and all ready to go with suitable power points in the cupboards.

In my kitchen I do a yearly review of appliances – sometimes I've bought into a fad and haven't used that amazing machine more than twice. It's easy to sell things online these days so there's no excuse for keeping anything you don't use.

Make sure that wherever you have your appliances there is room close by for the accompanying equipment. So, for example, the coffee paraphernalia is next to the coffee machine, and glassware next to where you make the drinks.

▲ When this kitchen is in action the doors are folded back to reveal the appliances, which are at a comfortable height to use. However, when the kitchen jobs are over, the doors close and the clutter disappears behind joinery.

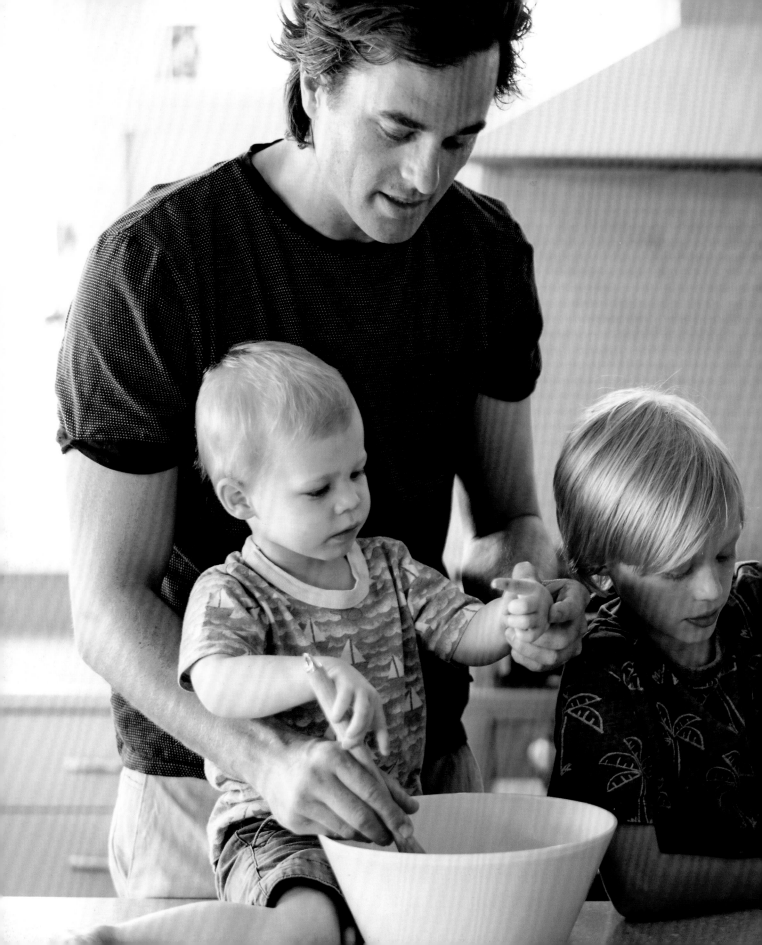

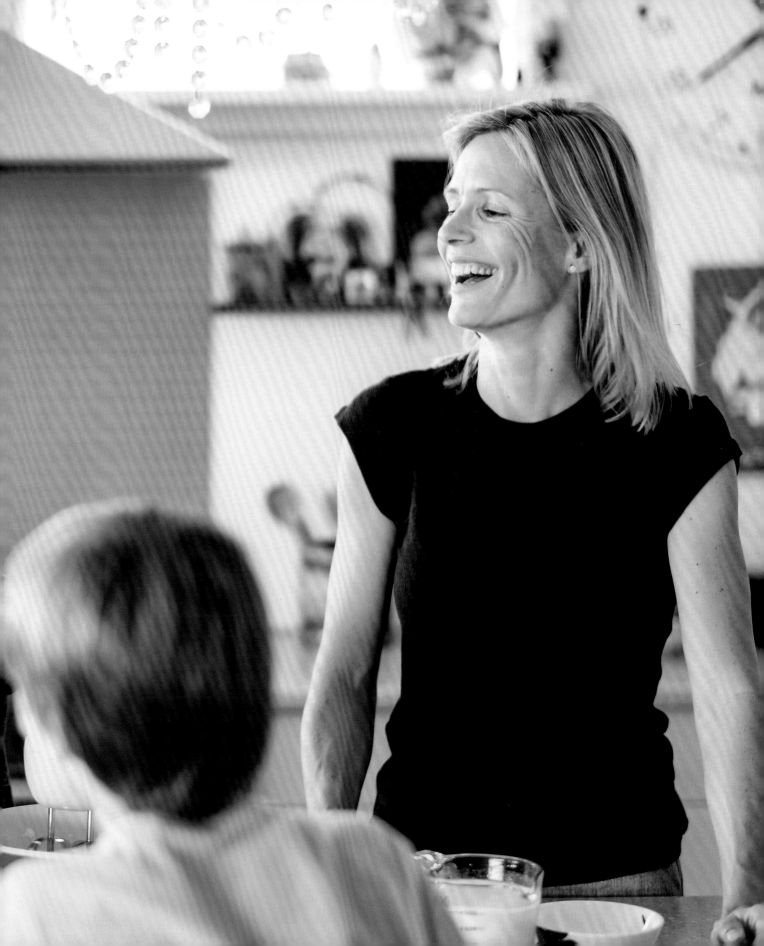

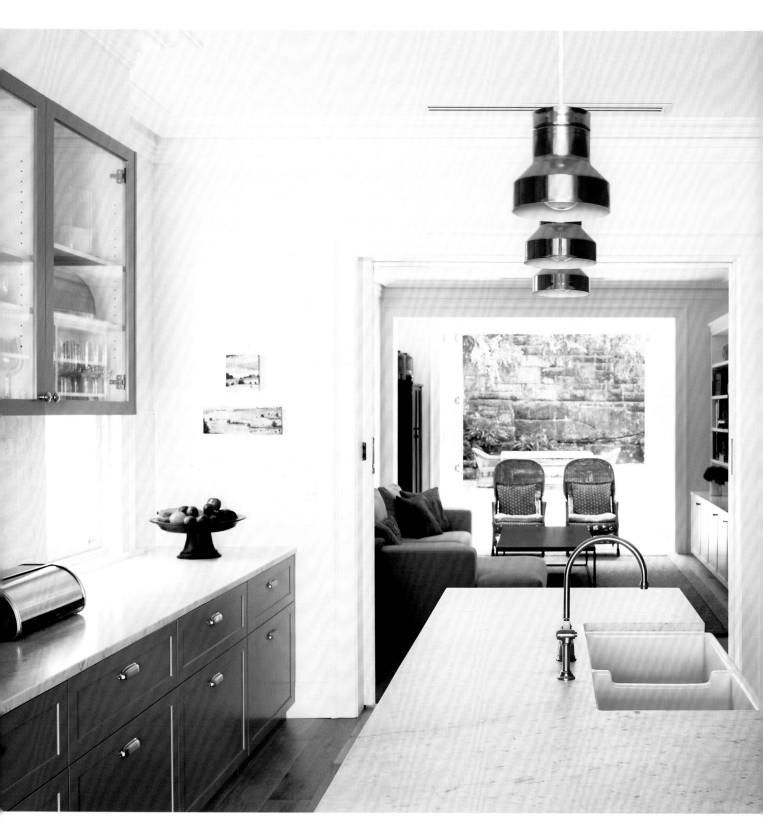

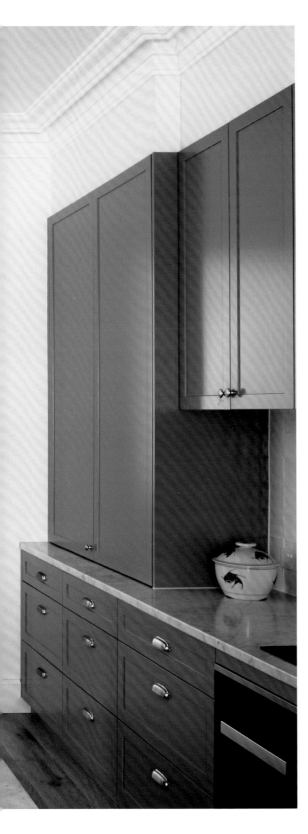

LIGHT

The primary role of a kitchen is the preparation of food and this is clearly a task that requires high-quality lighting over work benches. However, with the advent of open-plan living we also want our kitchens to be lit in such a way that the bright task lighting can be toned down, and in the evening the kitchen can become a lovely soft backdrop to our living space. No one wants to relax on the sofa with a commercial-grade lit-up kitchen in the background. So, ensure there are dimmer switches on your lights, or, even better, introduce different lights for different purposes. When the task of food preparation and clean-up is over, turn off those task lights and just leave the under-cupboard lights on to illuminate your splashback and nothing else. This will transform your kitchen from a task-lit space to an accent-lit space that becomes a visual asset to the living and dining rooms. You will find that this accent light is bright enough for you to go back into the kitchen during a movie break and make a cup of tea or grab a biscuit. Make sure this accent light is a warmer colour, rather than the cool bright colour of the task lights.

◀ These copper pendants provide quality task lighting on the island benchtop for the intensive work of food preparation, as well as being aesthetically beautiful.

▼ Windows directly behind a kitchen bench are not common but they can be fantastic for creating a bright and sunny kitchen, and even a sense of cooking outdoors. Note the appliance cupboard with its automatic light that comes on when the door is opened.

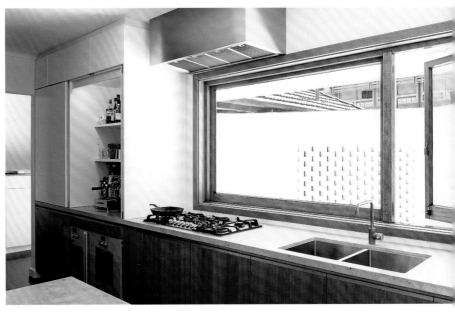

POOLS OF LIGHT

Remember to create lighting areas within the larger open-plan room – make sure you can turn off your living and kitchen lighting and just leave on a few accent lights. That way, if you are dining more formally, you can just light your dining area.

SUNLIGHT IN YOUR KITCHEN

There is something just glorious about sunlight glinting through water and I always think, well why can't we have that in our kitchens? I often design kitchen sinks to be below a window, so that the water catches the sun and also the view. Skylights can offer excellent ambient and task lighting during the day, which means you don't need any lights on to prepare food. There is also a healthy and hygienic feeling about natural light and kitchens. In fact, sunlight has been found to kill germs – so why not help yourself?

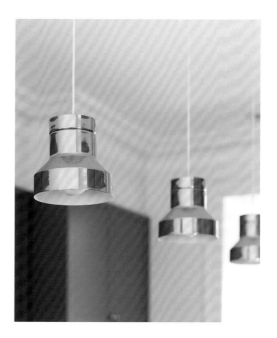

WINDOW SPLASHBACK

Natural lighting in a kitchen can also be sourced from a window – if you are renovating or building you could fit a long, above-bench window as a splashback. It can be a great look to have natural light and a strip of view coming into the kitchen between the overhead cupboards and the benchtop. The glass might need to be toughened, depending on how close to the hot cooktop it is, but as a splashback glass is easy to clean.

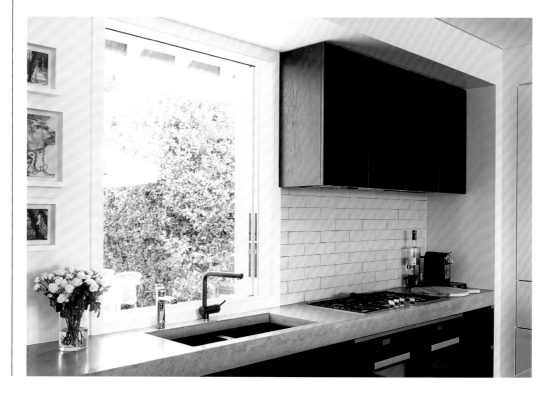

▲ Ensure pendant lights are at the right height for the overall space and are perfectly spaced, particularly if they are a major design feature like these shiny copper numbers.

▶ The range hood does not need to be a special feature; the upper joinery here houses a concealed range hood that takes a quiet back seat.

TASK LIGHTING: BENCHTOP

Over an island bench, the best task lighting is pendant lights. They give good light to the task, but hang low enough so that the light spill and glare does not bleed into the living spaces. You can also put in a ceiling downlight that gives off a tight cone of light, almost like a spotlight that shines directly onto the island bench. Make sure it is directional and that the light source is set well back into the ceiling, or has a diffuser fitted that directs the light and reduces unwanted light spill and glare into the rest of the space. Choose a cooler colour light for task lighting – closer to daylight colour; this is better to see food by and for concentration when doing task work.

Over benchtops that are facing the wall, the best task lighting is in a pelmet placed beneath the overhead cupboard, with the cupboard door hanging down low enough to conceal the light source, thus preventing light bleed. Design this so it is on a switch of its own and can come on as an accent light – this gives you a great opportunity to light the splashback only, creating a sense of depth and drama.

TASK LIGHTING: DINING TABLE

If you have an open-plan kitchen and dining table, then make sure you have enough light over the dining table to be able to see the food you are eating without lighting up the rest of the room. Design some low pendants to hang over the table, remembering to hang them at a height suitable for when you are seated, not when you are standing. It is always frustrating when pendants are hung too high over a dining table, as if allowing someone to walk underneath them – they become more intrusive in the overall space as they start to get in your eyeline if you're standing in the kitchen or living room.

Other than pendants over the table, you can use downlights that have a very narrow cone of light so that they only light the table. These should be either set into the ceiling or be equipped with a diffuser to prevent glare and light extending beyond the task of lighting the table.

ISLAND BENCH AS A LIGHT FEATURE

An island bench is one of the few built-in objects in a room that can be enjoyed in the round – that

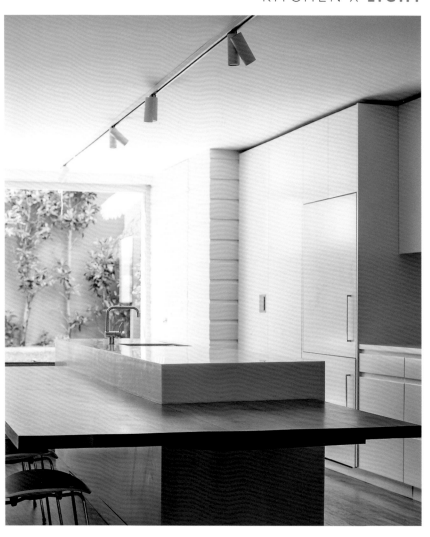

is why it is called an island. Most other built-in elements are attached to walls. So, here is an opportunity. With some clever lighting you can make your island bench a much lighter object in the space and even make it appear to float. Insert LED strips around the base and a halo of light forms that will blur the connection between the floor and the island.

OTHER LIGHTS

Remember also that your appliances often come with their own lighting. You should take into consideration what light they generate and make sure there are not too many blinking colourful illuminations as unnecessary attention-getters in your special kitchen. (Although the refrigerator bulb is always handy as a light source for the midnight snack.)

▲ Track lighting with spot lights allows you to direct the light and also to add more or take off lights as needed.

A wall of bifold doors lets this space become one with the outside area.

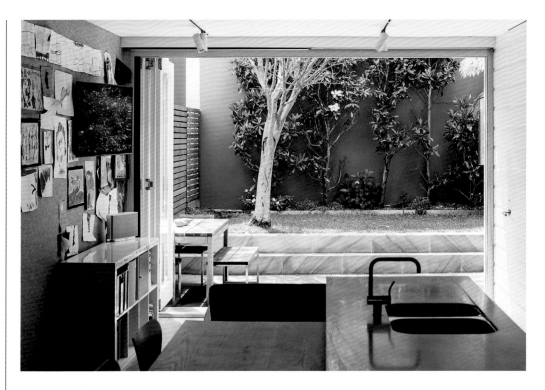

AIR

When I design a kitchen, I aim for as much natural air ventilation as possible. I am thinking much more open-air kitchen than in-a-box kitchen. There is something lovely and liberating about cooking in the outdoors, so why not bring a sense of that to your kitchen? There is no doubt that every kitchen requires excellent mechanical ventilation, but if you can couple that with the ability to throw open the windows and achieve cross-flow ventilation, it is a wonderful bonus. Windows in and around the kitchen are a great asset, in particular a set of louvres near the main cooking area if you suddenly need to aerate the space. An openable window splashback is a great option; consider a long sliding window or a set of louvres. But do ensure that you research toughened glass for this use – there are building regulations for glass that is near a heat source.

Remember your kitchen is a heat source and hot air rises, so some ventilation in the ceiling is a great idea. Roof ventilators, such as whirlybirds, are a good natural way to release kitchen heat and odours. Opening skylights or high clerestory windows are also a good option, giving the added bonus of light and a sense of the sky.

EXTRACT AND FRESHEN

The smell of cooking should waft from the kitchen and entice the household to the table. However, yesterday's cooking smells are not good. Excellent extraction is required. Remember that extraction not only sucks up air, but also steam and evaporated grease, so it is important to invest in decent technology – you don't want a grease patch collecting above your stove top.

There are many types of air extraction on the market but by far the best is external extraction, which pushes the cooking air outside. Range hoods that use filters do work, but you must change the filters fairly regularly. And there are more options now than just overhead range hoods – many brands have in-bench air extractors that pop up and suck the air down around your cooking area. Also consider placing any other devices that give off smells or steam near the range hood.

MUST DO

FRESH AIR AND FRESH FOOD GO TOGETHER WELL. MAXIMISE THE FRESH AIR FLOWING THROUGH YOUR KITCHEN AND IT WILL HELP INSPIRE YOU AND YOUR FAMILY TO SPEND TIME THERE, ENJOY COOKING THERE AND EAT HEALTHIER MEALS TOGETHER THERE.

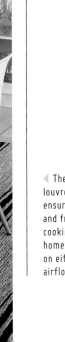

◀ The upper layer of clerestory louvres let in light and air to ensure this kitchen is bright and fresh as a daisy. If the cooking smells are strong, the home owners open the louvres on either side of the room and airflow freshens the space.

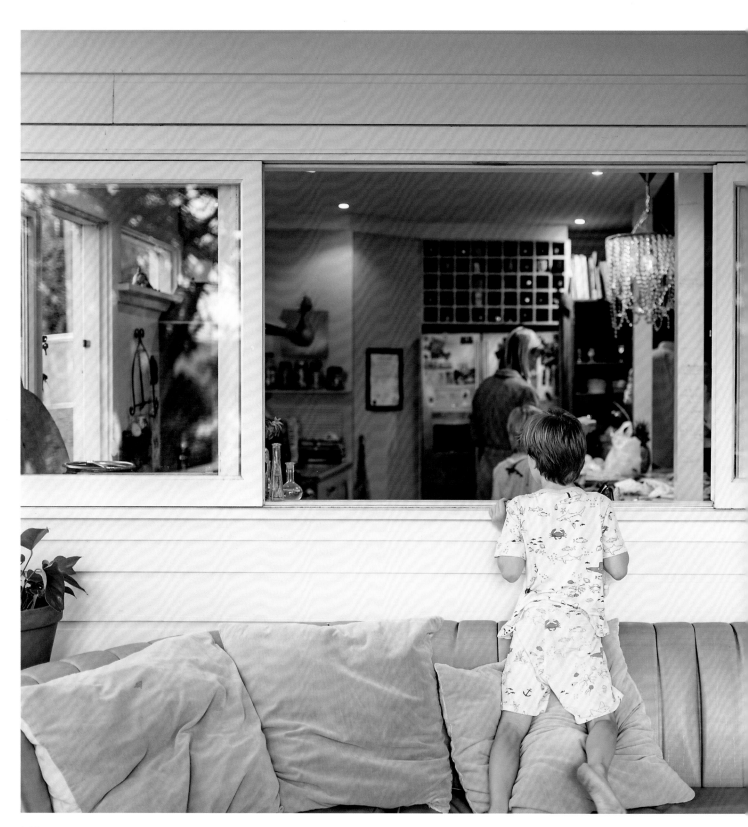

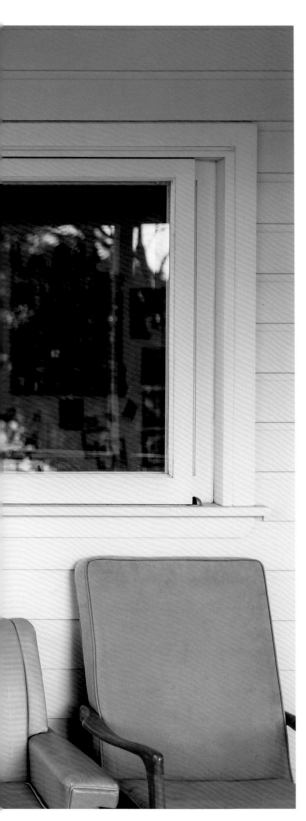

Do think about where your extraction fan comes out. Extraction must also be considered with regard to your neighbours, particularly in apartments. Have some courtesy and make sure your curry is not ruining someone else's day! There are a great many regulations for apartments, as you need to vent away from other people's homes, so you either need to tap into a ventilation system in the building or invest in a filtered range hood that is regularly changed.

FRESH AIR AND FOOD

Fresh air and food go together – so make sure your kitchen is naturally ventilated. In a new house I will often design glass louvres at either end of the kitchen to get the natural cross ventilation, and also consider other windows in the rest of the space. Skylights and a high ceiling can give a great sense of fresh air. In a renovation, consider the option of replacing the splashback with an openable toughened window to the outdoors – this will completely change your cooking experience. For a quick fix, change any fixed windows to openable. If you find you aren't opening windows because of insects, get flyscreens fitted immediately.

Consider introducing an air vent to the wall or ceiling; they require only a small penetration, are relatively cost-effective to buy and install, and can make a big difference to an otherwise stuffy kitchen. Any natural airflow is better than none, especially when you are using filtered extraction. And finally, just get into the habit of opening the windows every time you cook.

SCENT FACTORY

Everyone knows that freshly brewed coffee and baked bread will make your home smell great when you're trying to sell, but you can see your kitchen as a scent factory. Boil water and add fragrant ingredients, such as cloves and cinnamon sticks and slices of orange and lemon, to fill the air with seasonal scents. It's just essential oils, but on a bigger scale.

Invest in high-quality and beautifully scented dishwashing liquid. As the kitchen is one of the more frequently cleaned places in your home, splash out on lovely smelling cleaning products to make it smell great every time you clean.

These large windows are not only a great physical connection but they also aerate the kitchen, keeping it fresh.

SOUND

The kitchen should be located so that the sound of living spaces and outdoor spaces can travel to it. The person in the kitchen wants to be part of the conversation and not feel like a servant preparing meals and clearing up. Also, invariably, a parent in the kitchen wants to know if the kids are OK and being able to hear them is a big reassurance. But at night time, the location of the kitchen is important relative to the sleeping areas of the house. If you can separate the generally noisy kitchen from bedrooms (which traditionally used to be upstairs, while the kitchen was downstairs – not always the case any more) or at least have an acoustically solid door to shut off the kitchen, you will be more relaxed. It is impractical to have to creep around the kitchen early in the morning trying not to clink your breakfast bowl and wake up the household.

If there isn't any separation between kitchen and sleeping areas, I often design a large sliding exposed or cavity door that can be slid across when the kids have gone to bed at night, or when you are up early and everyone else is still asleep.

THE NOISY WORK OF FOOD

A kitchen is generally full of hard surfaces and can be a noisy place, with much bashing and crashing of kitchen crockery and equipment, humming of extraction fans and bubbling of pans and kettles. If you use fabric acoustic panels – such as you would use in a living space – to dampen and absorb sound, then these can fill up with cooking smells. So, to reduce reverberation of sound, use acoustic panels such as a perforated plasterboard or a series of drop-down panels that break up the sound but are not made of soft absorbent material.

There are many products on the market that are lightweight and designed to be installed either as a new build or retrofitted. If you have a noisy reverberating kitchen, seek advice from a professional who will advise what the options are and the quantity of acoustic panels that are required. Otherwise, you can experiment by implementing a few panels on the ceiling or on an unused wall and mark the change in the space. Importantly, ensure you install panels with a washable surface as the kitchen is a working space.

SOUND SYSTEM

Music is a great resource in the kitchen as it can make cooking and entertaining a memorable pleasure. Some speakers in the kitchen certainly won't go amiss and if you can have them connected to the TV then that can be a bonus. If you are keeping an eye on the living room TV while preparing food this saves the TV blaring across the area.

EQUIPMENT INTRUSION

Range hoods are generally loud beasts and unfortunately it really is down to management to control the noise level. Use the different settings so that you are not always on the noisiest high setting. There are some brands on the market that say they create 'silent' range hoods but you need to do your research. Just remember that often a showroom has quite a lot of ambient noise compared to your home, so the display range hoods might sound quieter than they actually are.

The good news is that dishwashers have improved a great deal. Frankly I have always found the sound of a dishwasher relaxing and even therapeutic – it signals the clean-up has been done and now the family can really relax. This is an example of the sound of home, with the dishwasher signalling the true end of day.

If you have to incorporate the laundry into the kitchen, then consider investing in some well-fitted doors to minimise noise, and find the most isolated spot within the open space; for example, as far away as possible from your comfy armchair. Having said that, you will never totally defeat the noise of a washer and dryer in your open-plan living space, so work out a timetable of when is best to put them on, such as when you go to bed or are out at work.

▶ Kitchens can be noisy spaces but the wall here, opposite the cooking area, is covered in soft grey acoustic panels that absorb and diffuse sound.

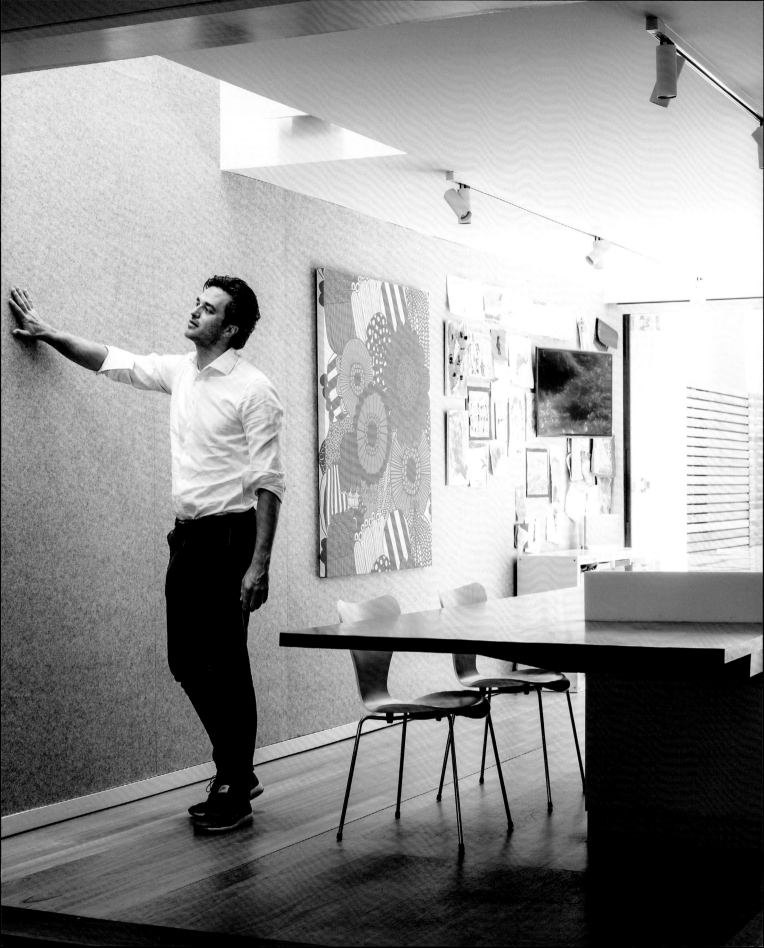

VIEW

Interestingly, a kitchen is predominantly a standing space – arguably one of the few intensively used spaces of the house that is. This means it should be designed as such, with views from the perspective of a standing position. For example, window sills can be higher than in other rooms. Also, as you are standing, you can 'borrow' views from other parts of the house over the top of living and dining areas. For example, you can be standing in the kitchen and look over the living or dining, both seated areas with low-height furniture, to the garden. This is why in open-plan living areas the kitchen is often designed at the rear of the space in relation to the garden. It is important to remember a kitchen bench is at 90 cm (35 in) – without even counting any tall cabinetry – so you won't be able to see over the kitchen area from a sofa or dining table unless you stand up, which isn't very relaxing.

KITCHEN SURVEILLANCE

The kitchen is often a central location of the home, from where you want to be able to keep an eye on everything: a little like the bridge of a ship. If you have young children, this is where you want to be able to prepare food and organise the house, while still being aware of what they are up to. It is important to get your views right in your home so that you can relax (as much as possible with kids running around).

With older children, it's nice for you to have a view from the kitchen to a space where they can do homework. Answering questions and helping while they do homework and you prepare a meal can be great family time. In a way it is about everyone doing their jobs at the same time – not a bad work ethic.

SPLASHBACK VIEW

If it's against an outside wall, replace the splashback with a window for an unexpected view, especially if it can look out onto some carefully planted green foliage.

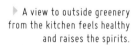

▷ A view to outside greenery from the kitchen feels healthy and raises the spirits.

▽ It is not all about external views. Create layered views inside your home and take advantage of your standing position in the kitchen.

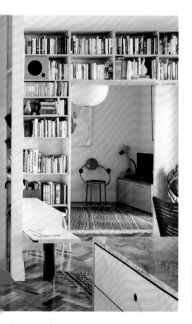

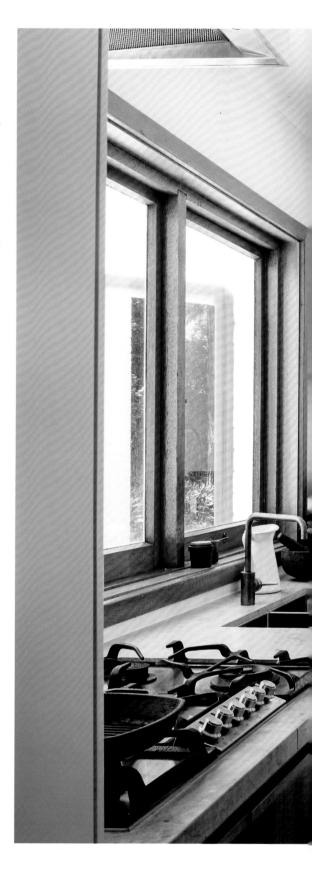

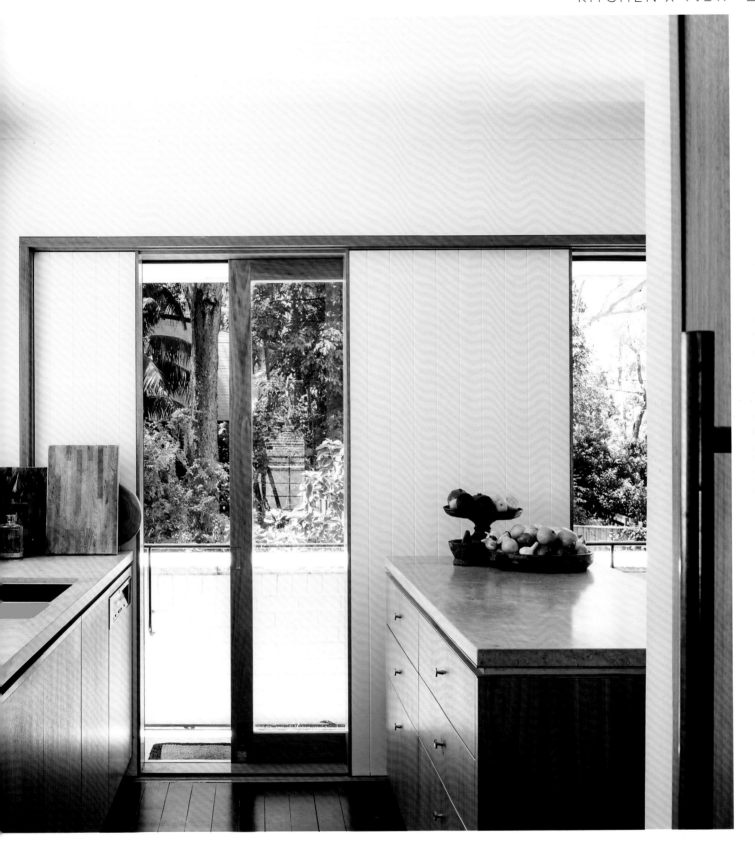

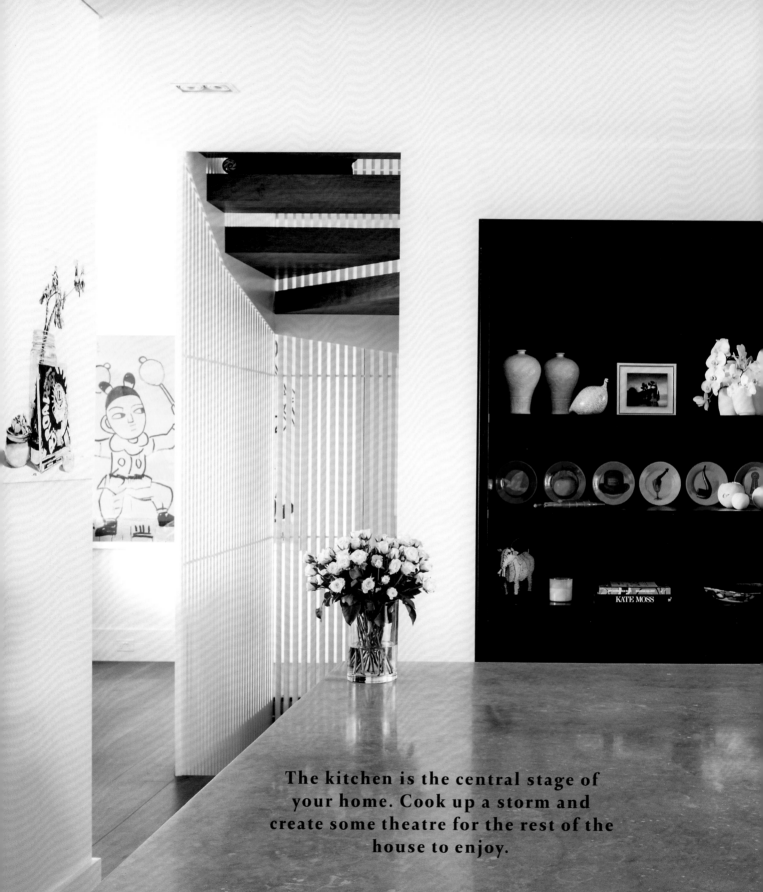

The kitchen is the central stage of
your home. Cook up a storm and
create some theatre for the rest of the
house to enjoy.

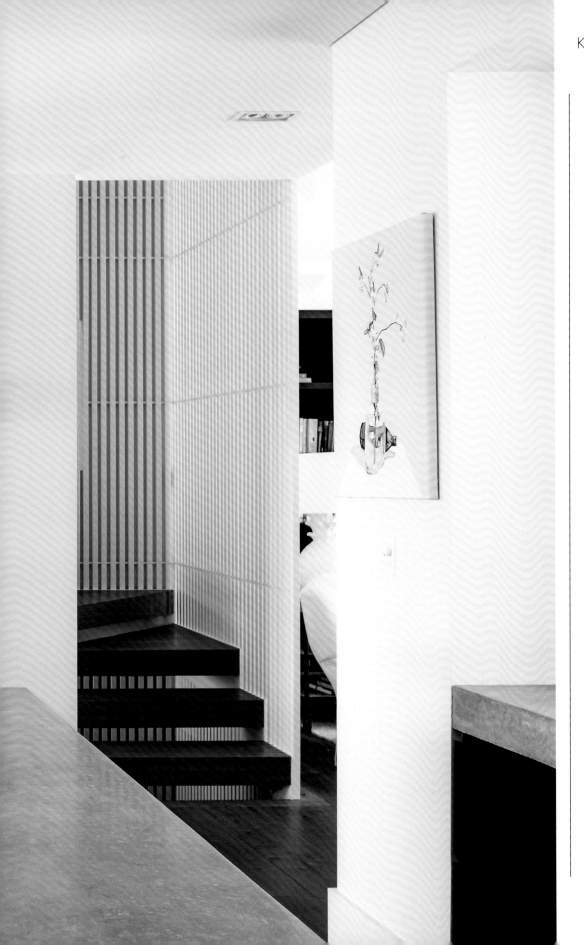

◀ These artworks have been perfectly framed by the dark shelving to provide an unusual internal view for anyone who is cooking.

5 X 5
KITCHEN X VIEW

▶ This long view connects a secondary living area to the kitchen. If the connection is not wanted, then a simple separating door can be closed.

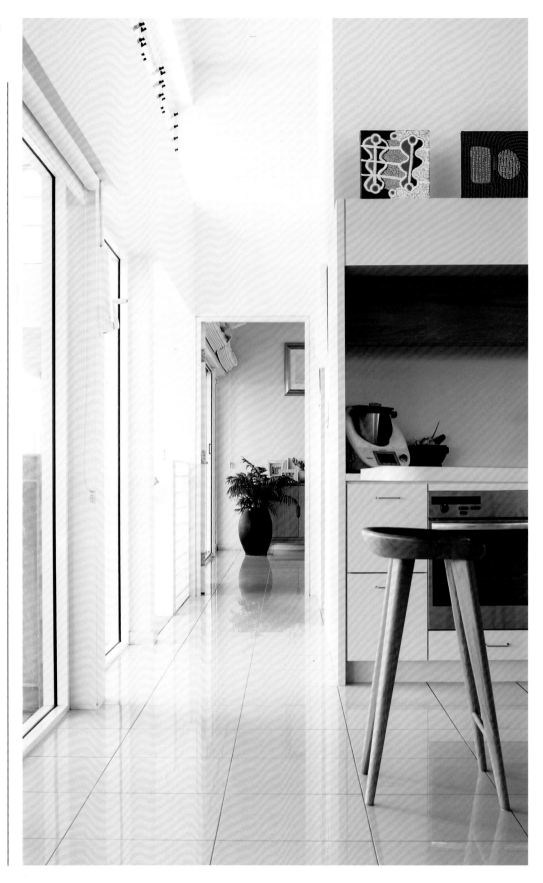

FIRE AS VIEW

Gone are the days when we used fire for cooking, but a hearth still feels good in a kitchen. Build a fireplace into a wall and line it with bricks as a focal point for the kitchen. Or design the kitchen to be separated from the dining area with a two-way fireplace; this is a dynamic divider of two spaces and adds a familiar sense of warmth to both areas. It's all about tapping into our deep evolutionary memories of fire being linked to the kitchen and food.

MAKE THE KITCHEN THE VIEW

Design your kitchen around the idea that it is something to view and enjoy from the rest of the house. The possibilities are endless if you have a clear goal of what you would like to see when looking at the kitchen from the living area. Remember that in a lot of ways the kitchen is the stage of your house; every night a performance is given and the audience is the living room and the areas around. For example, you could introduce a set of copper pots to add warmth and a sense of authenticity (it wouldn't be the first time a kitchen has been designed around a set of pots). Then bring the same metallic patina to your utensils and add hammered copper bowls. Consider a copper pendant light over the kitchen bench or a copper range hood. Or, instead of copper, consider antique brass, or recycled timber as the feature of your kitchen.

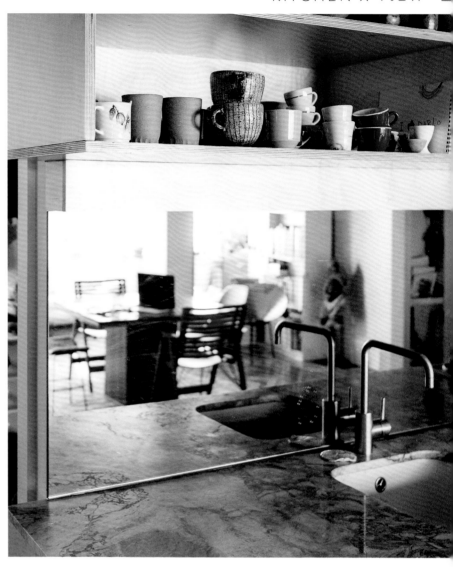

UNEXPECTED ART

Art is often not expected in the kitchen and so what better excuse to introduce some as a backdrop to the theatre of preparing food? There is a lot of creativity in a kitchen and art goes extremely well with that. Don't be afraid to put some framed family portraits in the kitchen, as well – sometimes it is nice to remind yourself who you are cooking for. Of course, you don't want to put your art or photos in the firing line of cooking grease, so find a wall that is away from the heat and splashes of the stove. As a precaution, put the artistry behind glass to allow for a simple wipe down. An expensive oil painting is probably not the one for the kitchen, but this should not stop you from adorning your kitchen with some character and colour.

MIRROR SPLASHBACK

Mirrors are sometimes used in restaurants to reflect the activity of the kitchen back to the diners; this can work well for the home kitchen as well. A mirror splashback that reflects what's simmering on the stove top into the living room can be a lot of fun, but do make sure that toughened glass is used if it is close to a heat source. In the same way, you can bring an outside view into the kitchen; perhaps the reflection of garden foliage from a particular angle? A kitchen often has many short and unexpected walls and cavities. Rather than leaving these bland and empty, consider using mirror to make corners disappear and bring connection to other spaces, such as a reflection of the living room.

▲ The mirror connects you to the living room even when your back is to the room. And the reflection adds to the theatre of creating a meal.

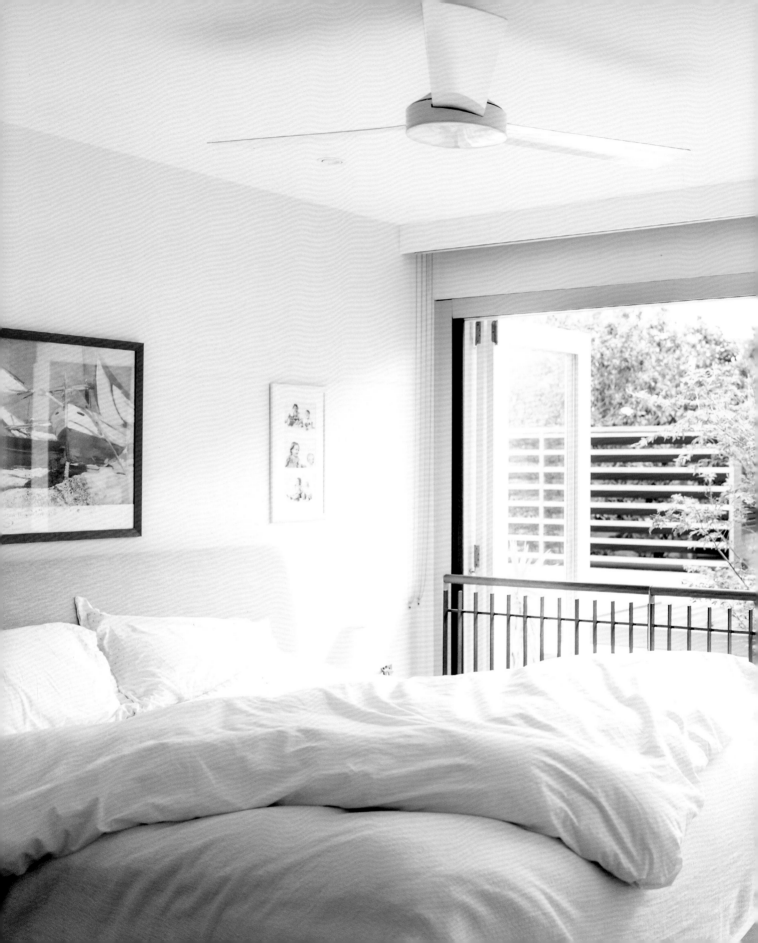

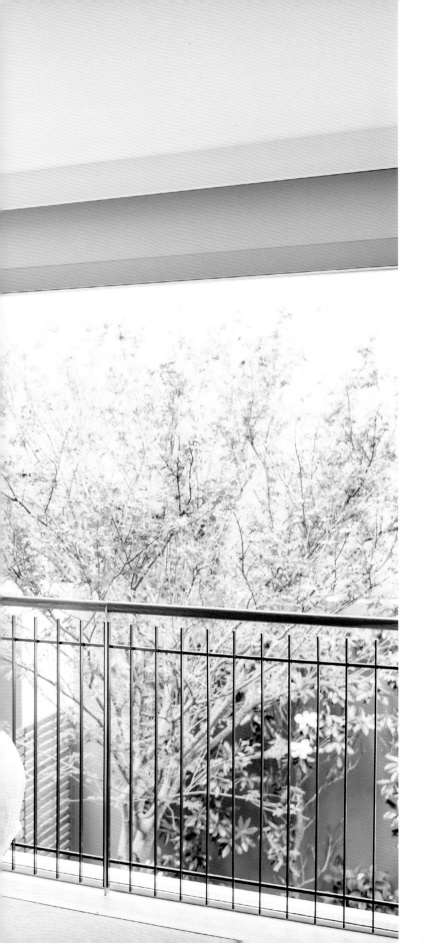

CHAPTER FOUR

BED ROOM

SPACE

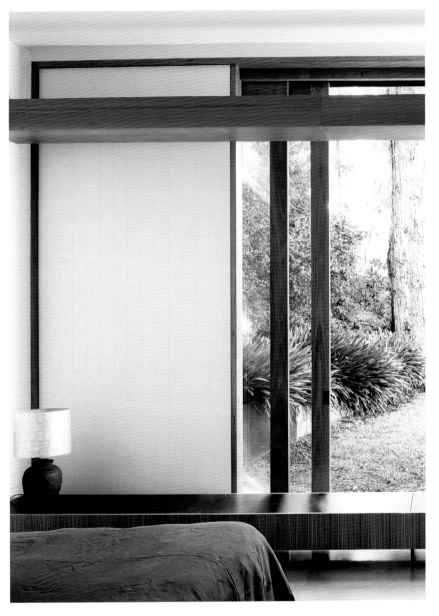

▲ This bedroom has a wonderful connection to the outdoor environment. There is nothing like sunlight to get our bodies going in the morning, so the more access you have to natural light when it's time to get up, the better.

First things first, where should the bedrooms be located in your home? Bedrooms have traditionally been seen as a 'destination', an end point on your journey through the home. The reality for most of us is that we usually only go to bedrooms to sleep or change clothes. The rest of the time they are pretty dormant spaces in a home. With this in mind, you would never give the sunniest spot in the building to the bedroom – that would have to go to the living room. And the same would be said for the view; best to share that with the whole household and not just one bedroom. However, most humans spend about a third of their life lying down, and that's not even the lazy ones! We all need to sleep around 8 hours a night, so it makes sense to be careful with the space we spend so much time in. It has to be a healthy space.

MASTER BEDROOM

Once you have sorted out the best spots for the living spaces, the next space on the hierarchy in many homes is the master bedroom. By its very nature, the master bedroom serves the owners of the property and they get dibs on the best location in the house for sleeping. However, there is much else to take into consideration when locating bedrooms, not least their relationship to each other and also to the main living areas. Generally speaking, in single- and two-storey houses, I design the master bedroom to be as far away as possible from the living space of the house, with any kids' bedrooms in between, in a way bookending the house. This is a natural solution, where the adults are at the 'outside edges' of the house, in a sense the least protected, with the children in the middle of the 'nest'. This generally works for young families where the parents don't want the kids' rooms to be too far from the living room or the master bedroom. Also, if older children are making noise in the living room it allows the parents to escape to the other end of the house. As children grow up, you may want to change this configuration to give a

THERE ARE TWO TYPES OF BEDROOM – the adult bedroom (and I'm including guest bedrooms in that) and the child's bedroom. Adult bedrooms don't generally change, so you can feel free to invest in something that will last a long time. Children's bedrooms, however, should be viewed as flexible – children change faster than you can imagine and it is generally unwise to spend the big bucks on their rooms. And these rooms will often end up as guest bedrooms when you become an empty nester.

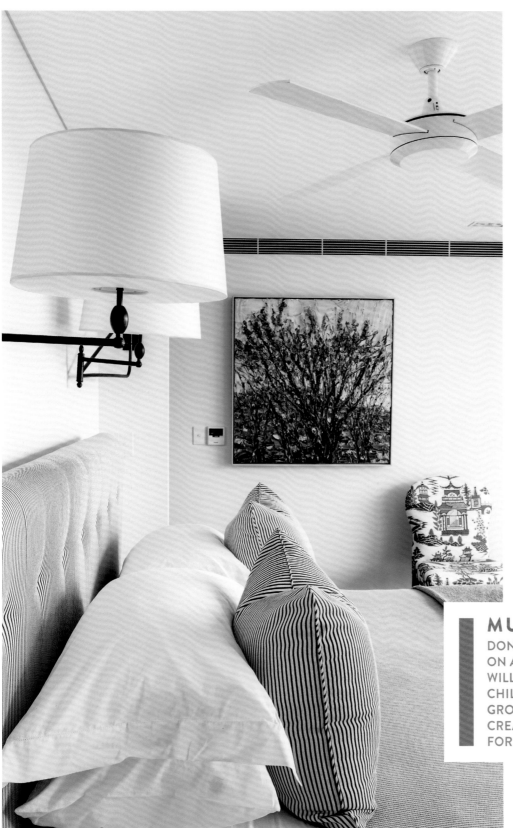

◀ The artwork you have on the bedroom wall is most likely the first and last thing you will see every day — so choose wisely.

MUST DON'T

DON'T SPEND A BIG BUDGET ON A KID'S BEDROOM AS IT WILL SOON CHANGE AS THE CHILD'S NEEDS AND TASTES GROW. INSTEAD FOCUS ON CREATING THE FLEXIBILITY FOR FUTURE CHANGE.

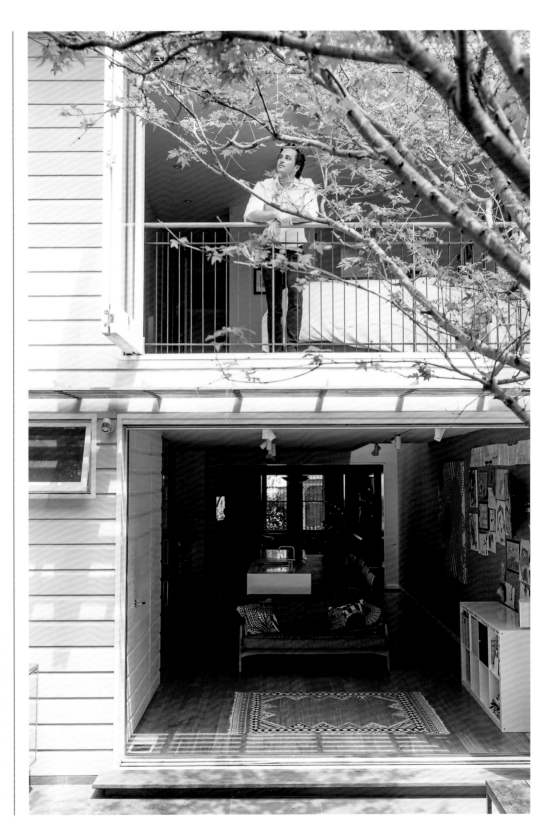

▶ The balcony balustrade here is on the inside of the bifold doors, bringing the outside world right to the bed. In some ways, decks can inhibit the view — you will often find yourself looking at the deck furniture, rather than the view beyond. Decks also require council approval because of privacy and shadowing issues, so a juliet balcony can be a win-win all round.

teenager more space and independence and allow them to be further away from the main living space for some privacy.

NOISE AND SLEEP

Usually, for similar subliminal reasons, bedrooms are not often designed to be right next to the front door. If you have a two-storey house then there might be the opportunity to give the master bedroom a similar location and view to the living room, by putting one on top of the other. In a two-storey house it makes sense that you would then group bedrooms together upstairs and have the noisier spaces, such as the living room, downstairs. There are, of course, many reasons to break these rules of thumb to suit the way you want to live. However, it is worth remembering the most common home layouts as there are usually reasons why they are popular.

BEDROOMS AND BATHROOMS

When laying out your bedrooms also consider the servicing of these spaces. It makes sense that the family bathroom is within close range of the bedrooms; it is not fair that anyone should trek across the living room in their pyjamas to get to the nearest bathroom. If there is room for an ensuite, then this is a great amenity for a master bedroom. Good planning would try to couple the family bathroom and ensuite so that they share a wall and therefore efficient plumbing services. Placing a natural buffer of bathrooms between a master bedroom and kids' bedrooms can be a good idea for acoustic reasons, as often these two parties are keeping different hours. In a two-storey house I work hard to make sure that the bathrooms are located above other similar services, such as kitchens and laundries, so the plumbing can run directly down in a cost-effective and efficient manner. This can have an impact on your bedroom layout.

CHILDREN'S SPACE

Usually the master bedroom gets the best location in terms of aspect, but sometimes that doesn't make sense when we spend hardly any time awake in the bedroom. This is in contrast to children, who might spend long stretches of time in their bedrooms playing, reading, doing homework or studying. Just a thought... Maybe they should get the best bedroom spot in the house for a while? As children get older and start to want their own space, it can be a nice solution to add a sofa and coffee table in a teenager's bedroom to give it a grown-up feel. However, if this means they might never emerge from their bedroom again, you may want to reconsider.

IN THE BEDROOM

When considering what to include in the bedroom space in a home, there are questions to answer. Is it also to be a retreat during the day, or simply a place to crash at night? Before you go to bed at night do you spend time there as an extension of the living room, reading a book or watching TV? If either of the above is 'yes', then it is worth considering including more than just a

▼ This bedroom has been extended into the ensuite bathroom, making the whole master suite feel much bigger. Now two partners can chat while getting ready for bed, or when one is already in bed.

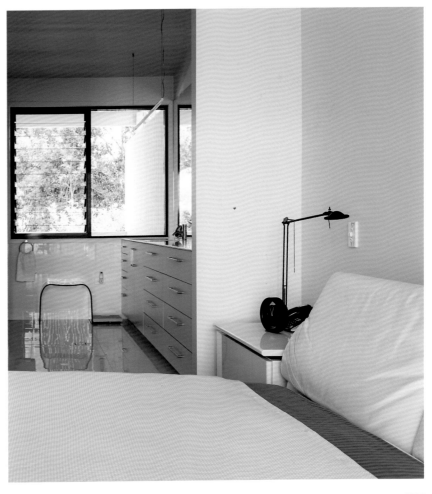

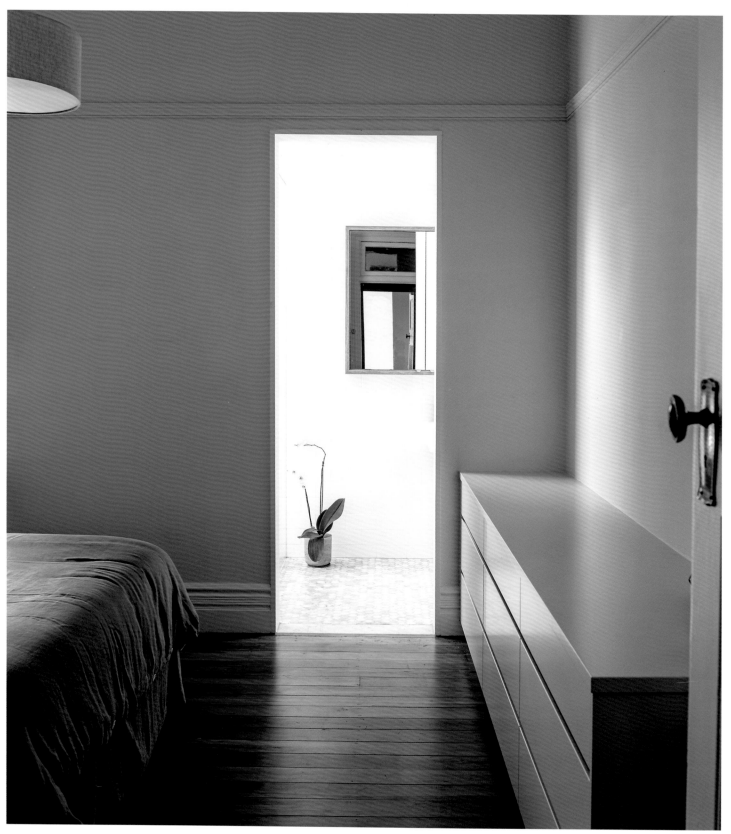

bed. Is there space to include a casual setting with a sofa and coffee table? This is quite a sophisticated thing to have in the master bedroom and gives you a way to escape from the rest of the house in the middle of the day, without having to lie on the bed. It means that you can sit up and enjoy a book or the telly in your own private space and have somewhere to put your cup of tea and your books. With couples, it is sometimes the case that one person goes to bed or gets up before the other; one might be in bed and the other on the sofa but you are both still able to share the space without disturbing the other. A master bedroom can be different to the rest of the house because it is truly only about you and not for the eyes of guests. See it as your sanctuary; a place where you can truly get away.

SHARE NICELY

A master bedroom is a shared space, and an intimate space, so make sure the planning of it allows for the movement and flow of two people and that it is not clunky and lacking in intimacy.

Ensure that in your design you have left enough room around the bed for two people to pass. If you have wardrobes in your bedroom ensure that you leave enough space for someone to pass while the other is selecting their clothes for the day. Little space considerations like this can make all the difference in a relationship as we rush around in our busy lives.

WHAT SIZE BED?

A bedroom is a relatively small room, so always imagine the space with humans in it – you will find it fills up pretty quickly. The bed is the biggest item in your room, so plan around it. In the early stages of designing, I will shape a room to take a king-size bed, minimum. Start with bigger objects to give you room to move if things get tight in your planning. It is generally a mistake to design a child's bedroom around a single bed, because one day that bedroom might need to become an adult bedroom. In terms of real estate, the real

◀ Extending the bedroom into the bathroom can make the room feel bigger, as long as you have plenty of privacy for the loo. The clever placement of the bathroom mirror here extends this bedroom further.

▼ Create room for a sitting area in your master bedroom so that it becomes a sanctuary, a comfortable escape from the rest of the house.

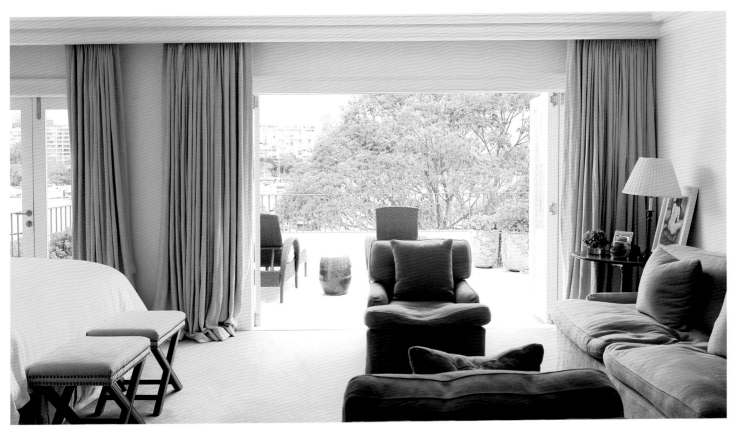

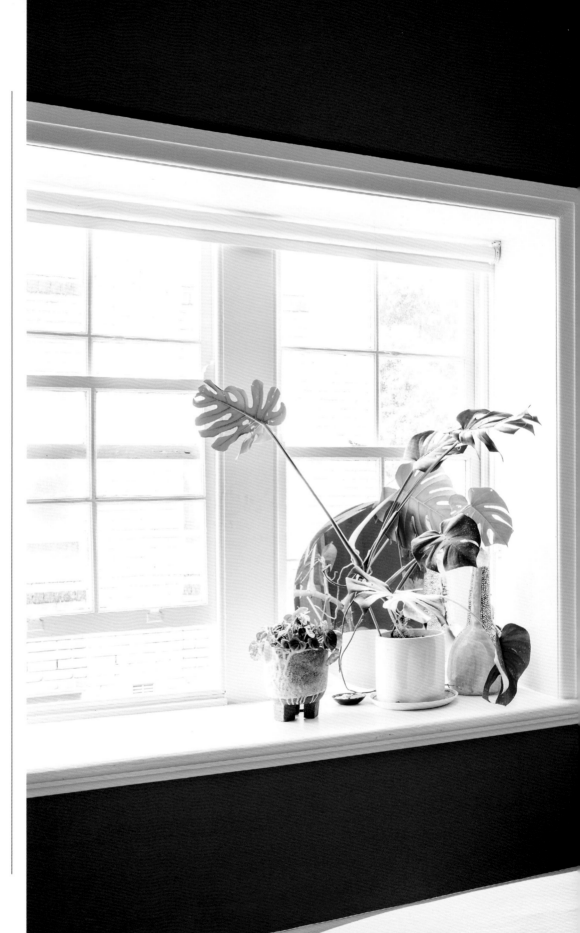

▶ This room has real character, with its dark painted walls and contrasting white window and architrave. The key to the space is the depth of the white window sill — deep enough to bounce around plenty of light, and also create a shelf that tells a story. Bedrooms can often end up with dead corners — make sure you create alternative moments in the space, to read a book or just put on your shoes.

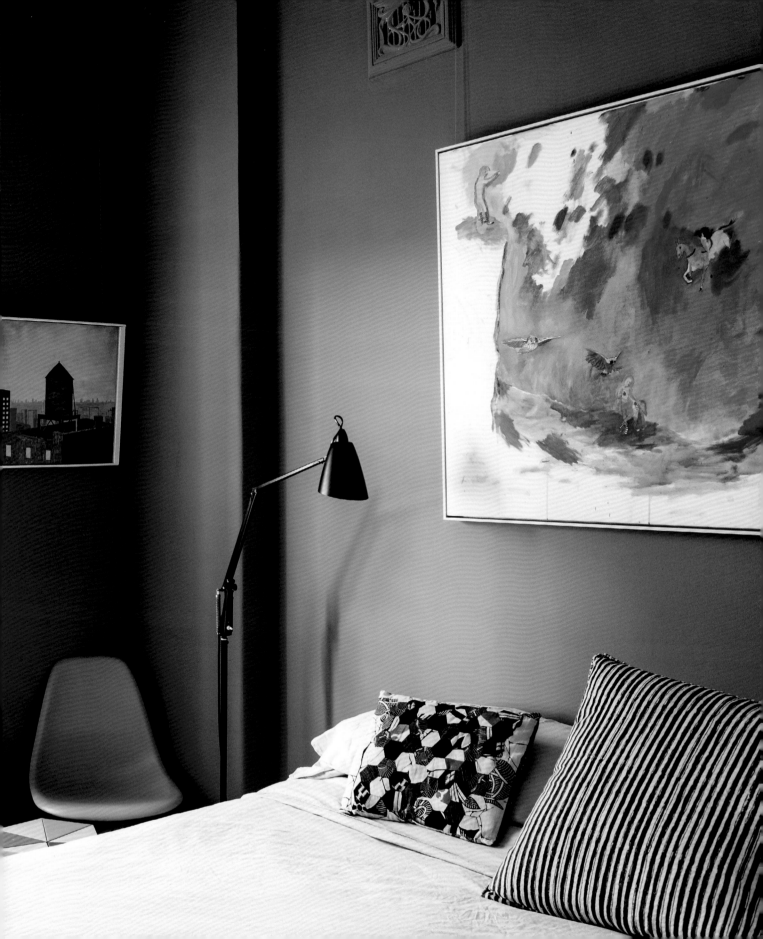

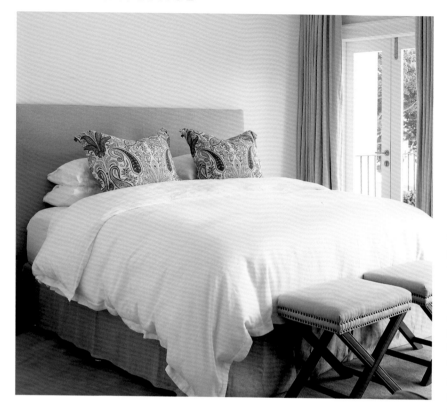

To create a sensuous room use soft furnishings and upholstery everywhere a human would touch. Moving around this room, it would be difficult to find a hard surface.

A bedside table only has to be big enough to hold the items you need.

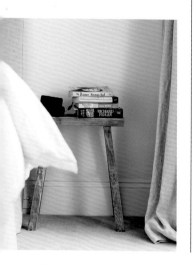

definition of a bedroom is that it comfortably takes at least a double bed. So, on those terms we will start by accommodating a king-size bed, knowing that if a smaller bed is chosen then the extra space around it is a bonus.

Making your bed and leaving it tidy should be your first job in the morning to get the day off to a good start, but you need space on either side of a bed to make that easy to do. You can get away with pushing a single bed up against a wall because you can reach across it, though I still find that uncomfortable. An absolute minimum of 60 cm (24 in) on each side of a queen/king is required for reasonable access, and 90 cm (35 in) at the base – this is about the width of a bedside table, which works out well. The orientation of the bed is also important if you want to wake up naturally with the sun – if the room has a window that will capture the morning sun, face the bed in that direction.

Don't feel you must share a bed with your partner; some loving couples I have designed for have two king singles in the master bedroom as they can't stand the disruption of sleeping in the same bed. In Scandinavian countries they get around this by sharing the same bed but each having their own single duvet – a clever idea, and one that I want to incorporate into our home as I always seem to lose the midnight duvet fight!

A regal four-poster can totally change the dynamic of a room, but only works if you have high ceilings. For an update, add ornate skirting boards, dado rails, picture rails and cornices, and then put in an ornate four-poster bed and you will create something special.

Extend your bed with a bench or blanket chest at the end to add style and functionality – especially when you're sitting down to put your shoes on! The bench should be slightly smaller than the bed to expose the bed corners.

SPACE-SAVING JOINERY

A bed is a big item if you have a small room, and one way to reduce its bulk is to partly nestle it into joinery. By designing your joinery to be part wardrobe and part bedhead you reduce the bulk of the bed, at the same time as providing good storage. You can store clothing behind doors around and above the bed and that joinery can also incorporate reading lighting, bedside tables and drawers.

If you are very tight on space you could consider a fold-down bed. The technology of these has vastly improved over the years and they can make a room so much more functional.

BEDSIDE TABLES

Wall mount your bedside tables – this will give you a greater sense of space around the head of your bed.

THE BEDHEAD

It is a very unusual feeling to not have a structure at the top of your bed. This has to do with a sense of security. Just like the theory of prospect and refuge, we feel more secure with protection behind us – in this case, a bedhead. That is why the tops of beds are usually placed against a wall and if they aren't then they need a substantial bedhead. It is not an accident that bedheads have become grand and stately elements in the bedroom. We are unknowingly constructing a shield to protect our head while we are in our most vulnerable state, asleep. Also, practically, if you don't have some kind of barrier at the top of your bed, you will keep losing your pillow over the edge, which is a touch annoying!

A bedhead and bedframe can instantly define the room in terms of style. Choose your favourite style of bed and then work from there to inform the decoration of the rest of the bedroom.

A bedhead can also be beyond a statement: it can be practical storage. I have often designed joinery that has drawers, cupboards and shelving on one side and on the other side it serves as a bedhead. This can be a great technique to achieve built-in bedside shelves as well, as you design them into the joinery on the bed side. You can add shelves for a bedside light or attach a small lamp for reading, and then also hide all the wiring in the joinery.

You can even create a library of bookshelves as a bedhead. If there is not the room for joinery, then a wall – even a low wall – can be a form of bedhead and give some privacy.

BEDROOM DECK

Decks off bedrooms are notoriously under-used, as there is often some effort involved in actually opening the door, brushing off the outdoor furniture and then enjoying the moment. If you're going to sit on the deck, you would often like to be accompanied by a cup of coffee or a glass of wine. Unfortunately, that means traipsing all the way down to the kitchen and back and then the moment is lost. If you have a deck off your master bedroom, try fitting a mini bar fridge, coffee machine or kettle nearby and I suspect you will suddenly find yourself using it much more. Make sure you don't overfill the deck; two chairs and a side table or two is all you need.

STREAMLINE

The idea of a few large items rather than a lot of small pieces applies to this room as much as it does to the living room. Try to declutter and

When you design your bedroom and position your bed, consider using screens to give you privacy without limiting your access to light and air.

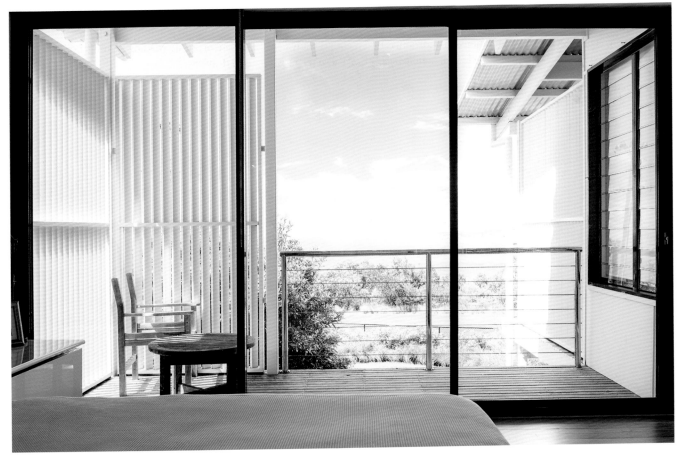

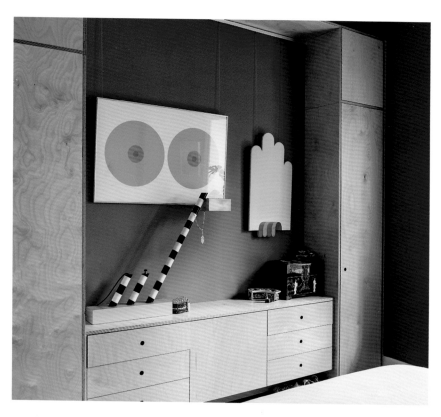

The master bedroom is your private space, where you can express yourself with objects and art that give you delight. I love how this joinery has been staged for the artwork — the storage aspect seems almost secondary.

For a classic style, think about symmetry and balance, as shown in this master suite. Though the style is classic, the family photos give a personal touch. The chair looks fabulous, but is also practical — exactly what is needed for putting on socks and shoes.

streamline. The bed is already a big item, and if you suddenly add another five objects floating in the space then the room begins to feel messy. Build joinery into walls and create alcoves and special spots for favourite pieces of furniture as much as possible.

Consider what furniture you want in a bedroom – a chair to aid you putting your shoes on, for example, a dresser, a dressing table with a mirror for makeup, a tallboy, or even heirlooms and somewhere to display them. Unless you have a separate dressing room, it's likely you'll need clothes storage. This might be a wardrobe or armoire and chests of drawers, but many bedrooms also incorporate built-in joinery. Houses with good built-in robes can be rented out for more money, if you think that might be a selling point for you.

THE WALK-IN ROBE

One of the most important considerations in space planning in the bedroom is how much clothing you have and where it will be kept. Another consideration is the storage of bedding

for the changing seasons. To reduce their volume and to protect them from the elements, bedding should be vacuum-packed away and stored in out-of-the-way spaces such as at the top of your wardrobes, under the bed or in the garage.

Clothes, like all fabrics, absorb dust and particles that are stirred up in the air around them, and can become a wonderful haven for dust mites. When clothes are disturbed, dust and particles can be shaken from them and contribute to allergies. A walk-in robe removes this issue from the bedroom and allows you to walk into a separate space and be surrounded by your clothes. Because the wardrobe is separated from the bedroom, you can have your clothes on show at all times. And, of course, by removing the clothes and shoes you have a much better chance of maintaining a simpler, less cluttered and more serene bedroom.

Apart from these practicalities a walk-in wardrobe is a grand experience. To have a space dedicated just to your wardrobe and the art of getting dressed each day is a great treat. If there is enough room, have a low table or flat day bed to lay out your clothes as you choose them.

There are two types of walk-in wardrobes: with and those without doors. I always like to introduce a separating door if there is room, and my favourite door type for walk-in wardrobes are sliding doors, particularly those that can be completely slid away so that the bedroom and wardrobe become one extended space when you want. Walk-in wardrobes without doors are usually extensions of one part of a bedroom. With these I usually introduce joinery doors to contain the clothes, protect them from dust and also to prevent the view of an often-cluttered space.

When planning a master bedroom, usually the wardrobe and ensuite are destinations from the bedroom. But that doesn't have to be the case; it is quite grand to create a journey from the door of a bedroom suite, to enter an open walkway space that takes you past a walk-in wardrobe and then past an ensuite and finally into a bedroom that captures the view. In a sense this reflects the journey of going to bed: removing your clothes, washing and then hopping into bed, and the reverse order in the morning. It is your private domain, so have some fun with it.

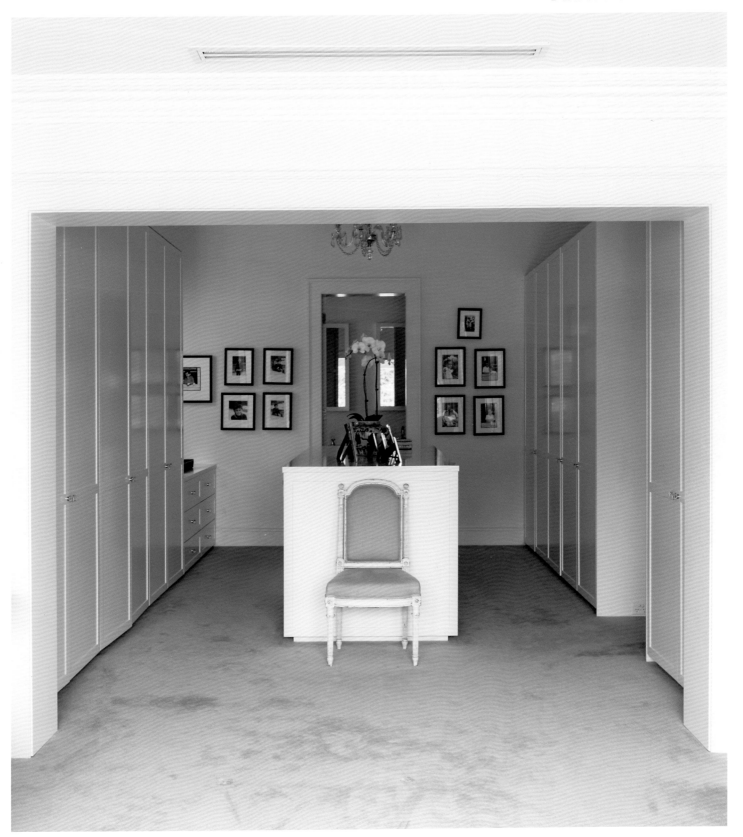

5 X 5
BEDROOM

▷ Instead of seeing joinery as a cupboard, view it as a wall. Once you do that, as well as maximising the storage capacity from floor to ceiling, you can explore different materials to use on the facade, such as this rich timber.

▼ These floor-to-ceiling wardrobes have shadow lines top and bottom and concealed finger pulls, all of which create a streamlined effect. Finished in white, they recede to become a wall of the room rather than obvious storage.

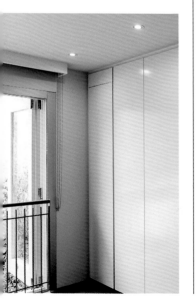

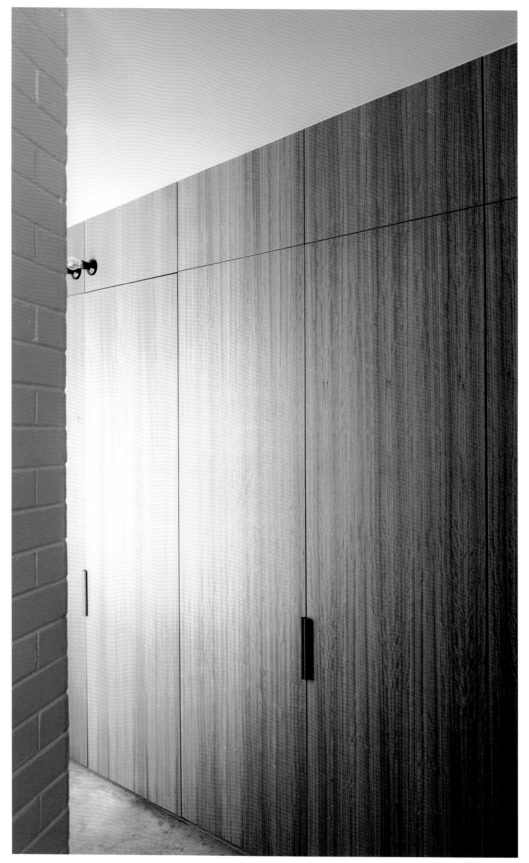

THE BUILT-IN WARDROBE

If you are going to store clothes and shoes in your bedroom, then you should definitely have a wardrobe with doors to remove the visual clutter of seeing them on display. A quick fix to update a bedroom is to get rid of old stand-alone cupboards and build fitted wardrobes instead. As well as being valuable in real estate terms, these maximise the space available for storage by utilising the whole area from floor to ceiling. The general depth of a wardrobe is 60 cm (24 in), which is based on comfortably hanging a coat hanger with a decent-sized jacket on it perpendicular to the door of the wardrobe; 60 cm is also a decent drawer and shelf depth. Wardrobes can start to take up a huge amount of square metres in a house and they need to be planned efficiently.

Some space planning tips are to design your wardrobe along one wall but then step it back enough to allow the entry door into the room. This is an efficient way of combining these two space requirements and putting less pressure on the overall width of the room – otherwise you end up having to take width from the room from the wardrobe and then a door.

Another space-saving tip, when designing two bedrooms, is to place them next door to each other and then split a wall of built-ins on their dividing wall. So, in one bedroom one half of the wall is wardrobe and the other half is wall, and then the opposite happens in the other room.

CREATING SPACE

If you have a bedroom so small that it won't fit a wardrobe because there is simply no room beyond the bed, look carefully at your floor plan and see if you can steal the 70 cm/27 in (60 cm/23 in wardrobe and 10 cm/4 in stud wall) from an adjacent room. I have managed to give a bedroom a wardrobe by putting the bulk of the wardrobe into an oversized laundry area, or into an oversized hallway, or even built a pop-out of the exterior wall to create the storage space. Achieving that wardrobe in a small bedroom turns it from a non-functional bedroom into a very functional and highly saleable one.

Think carefully how you want to treat the wardrobe, as it can be a large surface in the

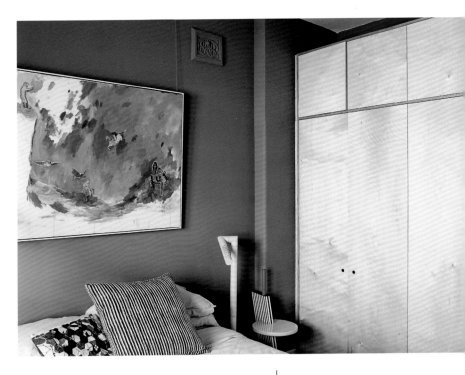

bedroom. If you give it a contrasting look to the rest of the room, it can become overbearing, especially in a small room. I would only use dark timber if you have the luxury of a very large room. I usually match the paint colour of polyurethane joinery to the paint colour of the walls to make it seamless and reduce the effect of its size on the room. Another option is to use mirror on the wardrobe doors – this makes the room feel bigger as well as providing a great dressing mirror right where you need it.

KEEPING THE CLUTTER OUT

Do a yearly review of your wardrobe – donate your clothes and clear the space. Have a donation bag in your wardrobe within easy reach, so that when clothes are no longer loved they go straight into the bag and not back on the rack. When the bag is full, donate.

Organise your life so that the out-of-season clothes leave your bedroom and go into other storage, such as an attic, or are packed and put away up high – you will be surprised how much this de-clutters your space.

Put hooks where you notice people drop things. Introduce a clothes horse or ladder for throwing clothes over at night – save that heap from

▲ This light timber veneer wardrobe joinery brightens the room and adds character.

building up on the bedroom chair. And bedside storage needs a drawer for bedtime necessities that you don't need to have on display.

If you think you haven't got enough clothes storage then make sure your wardrobes are using the full height of your room. There is some great technology out there from wardrobe hardware manafacturers, such as shirt hangers that sit high in your wardrobe out of reach, with a lever to pull and bring your shirts down to you – genius!

SMART HOME
BEDS WILL MEASURE OUR BREATHING, HEART AND MOVEMENT TO TRACK OUR SLEEP HEALTH. FANS AND AIR PURIFIERS WILL COME ON AUTOMATICALLY AND A PATH WILL BE LIT TO THE BATHROOM IN THE DARK.

▼ An ottoman at the end of the bed is a useful seat for having a chat or laying out clothes — even better if it can store pillows and blankets.

WINDOW SEAT
I always try to create an option for the bedroom to be a place to read a book during the day, but without having to get into bed. A window seat can work beautifully in this way. You can escape to your bedroom and curl up in total privacy from the rest of the house and enjoy a spot with a unique view to the outside world.

A window seat also creates a friendly warm view in a bedroom without cluttering the space, as it is built into the wall.

STUDY IN THE BEDROOM?
A bedroom can be an excellent space for a study if you are not able to provide another option, as it is under-utilised during the day and can be closed off for quiet concentration. The key is to build a nook for your study so that it is contained within a wall, rather than being a desk in the bedroom, which will start to feel awfully like a hotel room. Even better, create some shutters, doors or a pull-down screen to conceal your workplace when you are not using it, so that work isn't on your mind when you are trying to relax in your bedroom.

VANITY AND BATH
In master bedrooms in new houses, I am increasingly incorporating the bathroom and the wardrobe into the overall bedroom space. This gives a great feeling to the master bedroom suite without actually increasing its footprint, as you are stealing from the ensuite and walk-in robe and giving it to the bedroom. It makes the major space of your bedroom feel far more generous. If you and your partner have fairly similar schedules and tend to get up and go to bed at the same times, then consider bringing the bathroom

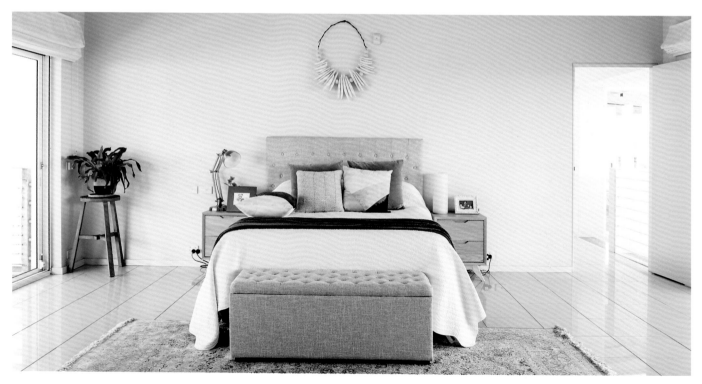

vanity and even the bath into the bedroom space. In this instance only the shower and loo are separated from the bedroom. This gives a strong feeling of a luxury hotel room layout and it's nice for a couple to be able to carry on a conversation as they get ready for bed.

BEDROOM FLOOR

There is a lovely sense of comfort and luxury in being able to pad silently around on plush bedroom carpet in bare feet. (Once again, though, if you have allergies, make sure you vacuum carpet regularly and especially under the bed – make sure your bed is easily moveable.)

It is tempting to choose a light carpet colour to make the room feel as large as possible. However, a dark carpet can be more sophisticated and 'earth' the room. Timbers and greys look especially good against a dark floor, so your floor colour can in turn lead to your styling and decoration choices.

For a relatively quick facelift to a bedroom get rid of old carpet and expose the floorboards below. Polish and seal them, whitewash them for a coastal look, or dark stain them for a sophisticated contemporary look. If you don't have floorboards underneath, you could lay timber boards. These are very accessible today, but avoid cheap-looking stick-on boards or laminate; instead consider engineered floorboards that have a relatively thick veneer. There is a great array of finishes and the bedroom is a low-traffic area, so you are unlikely to wear out the veneer, at least not for a very long time. I sometimes add a rug in winter and stow it away in summer to create seasonal change in a small space.

Tiles are generally felt to be quite a cold option in a bedroom, although there are now some very warm-looking tiles that can fight that effect; for example, timber-look tiles. If you provide a thick pile rug or sheepskin where your feet land when you hop out of bed, it can change the overall impression. Similarly, tiles take on a whole new character if you fit under-floor heating. It is only because we associate tiles with a cold touch that we think of them as stylistically cold.

One design feature I like to use in bedrooms is to carpet the floor but then have an area of timber floorboards in front of the window. This gives the feeling of a transition to an outside deck area, even when there is no deck. If there is enough space in the room, I make the timber floorboard area deep enough to fit two armchairs and a table. Suddenly you have created a lovely 'sunroom' in your bedroom just by a change of floor surface. It also creates a nice view from the bed.

NURSERY

One thing to consider also, which I know only too well, is that your master bedroom often becomes a nursery for the first months of the life of your child, so make sure you have room for a cot in the space if that is on the horizon. And then consider the relationship between bedrooms – I have not met too many parents who don't want their small children to be in a bedroom close by in their early years.

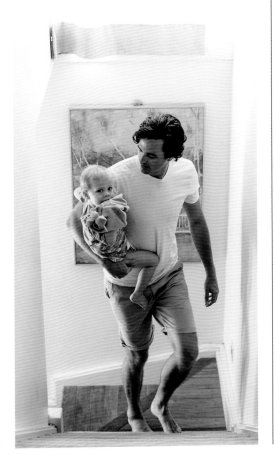

◀ Make sure your master bedroom has room for a cot; if you hope to have children then the reality is you will most likely be sharing with the little person for a few months.

Involve your child in designing and decorating their room. It teaches that they are able to control the look and feel of their environment.

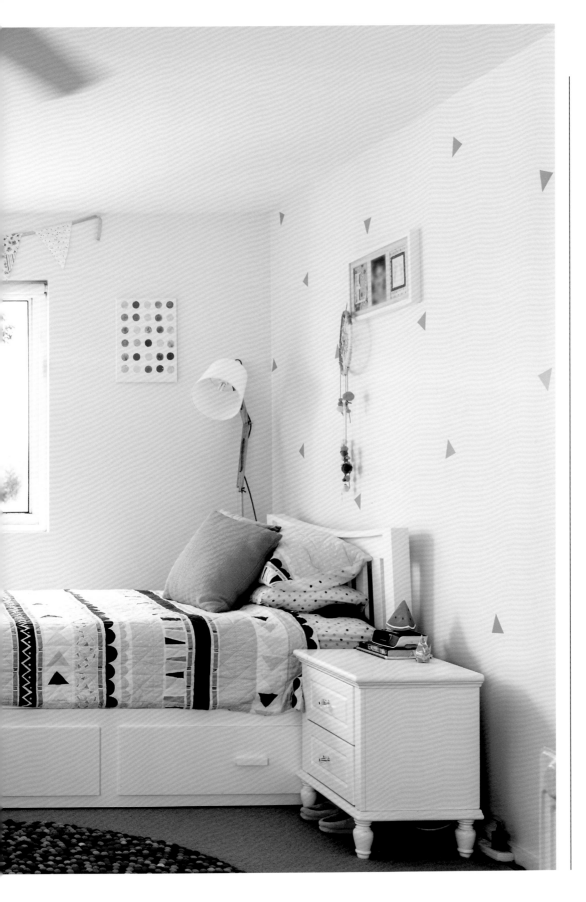

◀ This child's room is a simple space that is easy to decorate and, even more importantly, easy to change as the child grows up.

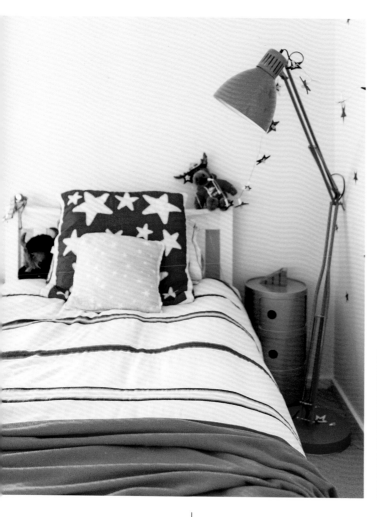

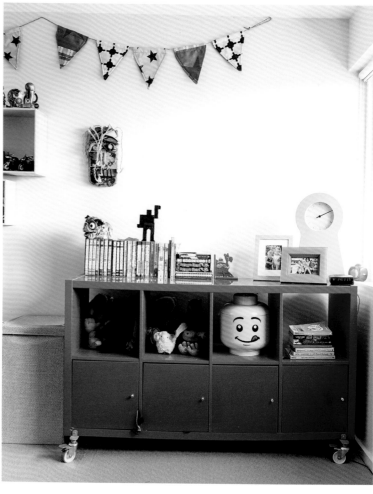

▲ Let the kids have some fun with their bedrooms — they need the room to change and grow as they themselves change and grow. I love this oversized reading lamp.

▶ Furniture on wheels is always a good idea for a child's room as it creates flexibility. This storage can be easily moved to make way for a train set or a sleepover.

KIDS' BEDROOMS

One of the biggest mistakes is to plan a bedroom for the age a child is now, and not factor in that they will change remarkably over the next few years. Make sure in your spatial planning that you allow for flexibility and the ability for the inhabitant to change and grow.

Involve your kids in designing their bedrooms. It's fun and educational and gives them a sense of control over their environment. Create a mood board – you might be surprised by their natural intuition, without all the preconceptions adults often have. They will respect the space more if they create it. Allow scope for it to change as they change.

Bedrooms for small children need to be as big as possible because play is usually carried out on the floor. When they are young, consider giving them the largest room of the house – they will use it more, and otherwise you will find the train set under your feet in the living room. Of course, as soon as they grow and your family changes, a redistribution of rooms can occur. That is a good excuse for a refit and to create some change.

Bunks are an obvious, and often fun, space saver in children's rooms, but make sure they are safe and conform to safety standards with guardrails and secure ladders. Children under six shouldn't be on the top bunk. Bunk beds are excellent for siblings sharing a room, and free up floor space for Lego and other activities. Beds with desks underneath are great when children are older: they are space saving and cater for the growing demands of homework. Or you could introduce a trolley bed, which slides under the main bed and is perfect for sleepovers.

Finally, the bedroom often ends up becoming a study once your child is in the later years of high school. They need a place of concentration, as well as a place to relax when it is time to go to sleep. If they are studying, give them a good chair – often you find they're using the one from when they were 10. Then, many students stay at home and the room might become a student bedsit and perhaps even include a partner.

Remember that the bedroom of the child/teenager becomes their home within a home and contains all the possessions that they deem to be theirs – forming an identity separate from everyone else in the household. So make sure you give them the space to express themselves with storage and ways to display their stuff. Introduce low-level pegs and rails for accessible storage and spaces the kids can easily access and control. Be careful with tall items that can fall over – they need to be fixed to the wall – there are some horror stories out there and you don't want to be one of them. Make display areas for showing off their favourite things – Lego models are the prize possessions in our house at the moment.

Remember to let them go crazy with their own decoration – it's just paint and soft furnishings, and they get to understand they can control their environment. Make it safe, though: no candles!

As you can see, the child's bedroom becomes a chameleon of a space – it needs to evolve and grow and change as its occupant does. Apart from built-in wardrobes for storage, I tend to advise that the non-adult bedrooms of a house are seen more as malleable spaces.

GUESTS TO STAY?

Unless you have people to stay for more than 75 per cent of the year, a guest bedroom is an under-utilised space in your house. It is much better to design the room with another function and allow it to be easily converted to a guest bedroom when needed. It could be a study, games room, or movie/sewing/yoga room... whatever, it doesn't matter. What matters is that the room doesn't lie dormant for most of the year. A good-quality sofa bed is a great way to instantly transform a room. And I say good quality, because if you wouldn't sleep in it then please don't offer it to your guests! Another space-saving

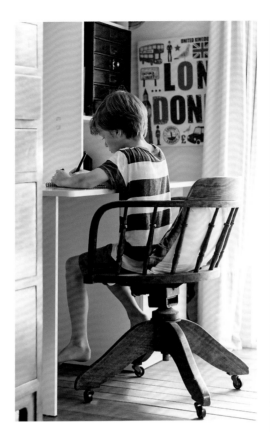

A desk in a child's bedroom can be an important space to allow them to develop as an individual. Don't forget to upgrade the chair as they grow.

option is a fold-down bed.

The key requirement for a guest room is comfort: make your guest feel at home. Provide clean sheets, a clean towel, soap and other items and be prepared with these things on hand so that the guest feels you have taken their arrival in your stride, and that they are not a burden. If there are house rules then don't be afraid to let them be known: this is far less awkward than dealing with annoyance later. It is a sign of respect to share these rules of your home.

And fight blandness; use colour or art to tell a story in your guest bedroom.

AND, OUT OF THE BOX...

Your bedroom doesn't have to be a box. Be brave and put your bed on a mezzanine that overlooks the living room. Use screens for privacy, not necessarily acoustic. Depending on where you are up to in life – hopefully there won't be a party happening in your house when you are in bed. Note to self: I have three sons – what on earth am I thinking?

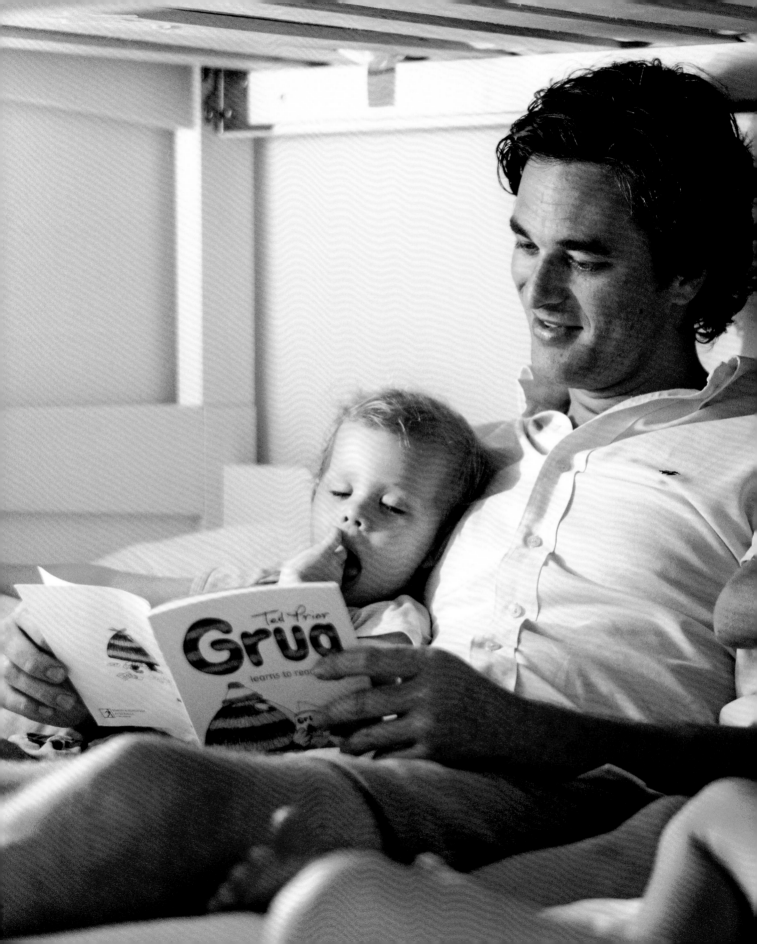

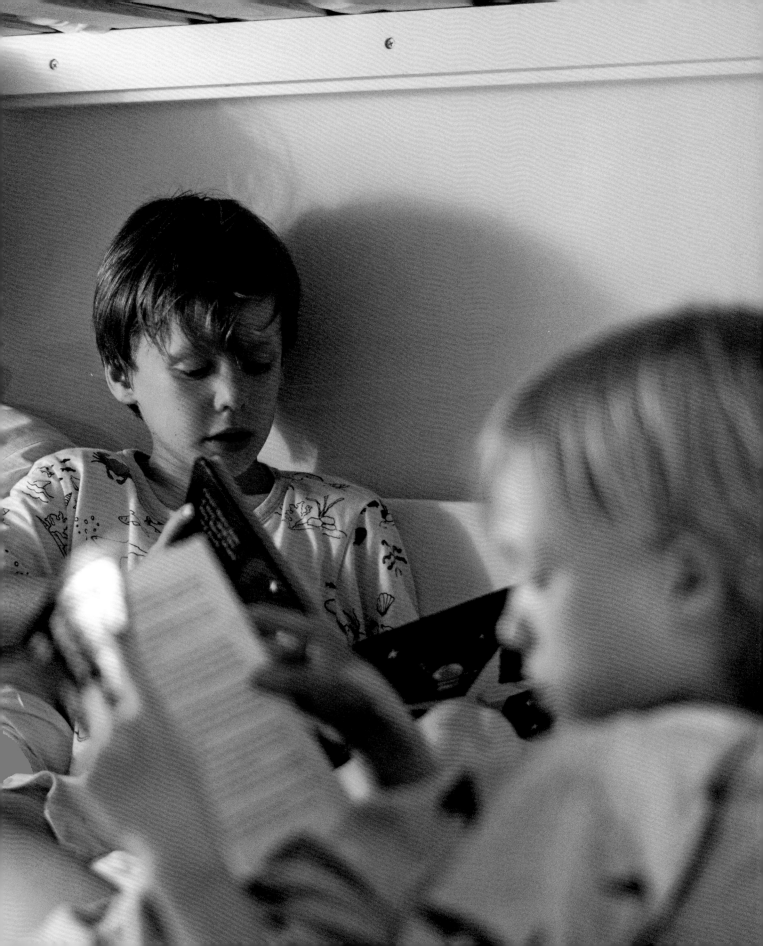

▶ Have some fun with your bedside lamps. And don't feel they have to match if that isn't your style. Already we can see that two different characters share this space!

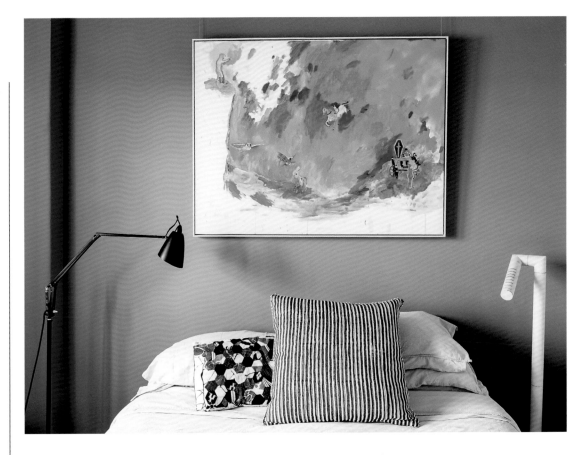

LIGHT

Bedrooms are often the forgotten part of our homes in terms of lighting. They too often have a dismal central light or, even worse, a grid of six downlights. A third of our life is spent in these rooms, sleeping. Once you are up you should be able to draw the curtains and let light pour into the room, so a bedroom that faces the rising sun is the ideal. With the light pouring in you will hopefully feel invigorated, your circadian rhythms are set for the day, plus some direct sunlight will prevent mould and damp in your sleeping environment.

On the other hand, when you're sleeping, your room needs to be dark with good-quality curtains or blinds, as in hotel rooms. A darkened room is a blank canvas in which to introduce new lighting and sleeping smart technology. This is especially important if you need to sleep in the day because of work shifts, or in the bedrooms of young children who still need daytime sleeps.

TASK LIGHTING

Do you read in bed? If so, make sure you have some over-the-shoulder light to illuminate the page while you are sitting up in bed. These days, reading in bed is often the only time many of us have to get into a book, so a good bedside reading lamp is imperative. I suggest a light that is close to you, has a small beam of light and is hooded so that the reader isn't disturbing a partner who is trying to go to sleep.

If you have a sofa or chairs in the bedroom, then make sure you have a floor lamp or dedicated downlight to illuminate that area specifically.

WARDROBE LIGHTING

If your wardrobe is in your bedroom, make sure you have lights centred in front of the wardrobe doors so that when they are open they light up to reveal the clothes inside. Lights within the actual closet behind the doors are also a great idea and can look fantastic; switching on when you open the door, they are a practical and efficient way of lighting up your clothes so you can make a good choice for the day. In a walk-in wardrobe with no doors, ensure that there is good lighting that focuses on the clothes. If you have a layout bench then make sure you have some excellent spotlights onto that. And be sure to light the area in front of a full-length mirror. I recommend also involving natural light in the area where you dress. (We have all noticed someone who has clearly got dressed in the semi-dark...)

AMBIENT LIGHT

With good task lighting in place for reading and dressing, the only reason you really need strong ambient light in a bedroom is to clean. Otherwise, bedrooms are places where most of us would appreciate soft and low ambient light. Of course, this ambient light should be cosy, never glaring: a warm white–yellow light is best. Introduce wall lights that cast a light upwards on the wall and ceiling and then bounce a diffuse light back down.

A tray or coved ceiling can be a lovely addition to a bedroom and give you a great opportunity to create concealed lighting that illuminates the positive and negative spaces formed. Or you could consider a ceiling rose and drop a pendant light into the room. You can do this in a heritage style or an uber modern way depending on your

taste. If you add a plaster moulded pattern into the ceiling it can also pick up the light in dramatic ways and adds interest as you rest your head against the pillow.

SPOT LIGHTING

With the ambient light hopefully down low, there is a great opportunity to bring some art and drama into your bedroom with a carefully placed spotlight on an evocative painting or sculpture. Choose carefully, as it will be one of the first and last things you see every day.

ROMANCE

Now let's be honest, we could all do with a bit of romance in our bedrooms, and dimmable, soft, warm lighting is key in that area. I don't condone candles in bedrooms – there are too many horror stories of people falling asleep and curtains catching fire. There are alternatives to candles on the market today but do research them well, as I have found there is a fine line between these being lovely or looking cheap and in poor taste. Another idea to consider is fairy lights.

NOTE TO SELF

SPEND TIME DESIGNING HOW TO CONTROL LIGHT IN YOUR BEDROOM. A BEDROOM NEEDS TO MAXIMISE LIGHT FOR PRACTICALITIES, BUT THEN ALSO MINIMISE IT FOR RELAXATION. EXCELLENT CONTROL IS THE KEY.

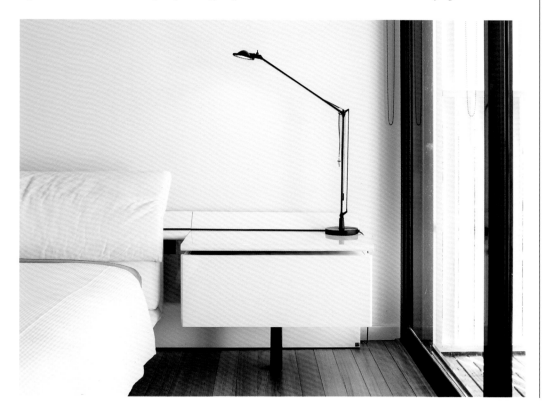

◁ Bedside lamps can be a wonderful accessory to a bedroom and come in styles and design to suit any room. The fact that they help you read in bed is a bonus.

These small points of light wrapped around a mantelpiece or window frame can bring a sense of occasion and wonder to a room.

I can't help but feel that burning any kind of fuel in a bedroom is a risk, so I am wary of a fireplace, even though it would be rather lovely. I rate the quality of air in the room where I sleep more highly than the romance of flickering flames; but if you do have a fireplace, check it is well fitted and is not smoking. Lighting can help the mood, especially when it's paired with sensuous materials; for example, a silky soft wall covering.

DECORATING FOR LIGHT AND SPACE

Avoid dark paint on bedroom walls unless you have a very large palatial bedroom – dark paint can make a room feel small and claustrophobic. You can make darkness with block-out blinds and low lighting – you don't need to paint dark colours onto the walls. I prefer a white ceiling so that I can reflect diffuse ambient light down into the space (no downlights), and then either back up the white ceiling with white walls or add a richer shade of white with more cream for warmth. White will make the room feel larger, and this also gives you an opportunity to create a white-on-white room with your bed linen, or contrast the white room with rich and warm textures in the bed linen and window furnishings.

Bedrooms are often small so don't over-pattern: you can use texture instead of too many overt patterns. Bring in a splash of colour to add a sense of vibrancy: a bedroom that is too blended is too bland. And remember that a shared bedroom should be a neutral space in terms of appeasing both users; no one should feel left out.

Although, as bedrooms are isolated rooms and don't affect other spaces, and are generally not large, it is relatively easy to change your bedroom decor down the track if you start to tire of it.

▼ A simple skylight can make an enormous difference to the quality and usefulness of a bedroom. This one turned a sombre, gloomy room into a lively space that notices the passing day.

▶ A stained glass window and shutters are the perfect combination to control light into a bedroom, as well as to create delight.

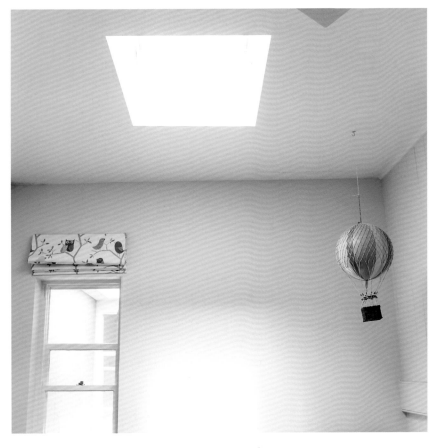

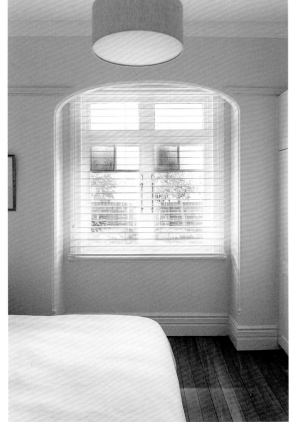

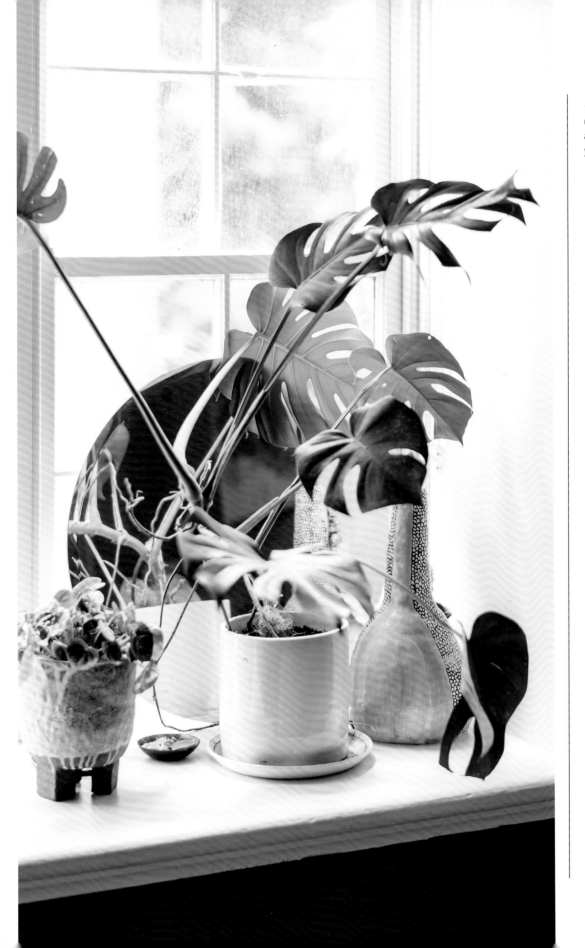

◀ Healthy plants produce oxygen — they are a perfect addition to the bedroom where you spend so many hours.

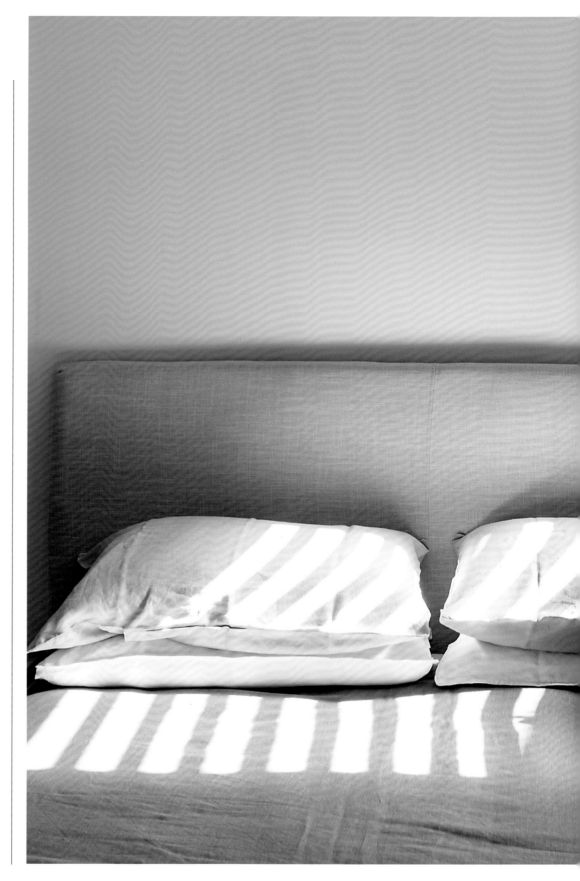

▶ Good-quality blinds and
shutters are a wonderful asset.
Fully opened, or completely
private, they are useful — but
when they really come into their
own is somewhere inbetween.
Sometimes you're just not
ready for a full blast of morning
light and this dappled
shade is glorious.

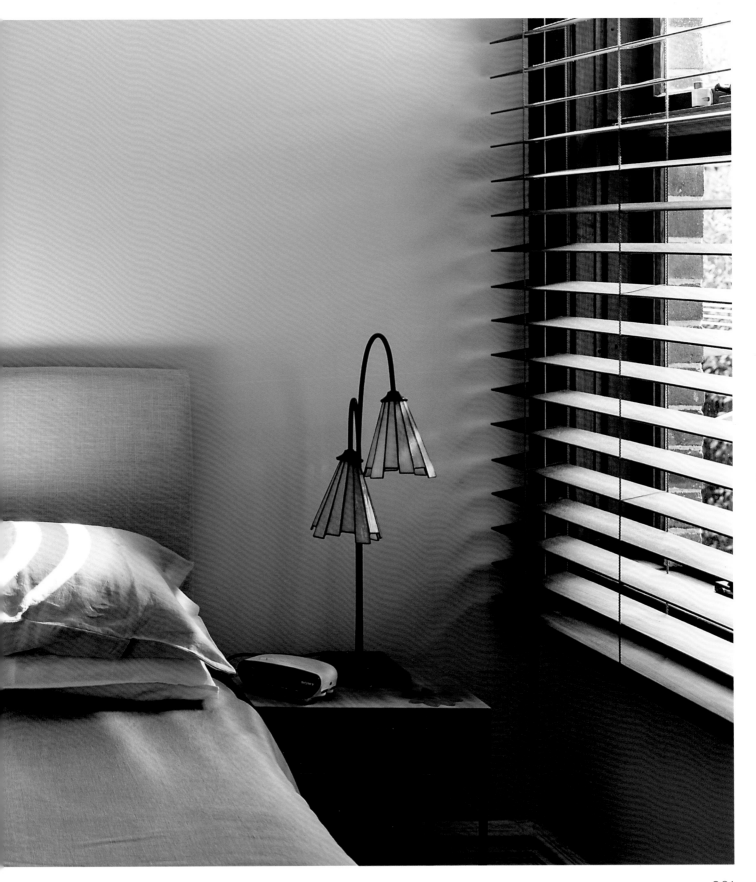

> ▷ Large sliding doors open up this bedroom to refreshing and invigorating sea air.

AIR

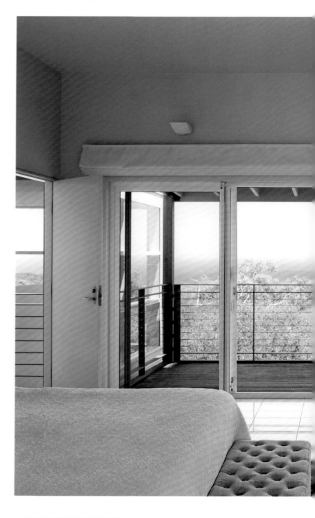

Considering how many hours we spend in a bedroom, healthy air and good ventilation are imperative. I always design a bank of louvres and a window in a bedroom to create some air movement between them. I often lean towards designing two smaller windows at opposite ends of a room rather than one large window in the middle of a room for this very reason. Louvres work well because you can open them partially if required and they can be fitted with fly screens and be secure. If your bedroom has only one external wall and you are struggling to get cross-ventilation, consider introducing a louvred clear light or fan light (a clear-glazed window above the door that allows light and sometimes airflow without opening the door). These were fitted in older houses for that very reason, but have somehow been forgotten in modern homes. By opening a window and the clear light you get good cross-flow across a bedroom.

Another solution is to leave your bedroom door ajar at night.

In winter, having open windows at night is perhaps not an option, so make sure you air the bedroom during the day with air circulation to freshen the space in readiness for closing it up in the evening. Or, open your windows when you get out of bed in the morning and then shut them when you head out to work or wherever.

CEILING FAN

Use a ceiling fan directly over the top of your bed and ensure you invest in a decent one that is quiet and has variable speeds. In most parts of Australia a revolving ceiling fan combined with an open window will get you through the warm summer nights.

Please, please, once again, do not buy a ceiling fan with a light in it. As they age they develop a wobble, which you would never notice except that there is a goddamn light in the fan that is now flickering over your walls.

A SIMPLE TRICK

Instead of, or as well as, a ceiling fan you can use portable floor or bench fans. These do a localised job, so are not as efficient at cooling a whole room in the way a ceiling fan can. However, there are some special things you can do. One trick for a hot, still night is to point your floor fan out of an open window. Yes, you heard me – point the fan out of the open window. What this does is create a negative air pressure in the room as the fan pushes air out through the window. Now open a window in another part of the room – preferably on the opposite side – and you will find that air is drawn in through there, creating the air flow across the room. This works even better if you can point the fan out of the window on the hotter side of the house and draw air in from the cooler side of the house. The key is to set this up as soon as the outside temperature becomes lower than the inside temperature. Also consider that, once

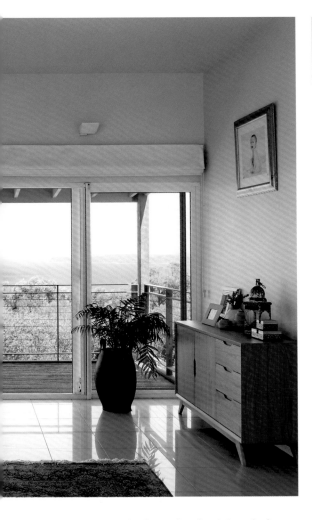

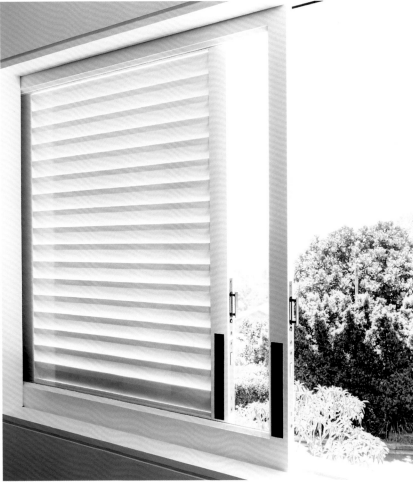

you have brought the cool night air into the house overnight, then in the morning you might want to keep your windows and doors closed so that you don't let in the daytime hot air.

AIR-CONDITIONING AND ALLERGIES

If you live in an area of high pollution, then I do recommend using an air-conditioner to filter the air and ensure you aren't breathing in pollutants while you sleep. It's an unfortunate sentence to have to write, but it is a reality of life for some of us. Air-conditioners can solve the problem short-term, but of course it would be better for all of us if the longer term air pollution was eliminated. A good air-conditioner will filter out dust and allergens, pet dander (skin cells and hair) and even pollen. Have the filters regularly cleaned and seek a lot of advice on the best system if this is why you are installing it. If you suffer from allergies, then install hard floors, such as timber and tiles, avoid carpet, and make sure your clothes are behind doors or in another room altogether.

Air-conditioners are great dehumidifiers. When the humidity is high and uncomfortable, the air-con will do a great job of sucking the moisture out of the air and creating drier air. High humidity inside is not ideal as it can lead to mould and general discomfort. However, you don't want air to be too dry – that is why you sometimes have an uncomfortable sleep in a hotel, where the air-conditioning can dehumidify the air so much that your sinuses dry out.

CURTAINS AND INSULATION

We seem to have forgotten that curtains were once more than a styling element in our homes. As well as for privacy, they were invented to retain heat in homes so that it didn't escape through the

▲ This clever system uses a sliding window and sliding shutters, creating many combinations to help control temperature and airflow.

203

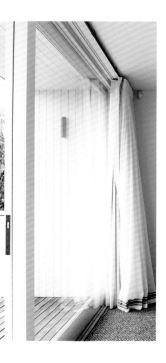

▲ Curtains are not just a styling element, they should be a functional piece of design in your home, keeping it cooler in summer and warmer in winter.

▶▶ This bedroom is prepared for anything, with openable windows onto the juliet balcony, ceiling fan and blinds to block out sun glare.

glass in windows. Curtains can be a crucial asset to the heating and cooling of the air temperature in your house. Glass allows a huge amount of heat transfer, both in and out of the house, unless an air cushion is introduced between two panels of glass (double-glazing). Unfortunately, where I live in Australia, double-glazing has simply not been embraced enough. In summer, close your curtains to parts of your house that are bombarded by hot sun – for me, that is east in the morning and west in the evening. In winter, close your curtains to keep out the cold.

Curtains should fit a window like a glove and form an air cushion between curtain and glass. The trick is to make sure the curtains are hung close to the window, that they are big enough to cover the window and long enough to reach the floor. Often you see curtains that fall short of the floor, allowing the cold air to come in through the window and drop down underneath the curtain and into the room. Curtains can indeed be lovely additions to your home – they can look luxurious and stylish and give the effect of warmth and cosiness. But if your curtain does not reach the floor then it is only there for aesthetic reasons.

Curtains can also become major dust collectors and are often quite dirty without our knowing it. If you ask an asthma sufferer, their pet hate is often curtains – especially in the bedroom. Tie curtains back away from the window and also up and off the floor. Also give them a regular shake down and vacuum so that dust doesn't build up.

Blinds are capable of retaining some heat in a room but are better suited to warmer climates where their main role is stopping sun penetration, especially in the early morning.

EFFICIENT HEATING

To further save money and help the environment, turn off the heating and cooling in the rest of the house and only heat and cool individual bedrooms that need it. Because they are such small contained rooms bedrooms are cost-effective to make comfortable.

(And, if you are worried about waking up to a chilly living room in the morning, then set your heating to come on 30 minutes before you get up.)

SAFE MATERIALS

If you are going to worry about any room in regard to air quality then it must be the bedroom as we spend so much time there. Do your research into low- and no-VOC (volatile organic compound) materials that won't pollute your living environment. VOCs are found in paints, floor finishes, wall finishes and such, and can be released into the air. However, many low-VOC products have now been produced – I'd advise you to research, source and implement these if you are doing a renovation or new build.

THE SCENT OF FRESH

A bedroom needs to smell nice – it should be a place you look forward to retreating to. The secret to a pleasant-smelling bedroom is cleanliness and freshness. But the reality is that there is a lot working against a bedroom smelling nice – they are usually relatively small and closed spaces, contain a lot of soft materials, such as bedding, carpet and clothes that capture dust and smells, and lastly, they contain us for long periods of time. Like it or not, we are not always as fresh as a daisy. The first line of attack is to open your windows and ventilate the room with air and sunlight – the enemies of odour-causing bacteria and mould.

Changing your bedclothes once a week is good practice. If it has been a hot night and you feel that the sheets need an airing during the week, then pull them back in the morning and leave the bed unmade while you get ready for work. Make your bed just before you leave the house, and the sheets will have had a chance to breathe. Flip the mattress every now and then to give it some air and to prevent uneven wear.

LEAF POWER

Bring in plants – but always near the window. Plants never look right in a dark corner away from light and air. They produce oxygen, which is great for helping with a good night's sleep and they are known to filter out toxins.

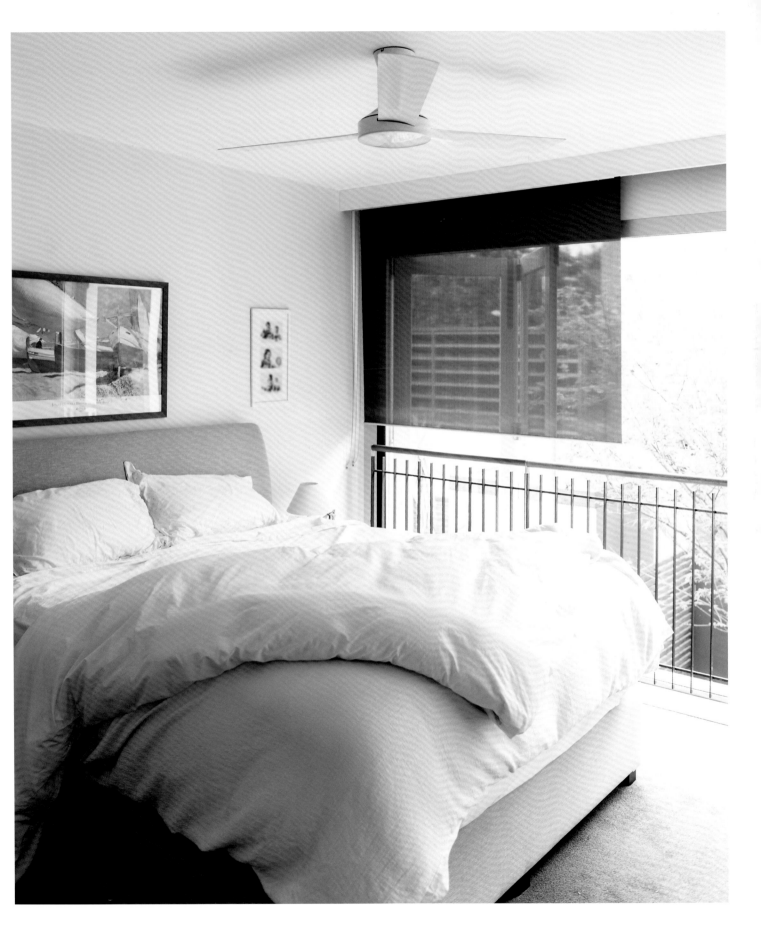

▶ A solid door that is well
fitted is a good acoustic option
for a bedroom. This charming
old door has been refitted
with new hinges to give
it a second life.

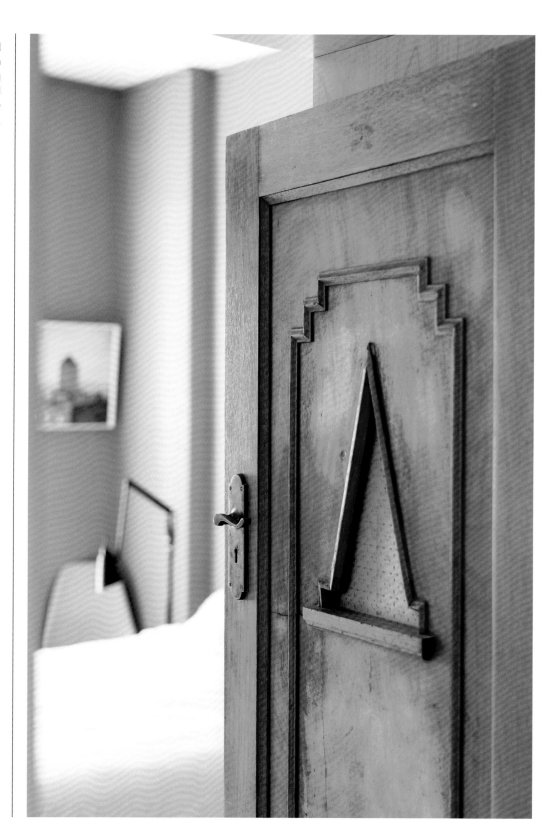

SOUND

Your bedroom should be a sanctuary in terms of sound, and have a quiet relaxing ambience. The last thing you want is for a bedroom to echo. I try to create a soft and plush sound, meaning you can hear fabrics slipping and rustling but there are no hard sounds. Your bed – layered with sound-absorbing materials – is a good acoustic start in the room, but for further dampening of sound, consider carpet instead of hard floors. Curtains are another soft material to bring into the space; you can even find special sound-blocking curtains, which particularly make sense if your windows let in traffic noise.

CHANGE YOUR CEILING

The ceiling is a great opportunity to change the acoustics of your room; if it is an untreated surface, then it is where much of the echo comes from. Design a ceiling that uses acoustic tiles or acoustic plasterboard. Some of the current styles are very contemporary and look amazing. Perforated timber acoustic panelling incorporates an acoustic insulation behind the perforations to absorb the sound. Another option is to clad a wall in an acoustic material. There are some brands now available that are made from recycled plastic bottles. If you batten it off a wall to create an insulating air gap it has great acoustic properties. And it has low-VOC emissions and so is fine for use in a bedroom.

SHUT OUT THE WORLD?

A good-quality well-sealed door is a great way to shut out noise from the rest of the house, so make sure it is a solid-core door and is well fitted. If you have an old-style door and it is a bit wonky and tends to not close properly, then please just get it refitted. You might find you need to replace the hinges or the latch, but you will be surprised at the new lease of life this gives it.

Interestingly enough, it can be a positive not to completely block out all sound from your room. Even when you are asleep you have an awareness of your environment and it can feel strangely uncomfortable to be in a completely silent muted space. If you are a parent, you want to be able to hear a child calling or crying; even some movement or something falling in the house. We have a primeval need to know what is going on in our environment. If you find the door is too much of a sound dampener, then leave it slightly ajar.

In other cases, maybe the best course of action is to get rid of annoying sounds that bother you at night. For example, if the fridge buzzes all night it might be time for an upgrade.

If you are on a busy road or under a flight path, you will notice a huge difference if you introduce double-glazed windows. The layer of air acts not only as a thermal barrier, but also as an acoustic barrier that dampens sound much more than a single layer of glass.

But at the end of the day you either have to stop noise before it gets to you or you have to drown it out with another noise. A water fountain bubbling away to cover distant traffic noise is the same as white noise for a tinnitus sufferer at night: not a solution, but a fix.

MUSIC – THE FOOD OF LOVE

A quality sound system is a great addition to relaxing when going to bed at night. Ensure you have the luxury of controlling it from your bedside, preferably with a dedicated control. Remember, we are trying to remove our smart phones from our bedside tables.

▼ Soft furnishings affect the sound of a room. Here carpet, bedding, fabric upholstery and curtains all soften the acoustics of the bedroom.

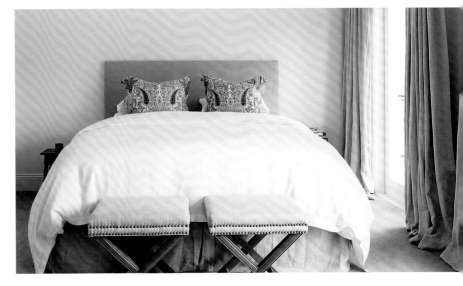

▶▶ Design your outdoor area to ensure you control and capture the view for your bedroom. Screen away neighbours and increase privacy with foliage.

VIEW

Because you probably don't spend too much time in the bedroom awake, and usually not during daylight, a view is less important here than in other areas of the home. However, it is definitely nice to have! Waking to a magnificent view is not to be sniffed at – just remember that it is something you are generally going to see in the morning or late at night.

LOOKING UP

A sky view is lovely from your bed in the morning; you can instantly start to read what sort of day it is going to be, and if you can have your blinds automated then you can start to appreciate the view without even getting out of bed. I will often recommend electric roller blinds on the windows.

A bedroom can often be suited to a secondary view; perhaps a small courtyard or a neighbour's tree or even a view over the street. Every room needs a window, so position it carefully to capture something worth seeing or, even better,

contemplating. If you don't have any view at all, consider adding some window sill planters or flowers. Or consider turning that blank wall outside into an artwork or even a vertical garden of foliage.

JULIET BALCONY

If you don't have a balcony or deck off your bedroom, then consider making the window more just than a window. Consider replacing it with a sliding glass door or a set of French doors (you will need the approval of your local authority). Then design a balustrade to provide safety. For a sliding door, the balustrade can be on the inside or the outside; for French doors the balustrade has to be on the inside. Flinging open the doors to let in the morning sun and breeze feels so much more of a celebration than just opening a window.

The balustrade needs to be well designed and add character to your room – think of wrought iron or timber hand rails, or glass to maximise the view. You can add window plants hanging from the balustrade to make it charmingly European, if that fits your style. Arrange chairs and a side table in front of the Juliet balcony and you have created your own 'outside room'.

▶ When you are thinking about bedroom views, remember what your main vantage point will be. If that is lying down, then make sure you can see the view from that position. Think, too, about materials used for balcony balustrades — this one is designed to not obstruct the view from the bed.

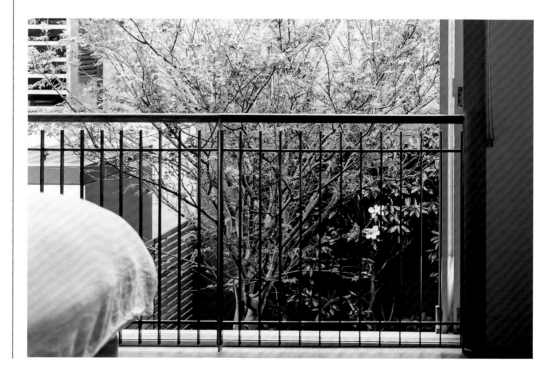

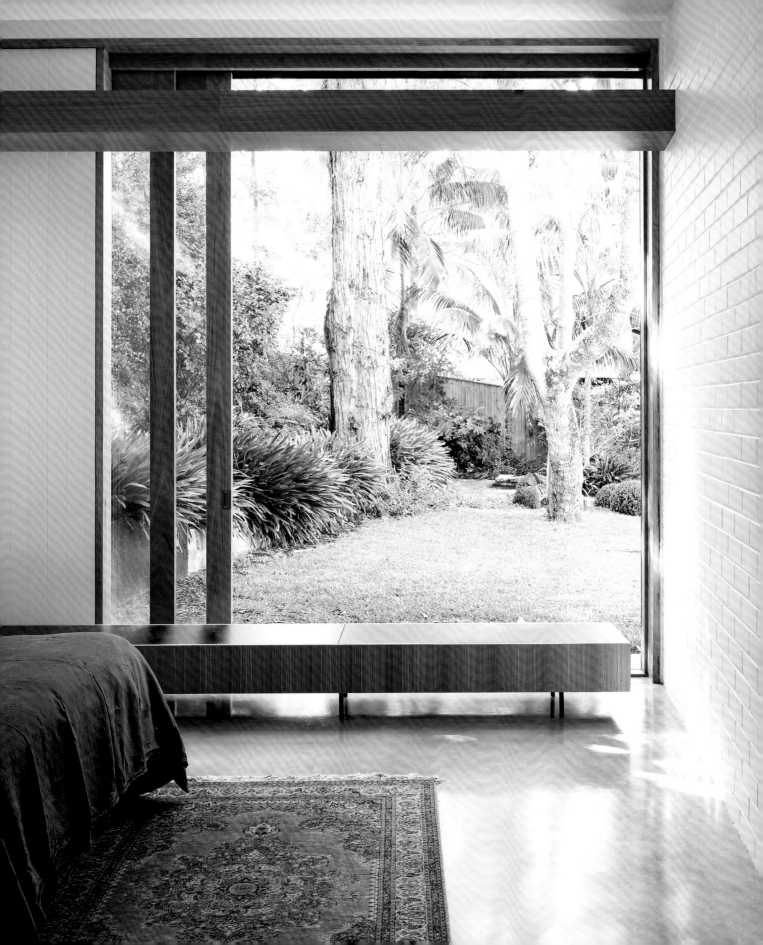

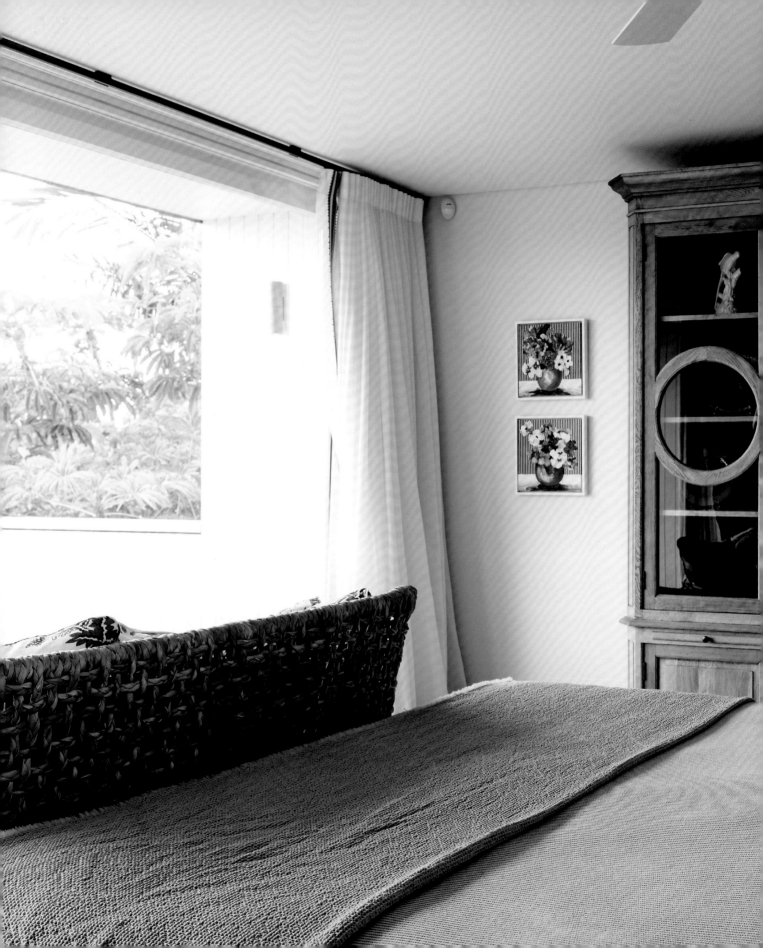

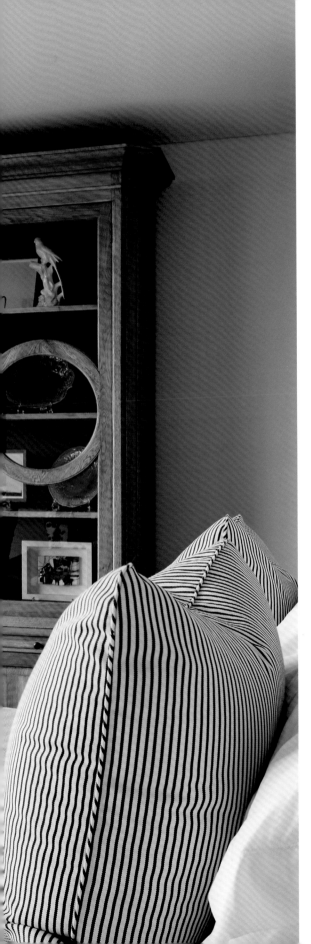

LOOKING OUT AND LOOKING IN

Every bedroom should have a full-length mirror. Make a feature of it – an ornate wall mirror, perhaps, or a New York mirror (one of those classic large lean-against-the-wall mirrors that is a simple minimalist rectangle with a thin black steel frame all around). In a small space, fit a tall slim mirror to the back of the door, or inside one of the wardrobe doors. Or give your wardrobe doors a mirror finish.

A mirror can capture light and a view outside your window but do remember your privacy – if you can see out, then people can see in. In a new build or renovation you could consider fitting higher sill windows in bedrooms – these allow you to walk around undressed and still have a sky view. In one house where there were privacy issues with an apartment overlooking the master bedroom, I designed high-level windows that allowed a view of a favourite tree from the inside, but stopped anyone being able to see people in the room.

Make sure you are aware of all potential sight lines into bedrooms from outside and within the house. This doesn't mean you create a room of walls; you can use shutters, parts of walls, screens and window films to block views and create privacy. Absolute privacy is not required all the time, so curtains and opening privacy screens are ideal for when you want to let in light and air.

INTERNAL VIEWS

Unless you have a city view that lights up, a window at night becomes black and creates a fourth wall in the room. Block-out blinds do the same thing. So, if you want a view at night, you need to create an internal view: consider 'borrowing' a view that you can then shut off when you require privacy, such as into an internal courtyard or over a void that looks down into the living space. One of the advantages of incorporating a vanity and a bath in the bedroom is that it creates an interesting inside view that prevents the room being a bland box.

◁ If you are lucky enough to have a lovely view outside the window, point your bed at it. These owners have doubled up with a sofa as well. And the reflection in the glass-fronted cabinet all adds to the experience.

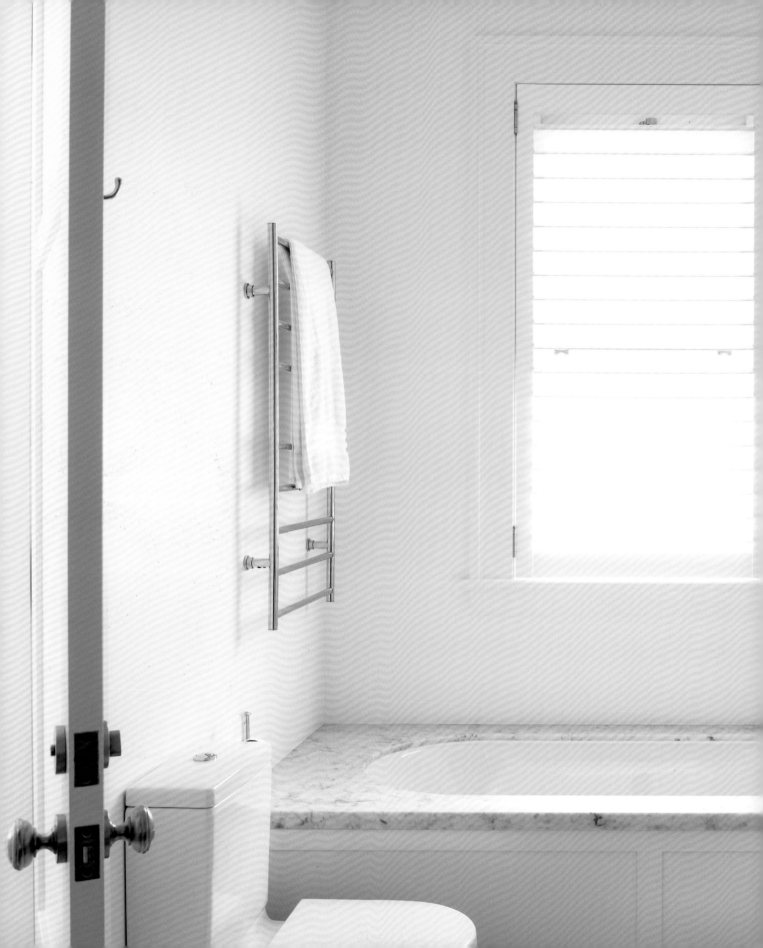

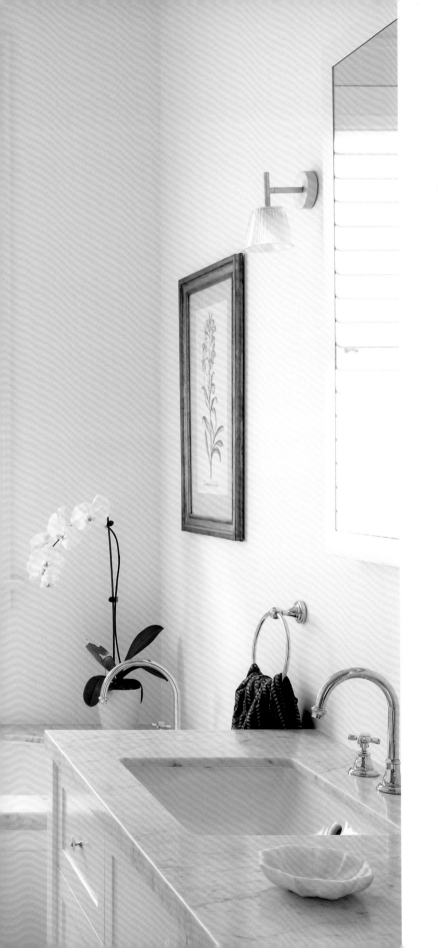

BATH ROOM

CHAPTER FIVE

▶ Have some fun with your guest bathroom and make it a talking point. This one is a play on the 'outdoor loo' with the exterior cladding of the house wrapping inside the house and around the guest bathroom. When the door closes the horizontal boards line up and the bathroom disappears.

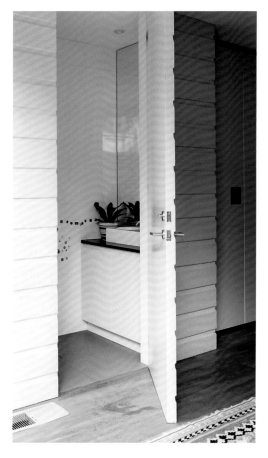

BATHROOMS ARE OFTEN TAKEN FOR GRANTED, but I view them as a vital piece of infrastructure in the home and a marker of our civilisation, no less. One of the most important leaps mankind has made is in the control and processing of human waste. Before our society worked out plumbing, disease was a major hand-brake on our progress. The humble water closet, pipes and sewers have solved this problem in many societies.

There are three general types of bathrooms that might occur in a home – the family bathroom, the ensuite and the guest bathroom/powder room. Each performs a different role and should be treated differently. If bathroom planning is poor, then the space can be an absolute failure – think shower doors hitting wash basins, doors that open unexpectedly to display you on the loo, or bathroom noise that can be overheard from the living room. Get the planning right and a good bathroom can add a whole new dimension to your home and your quality of life.

▶▶ Raise your bath to the air, light and views. If they won't come to you — take your bath to them!

SPACE

If you are building or renovating, then the minimum you want to aim for in the home is a family bathroom and an ensuite. If you can't achieve this, then at least put in a second loo – that is a must in a busy family household. In a two-storey house, with bedrooms and bathroom upstairs, a powder room on the ground floor is increasingly considered a necessity so that visitors don't have to traipse upstairs and wander into private family areas.

A bathroom is arguably one of the most difficult spaces to design well: it usually has a number of functions and is often squeezed into a tight space.

PRIVACY? OR FAMILY TIME?

The family or general bathroom is foremost a utilitarian operation. Often catering for multiple people rushing in the morning and evening, this bathroom needs to be as spacious as possible with plenty of room to move.

However, much as it's a cliché that we've heard a million times, it is true that the bathroom should also be a sanctuary. Where I would like to expand that conversation, however, is that the bathroom is often talked about as a sanctuary for one: a place to get away from the rest of the family. I am a huge supporter of this, and work hard to provide personal sanctuaries in all the homes I design. However, if you share a home, as many of us do, the bathroom can be a great connector within the family and, in particular, your relationship. In times past, bathing was a decidedly communal activity and it still is today in the form of Turkish, Japanese and Korean baths.

So, when you design your bathroom you might want to consider it as an inclusive experience. Of course, the loo needs to be separate, but everything else in the bathroom can be shared to varying degrees depending on who is in the home.

Some of the funniest moments in our family are when my three boys and I are all in the bathroom brushing our teeth – there is invariably uproarious laughter and great hilarity, all captured and reflected back to us by the bathroom mirror.

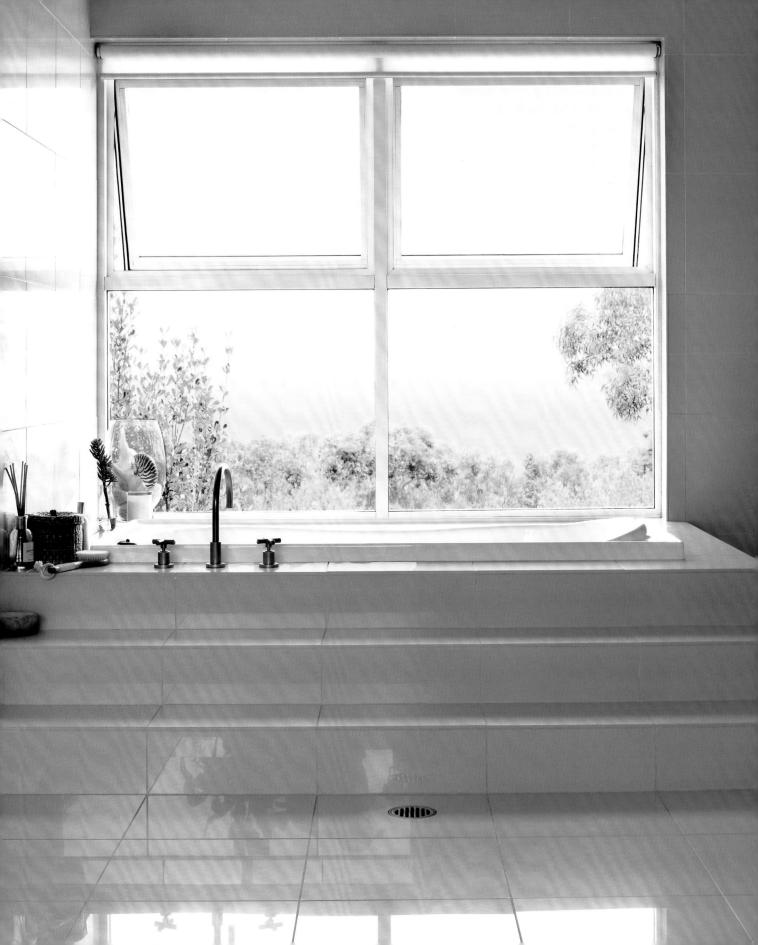

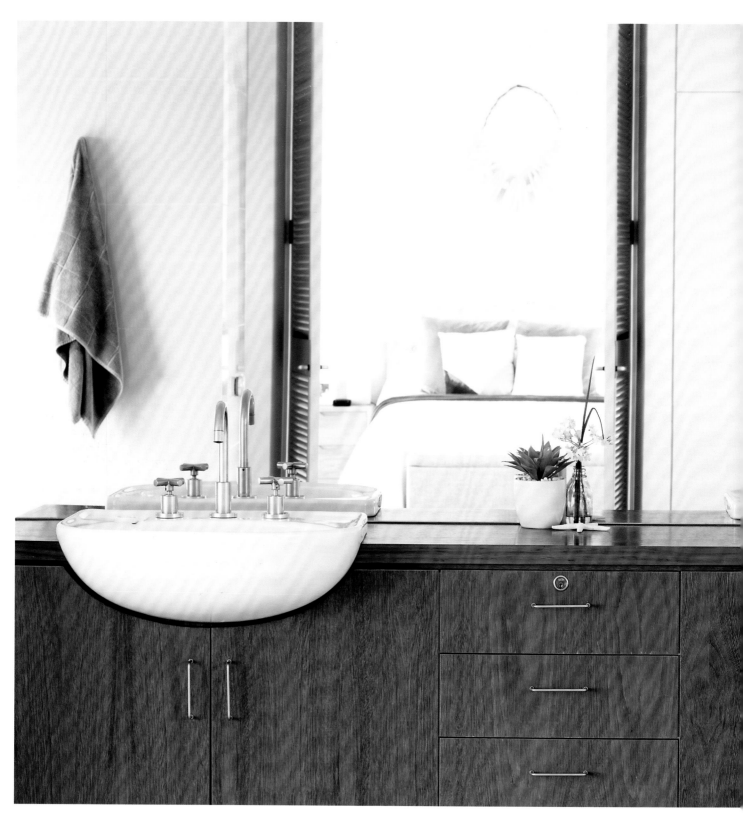

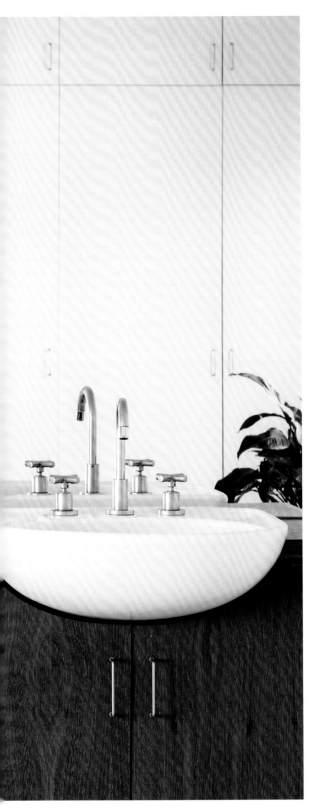

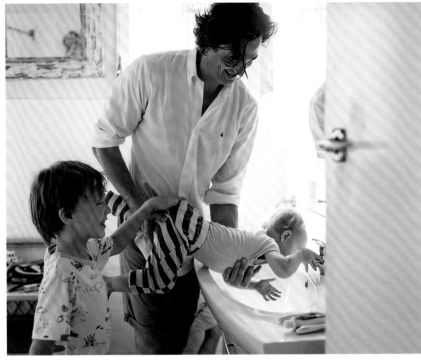

There is a sense of theatre, and there are few times in our lives where all members of a family, across all ages, are doing exactly the same job. I have similar memories from my childhood with my siblings.

Understanding these precious moments is important to the design of your home. I design long vanity benches, not only for a sense of space and a place to put your toiletries, but also to allow a number of family members to line up and brush their teeth. Once you have a long vanity, then you have the opportunity to run a mirror along its full length to reflect the moment, as well as to bounce light and views in the room.

Many families of young children also have a huge amount of fun at bath-time. It is a wonderful thing to have all the kids in the bath when they are that age, for all family members; it might have been a tricky day at work, but it's hard to dwell on that when you are watching the calamity of bath-time! These are good times, which don't actually last that long, and they are what life's memories are made of. So, if you have young children, or are hoping to have them, design for a bath somewhere in your house that will allow you to get the most enjoyment from this time.

◀ A double vanity allows a couple to be together, but not get in each other's way. Isn't that what every relationship needs?

▲ Peter didn't have his bathroom step-stool, so he needed a bit of help reaching the tap!

SEPARATE LOO

Separating the loo from the main bathroom space into its own compartment aids togetherness in the rest of the bathroom. In the days when we had an outdoor lavatory this was not an issue; we all once washed together in a communal space. However, with modern plumbing we were able to bring the loo inside the house, into the bathroom, and this forced us into more isolated activity in that room. So I suggest we bring back the idea of the outdoor dunny, only inside in the house, so that we can turn the bathroom back into a more communal wash area.

TWO PEOPLE, TWO BASINS

Still along the same lines, I have had many couples question me when I have designed their bathroom (especially an ensuite) to incorporate two basins. It is more opulent and it does take up more room; however, it does something else that is important to me as an architect – it encourages conversation and connection. When you have one basin, one of you, often without realising it, is either getting in the way or having to wait. With two basins, you have your own spot in a shared space; suddenly, where you were forced into separation now you are together. Washing, cleaning and preening is in our DNA as a social activity; you only have to watch the behaviour of other primates. Yet our modern circumstance has broken that down. In our increasingly busy lives, if I can get a couple to have a chat while brushing their teeth and getting ready for bed or work – not waiting for the other, not getting in the other's way, not disrupting the other's routine (so annoying!) yet still close together in their own spot – then design is doing a good job for that relationship. For me, two basins can be more

▼ Mirrors should complement the styling of your space. Here the black frames match the black taps. Just as a window frames a view and alters the experience, so too does a mirror with a frame.

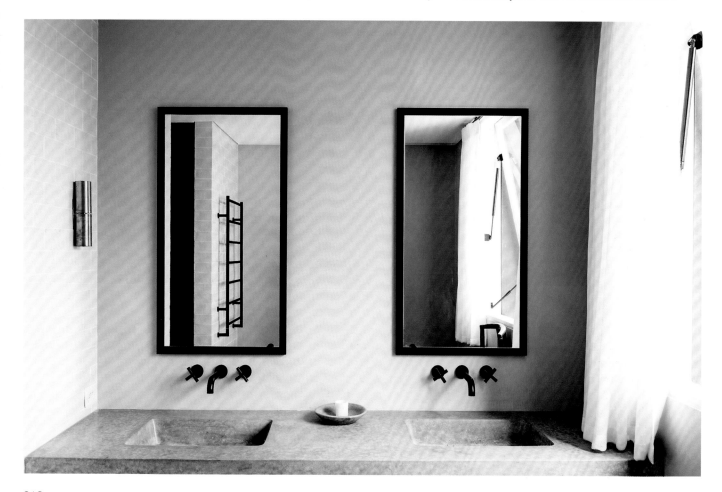

important than a bath, because of the freedom they give people to spend more time together.

In the same way, I have introduced two showerheads in a shower. How many times have you found yourself waiting for your partner to shower, when instead you could be sharing a chat about the day ahead? If you're not careful, it could lead to relationship bliss.

CAN A BATHROOM BE TOO BIG?

Sometimes a house will have one very large family bathroom that is obviously an inefficient use of space. Consider turning it into two bathrooms. If you have the space it makes a lot of sense, as all your plumbing services for the bathroom are already in one area. In a recent project I created a new family bathroom in another more convenient part of the house and then converted the existing large family bathroom into two rooms: a guest bathroom, and an ensuite for a bedroom. The home went from a one-bathroom house to a three-bathroom house in a relatively cost-effective way. When renovating, it is a big and often expensive decision to relocate bathroom plumbing. Best to try to work with existing water and waste locations if you can.

Another option is to split a large family bathroom into three rooms: the vanity and mirror, the shower and the WC. The WC should have its own small hand basin so that it can operate separately and so cater to more people. In a family environment this set-up would cater for up to three people at a time (hence I call it the three-way bathroom). It is a great option for a household with multiple kids and no other bathrooms. The downside is the required circulation space to allow for all the different doors and access.

... OR TOO SMALL?

The smallest (reasonable) bathroom that contains a WC, decent vanity and shower is a minimum of 1.5 x 3 metres (5 x 10 ft) and must be accessed by a side door, either opening outwards or a cavity slider. The side entry is key here because it allows the entry into the bathroom to be in the space in front of the vanity, which then allows access to the loo at one end and the shower at the other. This is the bare minimum and is all

about effective use of space and efficiency. You can go smaller but it starts to get ridiculous. If you have to create a long skinny bathroom, consider making one whole wall a huge door. This can slide back and be an extension of your room for most of the day, only sliding closed if privacy is needed, which is not that often. The minimum depth for a vanity with a semi-recessed basin is 40 cm (16 in) and with a contained basin it is 60 cm (24 in). The minimum shower space is 90 cm (35 in) square; however, I prefer to start with 1 metre (40 in) square and most showers I design are bigger than this. The minimum placement for a WC off a side wall is 45 cm (18 in) to the centre line of the loo. If you are enclosing a WC on both sides, then allow a minimum space of 90 cm with the WC in the centre at 45 cm off each wall.

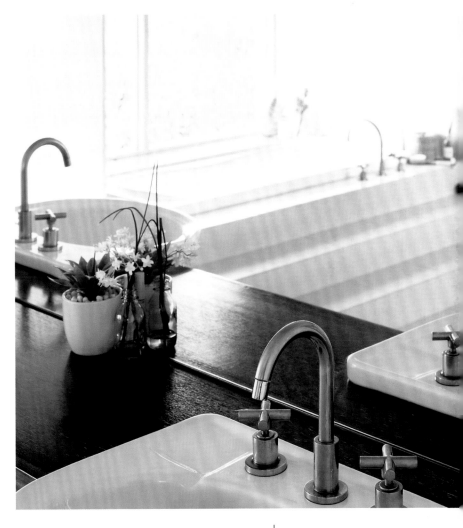

▲ Mirror is a practical feature of a bathroom, so take advantage of it; use mirror to extend the room and make it feel bigger, as well as to reflect and increase light.

▶ Bathing options give a sense of opulence, even if you don't always get the chance to use them. No doubt the shower is used far more often than the bath in this room, but it is the bath that adds a touch of luxury to the space.

▼ Elegant tiles and the dark wooden stool set the tone for this bathroom.

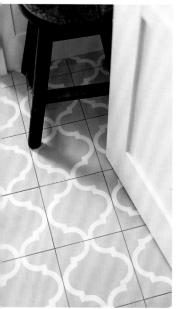

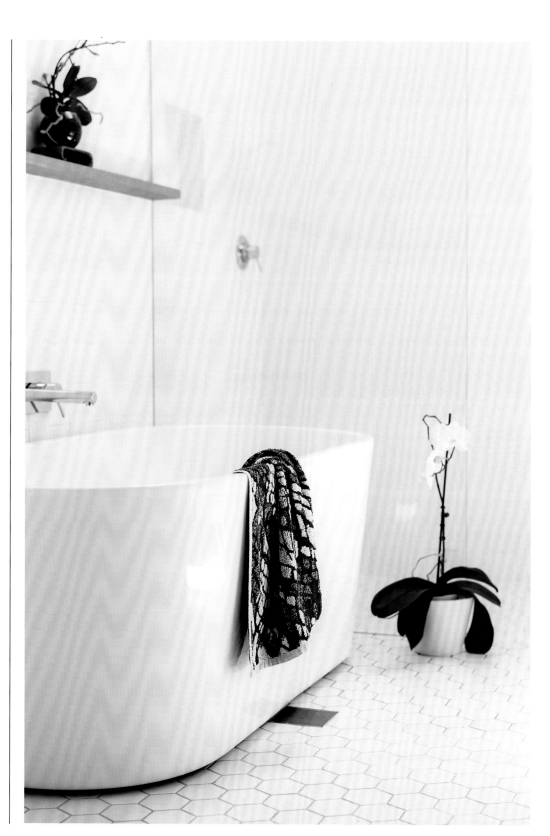

ONE-STOP BATHROOM

The opposite solution is to make the family bathroom as big as possible with loo, shower/bath and vanity all in one room. This certainly makes the most of the space available as no extra walls and doors are taking up room. I often fit laundries into large bathrooms to make the space even more efficient in regards to the overall home. As the laundry is often used outside peak bathroom times, this can be a good compromise – and on a low budget it can be cost-effective to bring all your services together in one wet area. You can even combine the laundry tub and the washbasin into one by choosing a deeper basin.

NOBODY PUTS JOE IN THE CORNER

When dealing with small rooms, corners become crucial; you need to deal with them cleverly and efficiently. The key point is to never put a person in a corner unless it is for a very defined job. Putting a loo in the corner is OK, because that is used for a very defined job and, anyway, if you are there for any amount of time you are probably looking out into the room. Putting a shower in the corner is OK because it also has a very defined job to do, as does a bath, which also should be orientated so that you are facing a view or out into the room. However, as much as possible, I avoid putting a washbasin in the corner. There is something that just sucks about standing in the corner of a bathroom, staring at the wall and brushing your teeth. You certainly don't feel like you have made it. Instead I work hard to get the vanity along one wall and position the person in the middle of the room to do the many undefined and varied jobs of using the basin and mirror.

BATH, OR NO BATH?

If there is room, installing a bath can be a great way to completely change the look and feel of your bathroom. Ensure the floor can take the weight of the bath full of water and people. The ultimate layout would be to have a separate shower and bath; however, you can combine both these into a shower bath, which is more cost-effective and space saving. If you are using a bath as a shower bath, then make sure you fit one that has been designed for that use. They have flatter bottoms that have been designed to stand in. They are sometimes not as comfortable as a normal bath to lie in, but often the shower is used much more than the bath, so it should win out in terms of compromise.

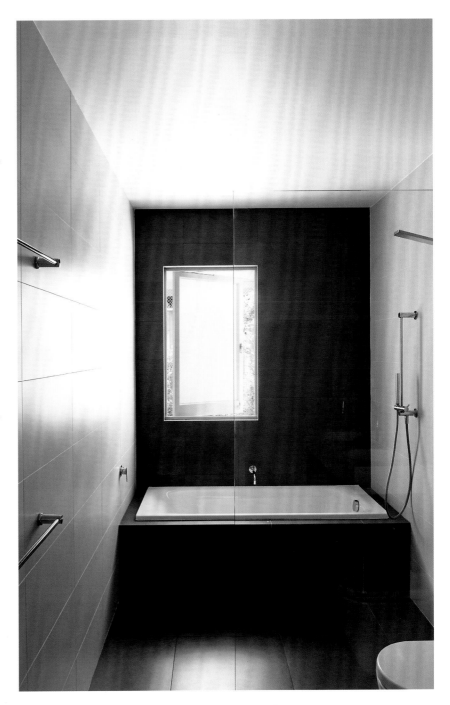

The dark tiled floor wraps up the bath and onto the far wall, making it appear to recede. The glass shower blade is barely visible, giving the illusion of spaciousness.

5 X 5
BATHROOM

▶ Separate your shower and loo from the public vanity area — that way several people can use the room at the same time. The window and veil wall combination lets in light while providing privacy.

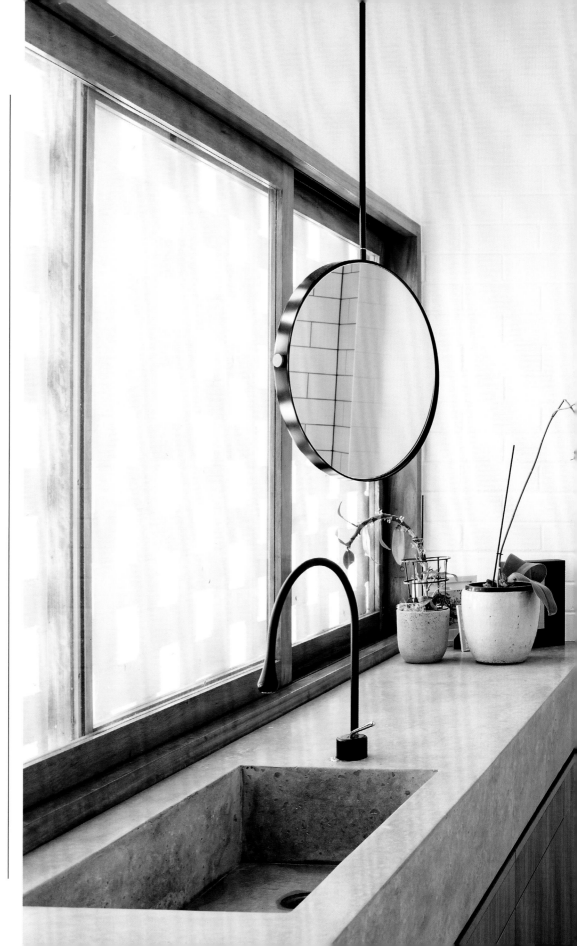

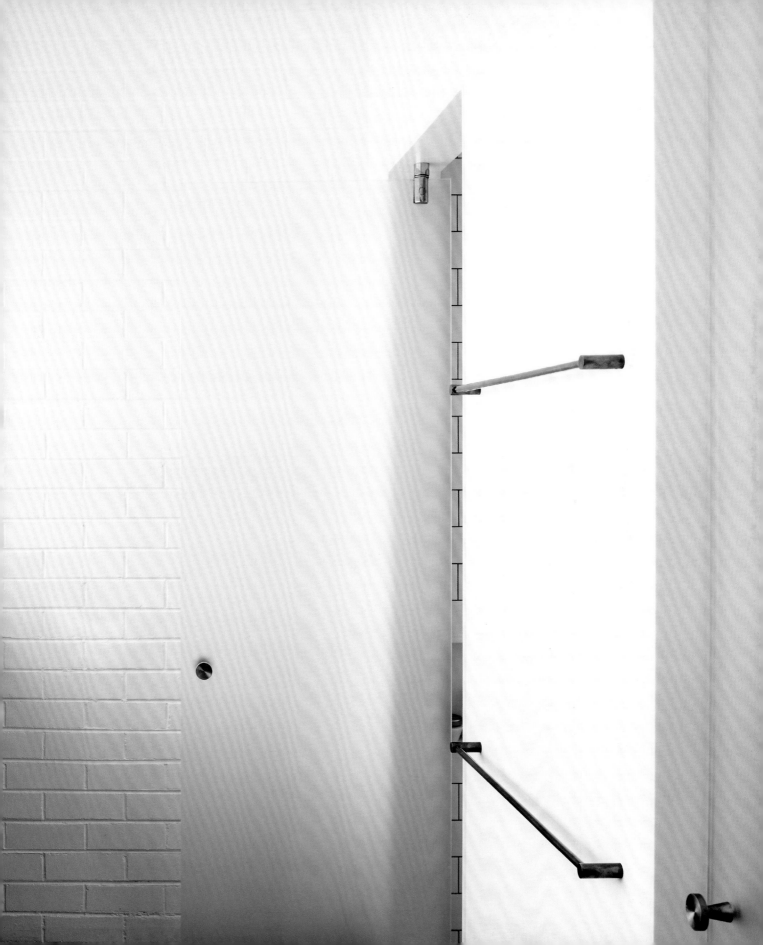

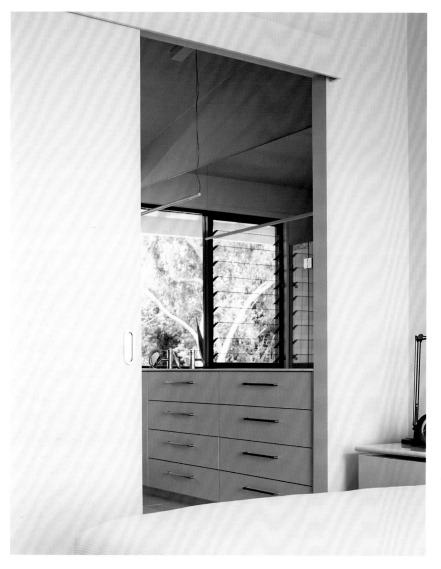

▲ By separating the loo and shower from the main area of the bathroom, you can extend an ensuite into the bedroom — this makes both spaces feel bigger and more connected.

CAVITY SLIDE DOOR

This style of door has saved me so many times. It is a great space saver: in smaller houses or apartments, you are always chasing space in a bathroom and a swing door can get very awkward as it bashes into loos, showers etc. A relatively easy fix that makes a big difference to your internal space is to replace your swing door with a cavity slider. You should invest in one that is solid and has a good seal, as they can be poor in terms of acoustic separation. If you can't do this, at least re-swing your door so that it opens into the room, giving you privacy until the person gets around the door – this works for loos as well.

PSYCHOLOGICAL SPACE GAINING

If you want to create the feeling of a big bathroom, despite the small size of the room, maximise the run of your floor tile. Make sure that it runs to every corner of the room. Lift the loo off the floor and wall hang it, so the floor tile runs to the wall. Wall hang your vanity basin and joinery and make sure you can see the floor hit the wall. Don't use a shower cubicle; instead allow your floor tile to run into the shower and separate the shower from the bathroom with a blade of clear glass. Use a claw foot bath and let the floor tiles run underneath it, or build in a bath and let the floor tiles wrap up and around it so that the floor continues. All these design techniques allow the floor to flow and give the sense that the bathroom is bigger than it is.

THINK HORIZONTAL

If your bathroom is a relatively small room, as they often are, work to enhance the horizontal rather than the vertical. By introducing horizontal elements, you elongate its breadth and make the footprint of the room feel bigger than it really is. If you emphasise the vertical in your bathroom, you are elongating the space upwards and making the footprint seem even smaller. If you use wall tiles, choose a rectangular shape and lay them horizontally. This will instantly make your eye run along the wall, rather than up it. It is no accident that subway tiles are so popular.

Add to this by designing a long edge of joinery for your vanity, or by emphasising the long edge of your bath, or fitting horizontal accessories, such as towel rails.

You can go further by introducing a horizontal dado tile or a feature colour band tile. The dado tile is interesting because it can be traditional and contemporary at the same time, and importantly it emphasises the breadth of the room. This also creates the opportunity to have some fun with the tiles below and above this line. Consider dark tiles below and light tiles above; this will ground the room and make the upper, lighter area 'lift'. Or keep it white below and bring in a rich colour, such as duck egg blue, above – then the space starts to get interesting!

In the same way you can consider a cove tile (much like a skirting tile) around the base of the wall, a picture rail tile and an upper tile (like a

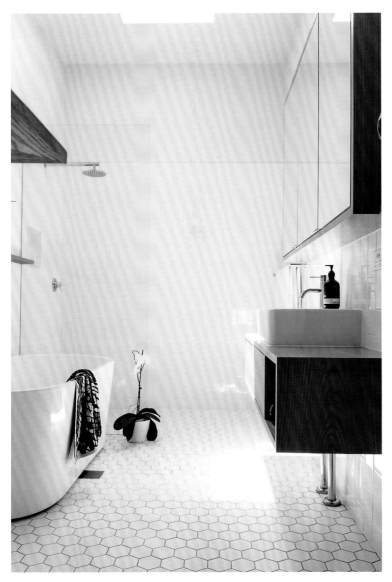

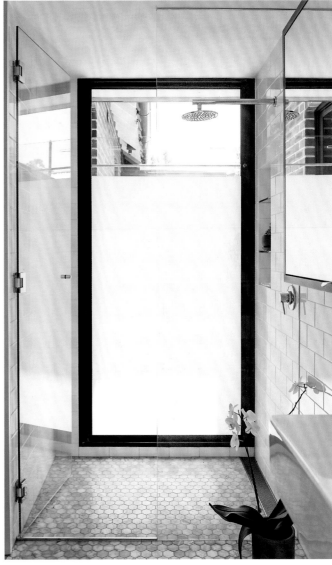

cornice) if you want to create an ornate look. The key is to create horizontal bands.

HOW TO TILE

Where bathrooms often go wrong is with too many arrangements of small tiles, which create a cluttered feeling. It is much stronger and cleaner to use a larger tile as the major tile. Once you have this larger tile in place, bring in a smaller tile as a feature. Small tiles work much better as a block – it gives them more power to stand alone in a space. With the bigger tile as background, make one wall a feature tile of coloured, or mirrored,

mosaic and it will truly sing off the foundation of the bigger tile. It draws your focus to the feature tile and takes the pressure off the rest of the room. The bigger the tile, generally the cheaper it is – especially 60 x 30 cm (24 x 12 in) white tiles, which are very popular.

Rather than spending your money on expensive smaller tiles all over the bathroom, just concentrate your budget on one feature area. Perhaps introduce the smaller tile on the back wall of the shower or to cascade down the wall and over the bath, both of which celebrate the more sensual parts of your bathroom.

◀ Elevate the vanity unit off the floor and allow the tiles to run underneath all the way to the wall. This tricks your eye into feeling the room is bigger.

▲ Use opaque films and screens to maximise light while maintaining privacy.

MOSAIC TILING

Now, you might be thinking that some bathrooms are completely covered in mosaic tiles and still look good. Well, you are right, and they are some of my favourite bathrooms. However, what the designer is doing there is treating the mosaic as one singular block of texture and colour. In that instance, you don't read the mosaics as many small tiles but as one blanket of colour. Of course, if another size of tile is introduced as well, then the illusion is broken and suddenly the mosaics look overdone and cluttered.

Mosaics are generally quite costly per square metre, so when designing your bathroom use mosaics in small but powerful ways, such as to highlight a recess or as a splashback to a vanity.

To reduce costs in your bathroom, reduce the tiles used. Many people think a bathroom needs to be fully tiled, as it is a wet area; however, this is not the case. If you have a tight budget, use a skirting tile in the bathroom and leave the wall in plasterboard except for in the shower, where you should tile up to 210 cm (83 in) – this should line up with the top of a standard bathroom door and the top of the shower glazing. If you have a bath, you need to protect the surrounding walls with tiles to at least 40 cm (16 in) above the bath. You could look at another line to give you a neat tile height above the bath – perhaps 90 cm (35 in) to line up with the top of the vanity.

If you have a larger budget, you can extend that skirting to dado rail height, and then after that you can go to the standard 210 cm all round, which will line up with the top of your door. A large wall mirror is cheaper than tiles, and a mirror will always make a room feel bigger and more glamorous.

GLOSS OR MATT?

When choosing tiles, take some time to consider whether to use a gloss or matt finish. If you choose gloss, your bathroom will have a more sparkly feel as the light is reflected – but, maybe, if you are not careful, it will also have a more 80s feel! Matt can be a more subdued look and it can come across as more sophisticated – the risk is here that it can seem bland. I often mix the two textures. For example, I create a background of matt white tile and then introduce a gloss black penny round mosaic to give an extra bit of punch.

MODERN COVING

A coving tile around the base of your bathroom walls is a very practical solution for water protection and cleaning. The cove gets rid of a sharp corner where dirt can gather, and creates a seamless surface between the floor and the wall. Aesthetically, coving tiles soften the corners of the room, which can be frustrating if you are trying to create a clean, sharp-edged modern look. If you like them for practical reasons but want to maintain a sharper look, then fit gloss black coving tiles that contrast with the rest of your tiles and form a band in the edge of the floor.

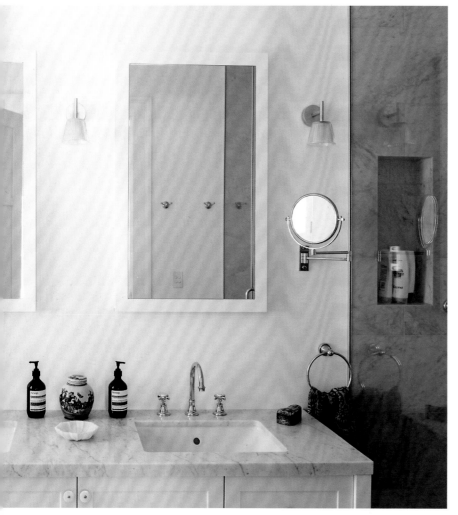

In this bathroom, stone has been used in the shower space and on the vanity benchtop. It is a clever way to tell a story without covering the whole bathroom in stone.

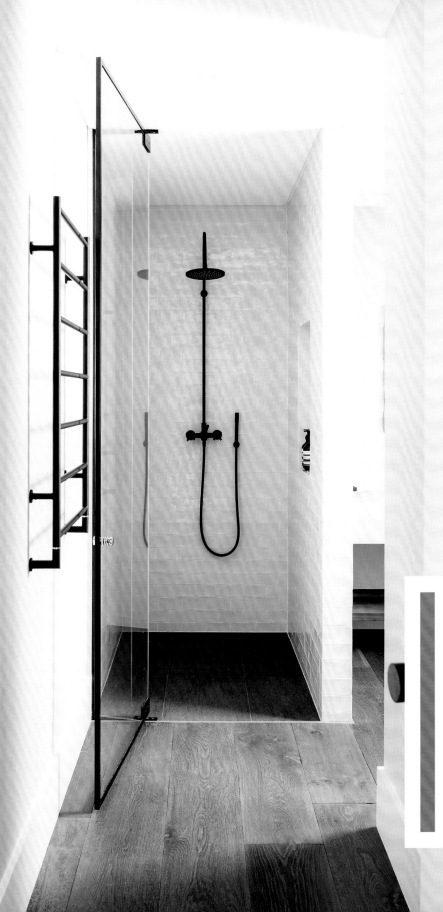

◀ Full—height but clear glazing to this shower ensures it is not shut off from the rest of the room. The shelf is recessed, which provides practical storage but means you don't bump into it every time you turn around in the shower.

SMART HOME

IN THE BATHROOM THERE WILL BE SHOWERHEADS WITH BUILT-IN SPEAKERS, MIRRORS THAT LIGHT UP AS YOU APPROACH AND SIMULATE SUNLIGHT, AND HANDS-FREE TOILET FLUSHING THAT WILL MEASURE YOUR PERSONAL WASTE TO ADD TO YOUR HEALTH FILE. A MOISTURE SENSOR CAN DETECT A PIPE LEAK, SEND YOU A WARNING AND RECOMMEND PLUMBERS WORKING IN YOUR AREA.

5 X 5
BATHROOM

▶ This bathroom moves from warm to light, from floor to ceiling: timber-look floor tiles, stone, warm white on the walls and then up to a white ceiling. The white skirting, curtain and bath bring crisp freshness.

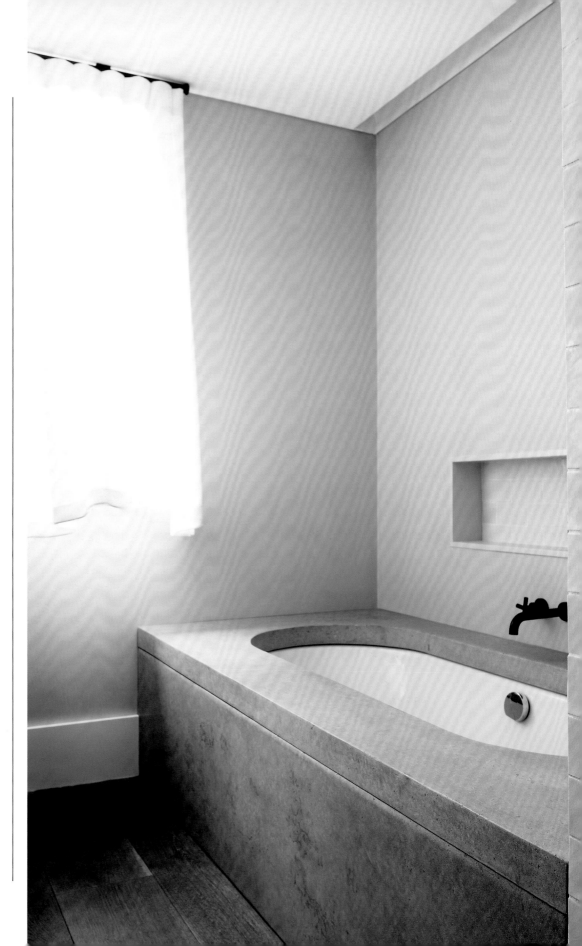

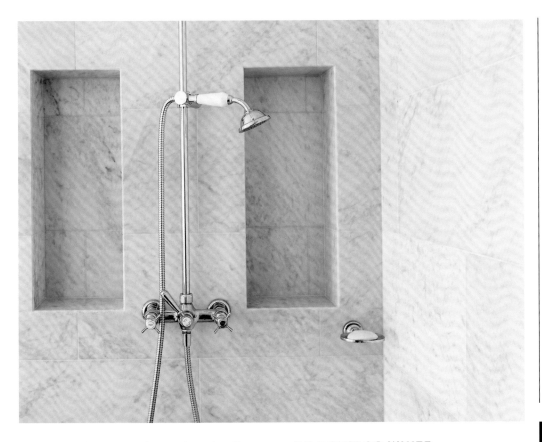

Plan recessed shelves when you are designing the room. Here the recesses are classically symmetrical in the space and the continuous stone tile forms a seamless background. This creates a shadow and shows off the heritage-style fittings.

You will lose the curve and instead get the effect of a black skirting which sharply draws the join of floor to wall.

GO WHITE...

We associate white with hygiene, cleanliness and sanctuary, so a fresh white look is perfect for a wet area like a bathroom. One of the easiest and most cost-effective fixes to a bathroom is to 'go white', and I mean white everywhere. Take that old bathroom, get rid of the old cream tiles and daggy grey floor tiles and replace it all with white. Use a matt white 60 x 30 cm (24 x 12 in) square-rectified wall tile (these have sharp square edges that reveal only a little grout, giving a cleaner look) and a white 30 cm or 60 cm square floor tile. Your ceramic elements such as bath, basin and loo should be white, complemented by a white joinery vanity and white shelves. Add a large mirror and a glass shower blade to reveal and reflect all that white. Suddenly you will have created a very fresh space. If you want to add some colour, do it with your accessories.

...OR DON'T GO WHITE

These days there are options of many colours for your sanitary ware. Gone are the days when you wanted to create a sleek black bathroom but still had to stick with a white loo and vanity basin. Now you can truly go all black with some beautiful black vanity basins and all-black loos. And with this comes all-black accessories, once only a high-end option, now you can get your taps and bathroom accessories right down to your toilet roll holders all in black in mid-price stores. An option I often go for is an all-white bathroom with all black accessories, which looks sleek and has an industrial feel. And then on top of this you can now go out and buy bright red, yellow, blue or green taps and fittings. Some of the most exciting bathrooms are those that have slipped in a bright yellow tap as an unexpected splash of colour.

NOT SO RECESSIVE

Recesses are a great way to increase both practicality and beauty in a bathroom. Examples include a shower shelf recess in your shower or

NOTE TO SELF

GAIN INSPIRATION FROM THE NATURAL ATTRIBUTES OF YOUR BATHROOM, ITS SHAPE AND WHERE THE LIGHT IS COMING FROM. RATHER THAN RELYING ON THE LATEST TREND, HAVE CONFIDENCE THAT YOUR OWN PERSONAL STYLE WILL ALWAYS COME THROUGH.

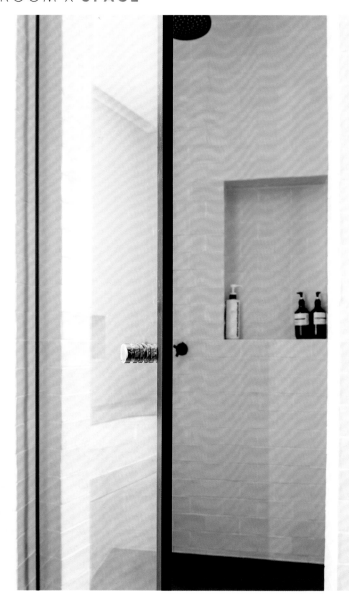

△ An all-white bathroom with crisp black fittings will always be a winner. Don't clutter the space.

▷ This simple bathroom has everything in its place and room to move. Note the timber cabinet frame that introduces warmth to the space.

bath, or a shelf recess above your vanity, or even a random recess in the wall above the towel rail that has been designed to hold a vase and flower. These recesses take advantage of the gaps between wall studs in lightweight walls. They are easy to create in a new building, as you can design the wall studs to create the recesses required. However, for a renovation you will need to locate the wall studs and carefully design the recesses to fit in them. Of course, you need to make sure that the recesses work for you in a design sense; I have seen recesses that are strangely placed in the room and I know that's because of where the wall studs are.

WALL CABINETS

In the same way, you can fit wall cabinets in the recesses between wall studs. This enables you to keep a flush wall and then reveal the recess when you open or slide the cabinet door. It is a great way to achieve surprising storage. And, just like exposed recesses, you can surprise with a feature material at the back of your cupboard, such as a rich timber, mirror or even a colourful mosaic.

WHICH LOO?

You can make a big difference in your bathroom by updating your loo – the technology has come a long way, especially in their water efficiency. Aesthetically speaking, the less loo there is, the better. I would always choose a wall-hung loo with a concealed cistern in the wall. This is the cleanest and most sophisticated look and it makes the bathroom spacious as there is no bulky cistern in the room, and the loo is up off the floor. There are two options for the in-wall cistern: put it in a wall, or put it in joinery. I often create one long piece of joinery in a bathroom to house both the basin and the wall-hung loo. It gives great design strength to the joinery because it is doing a few jobs.

Don't forget to spend some time thinking about the flush button – in a wall-hung loo situation it becomes quite a visible feature, like a little disconnected picture on the wall, and it needs to be elegant and beautiful.

If you can't incorporate a wall-hung loo then the next best option is a floor-mounted loo with an in-wall cistern to hide the cistern bulk. If you need to go for an exposed loo and cistern then always choose a model that is wall faced, meaning it allows for a flat edge to the wall, which prevents those weird cavities around the back. This looks better and is also much easier to clean. The less time you spend cleaning a loo the better, and it is never pleasant getting in behind a loo and cleaning areas that would be better off not being exposed to gather dirt in the first place.

SHOWER SHELF AND BENCH

If possible, every shower should have a shelf. It can be proud or recessed but either way it should be big enough to handle the family's needs. The shelf should not be hit by direct water – it is so irritating to get in the shower and find the soap

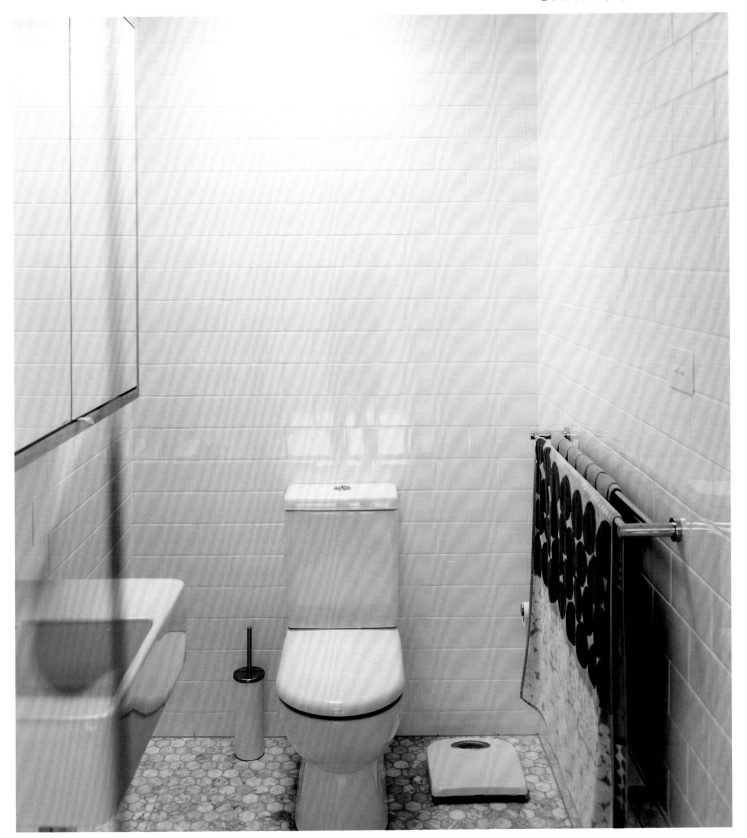

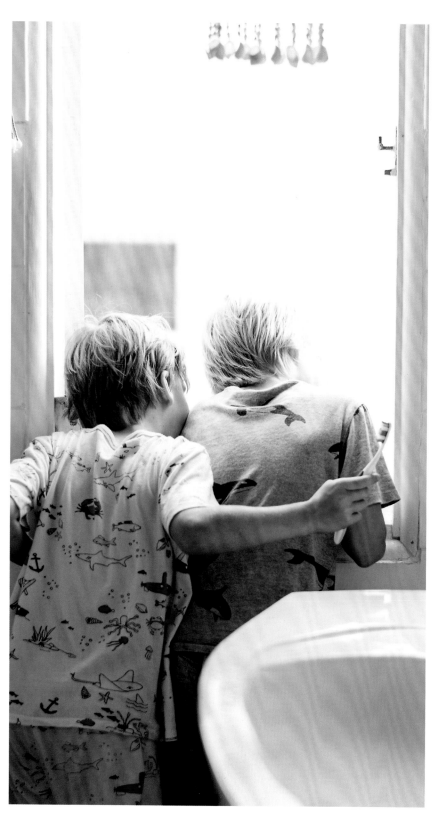

has been sitting in a pool since your last shower. Don't clutter the shelf: only have what you really need in the shower.

Also, if you can fit it in, introduce a bench in the shower. A bench design that is an extension of the wall and is fully tiled can be very luxurious and practical for the various jobs that need to get done in the shower, such as shaving. It is also a smart move in terms of real estate – with an ageing population a shower bench is a very attractive asset in a bathroom.

ENSUITE BATHROOM

There is no doubt that the ensuite has become an extremely sought-after element of the modern home and adds a lot of value. Previously reserved for master bedrooms, ensuites are now creeping in for the other bedrooms as well. In fact, it is often quite efficient to introduce two smaller ensuites back to back with each other to share plumbing. I have converted many second family bathrooms into one or more ensuites to take advantage of the kids leaving home. You might even find you can lose a bedroom and create more convenient guest bedrooms with appropriate ensuites. When you are renovating, the key is to locate the services and look for opportunities to move walls. You might find that an ensuite is no further away from a bedroom than knocking a hole in a wall into an old laundry or similar. Also the ensuite may not need to be as big as you think – you only need to provide space for a separate loo and shower and then include the vanity basin in the bedroom space.

THE GUEST POWDER ROOM

A guest bathroom or powder room needs to be located where access is easy from the main entertaining spaces such as the living room, kitchen and dining room. However, please work hard to ensure the door to the powder room is not so visible that it broadcasts to everyone that you have just been to the loo. A little bit of privacy around entering and exiting the guest bathroom is simply polite. At no point must the loo in all its glory be in line of sight from the dining table, sofa or, for heaven's sake, the front door.

The internal design should be very simple and easy to understand for any guest – usually just a

WC and a vanity. Two other imperatives are a hook to hang your coat or jacket, and a shelf for a handbag, phone or wallet.

Guest bathrooms are often in tight spaces, but make sure the door is designed to allow reasonable movement so that there is not too much fumbling on the way in or out. It is always unpleasant to press yourself up against a toilet just to get the door closed around you, not to mention finding yourself hitting your head on the sloping ceiling in a loo under the stairs.

In a guest loo you can go wild with your aesthetics and materials – these are not usually big spaces. However, your guests will notice, and mention it, if you put some passion into the space.

EASY-FIX CHANGES

Just as in the kitchen, you can make a big change in the bathroom by replacing the benchtop of the vanity. Upgrade that old melamine with a piece of marble or man-made stone. A bathroom benchtop is usually not a big area, so it should not be too expensive. Just make sure that the joinery below can support its weight.

A luxury upgrade option is to replace the shop-bought vanity with a custom piece. By custom-making a piece of joinery you not only get the drawers and storage that you want but you can also choose the benchtop that goes on top.

Failing that, sand back and give your joinery a new life – or replace the cupboard doors. If they were gloss before, try a matt finish. Or simply paint your vanity to liven it up. Change your cabinet handles for a freshen up. If you can introduce a minimalist look it will transform the way the bathroom feels. Add storage so that you get the mess off your bench. Replace cupboards with drawers and you will fit a lot more in, similar to the kitchen. And put organisers in the drawers, as you do in the kitchen, to stop everything rolling around. Divide your things into on-show items and non-show items – then fit enough storage to hide and to show off. Most of us aren't pure minimalists, so having something on show is usually more friendly than absolutely nothing – but choose what it is.

Introduce furniture for the things that you do in the bathroom. For example, if you constantly find yourself needing somewhere to raise your foot –

then find a foot stool that is the perfect height. Make a spot for it to slide away so it is not left out in the space. If you like a glass of wine in the bath, or to listen to your smartphone while having a soak, then invest in a small table that puts it comfortably within earshot (making sure it can't fall in the bath). These little things personalise your bathroom to service your individual needs.

Sometimes for a big family with five lots of towels, a coat rack might be better than two towel rails. Or use a ladder as a towel rack. Consider a clothes horse in a shared bathroom – depending on the living situation many of us get changed in the bathroom. If you have a long shower space, you can put shelving at one end for towels if they are far enough away not to get wet.

If you have a bathroom that is not quite big enough for a conventional bath then consider introducing a floor plan-efficient plunge tub under the eaves or in an awkward corner. It will feel luxe.

◀ Design your bathroom well and it will be a shared space where your family lays down happy memories.

▼ Don't hold back on the guest bathroom. It's not a room where anyone spends very long, so give it some personality.

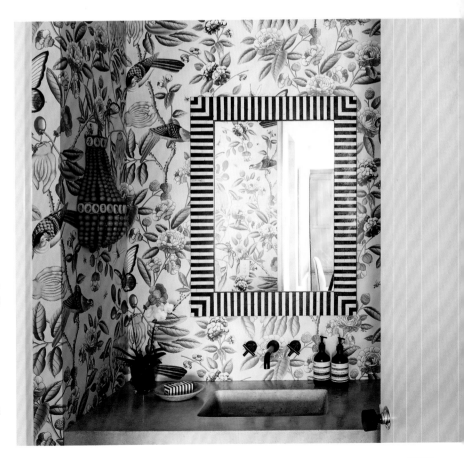

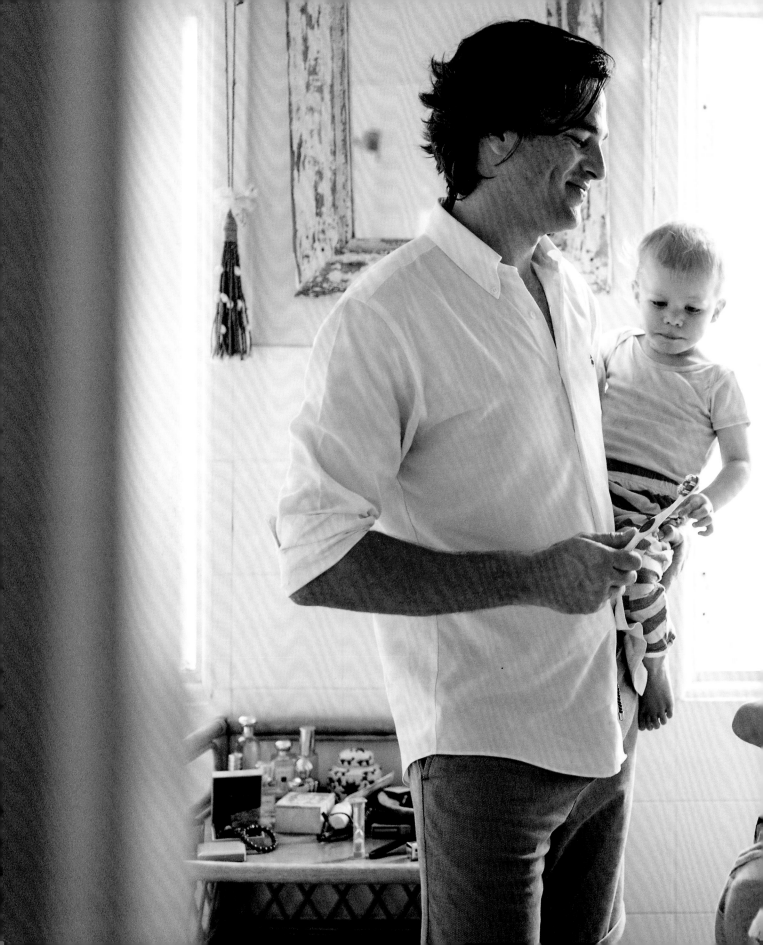

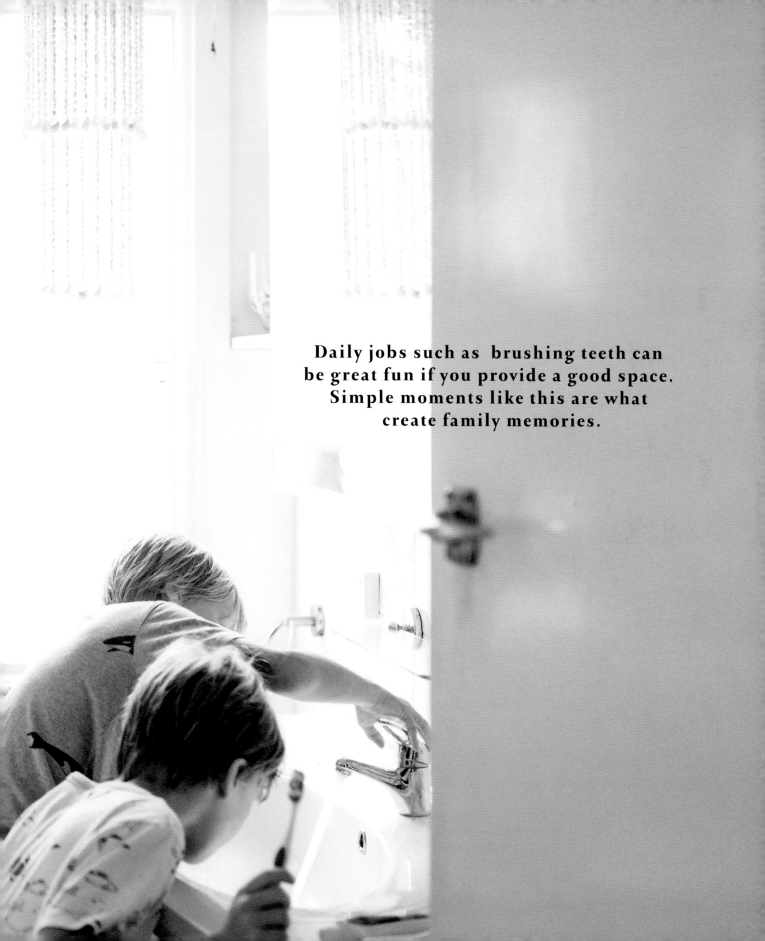

Daily jobs such as brushing teeth can be great fun if you provide a good space. Simple moments like this are what create family memories.

5 X 5
BATHROOM

▷ This light white bathroom feels clean and hygienic. The shutters at the window let in light while providing privacy.

▷▷ The fundamentals of this renovated bathroom are good because it has been designed around an existing asset: the window. Sunlight, air, water and green vegetation always work well together if you harness them properly.

NOTE
TO
SELF

CHASE SUNLIGHT IN YOUR BATHROOM. IF YOU DON'T HAVE ANY, WORK OUT A WAY TO FIND SOME, USING WINDOWS, SKYLIGHTS, SUN TUNNELS OR STEALING FROM ANOTHER ROOM. IT WILL BRIGHTEN YOUR DAY.

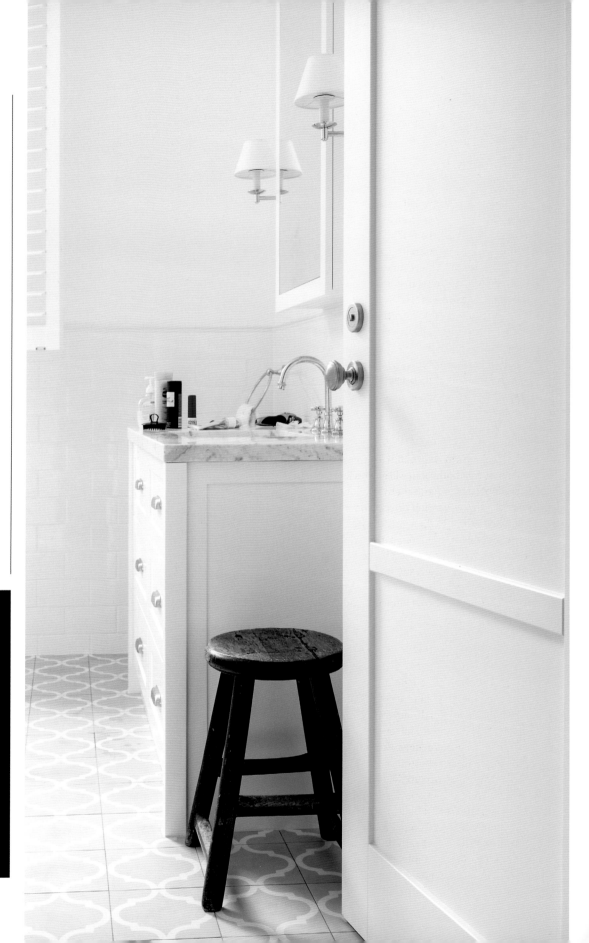

LIGHT

Water and light: there are few more uplifting combinations in the world. I spend a great deal of time working out ways to ensure that natural light passes through a stream of water, whether that is from the basin tap, the bath spout or the shower head. This is such a basic fundamental human pleasure and designing to capture it is one of the joys that can be considered in your bathroom.

Imagine placing a skylight that captures the morning sun and lets it stream through your shower every morning. That's not a bad start to the day and I guarantee it will get you going with energy. In the same vein, place a mirror behind your vanity basin tap and reflect light through the water as it runs.

WINDOWS, WINDOWS, WINDOWS

One of nature's most prolific cleansers is sunlight and so a sunlit bathroom will always feel cleaner. I invariably introduce as many windows as possible, always bearing privacy in mind. I often also introduce skylights – these are great for giving a sense of light, even early in the morning when there is not much light in the sky yet. If a skylight is not possible, sun tubes are a great resource in the bathroom. Their mirrored insides snake through your roof internals and bring in reflected sunlight.

BORROWED LIGHT

Many ensuites are land locked; they have no external window to let in natural light. If this is the case, and you can't put in a window to outside, try to borrow light from the adjacent bedroom by knocking a hole in the wall (or removing it completely) and screening with sand-blasted glass or plantation shutters.

One reason to open up the main part of your bathroom to a bigger space, such as the adjoining bedroom, is not only about space but also light. By not enclosing the room, you have an opportunity for light to spill both ways. The room doesn't have to be completely open; instead it could have a large sliding door or a bank of

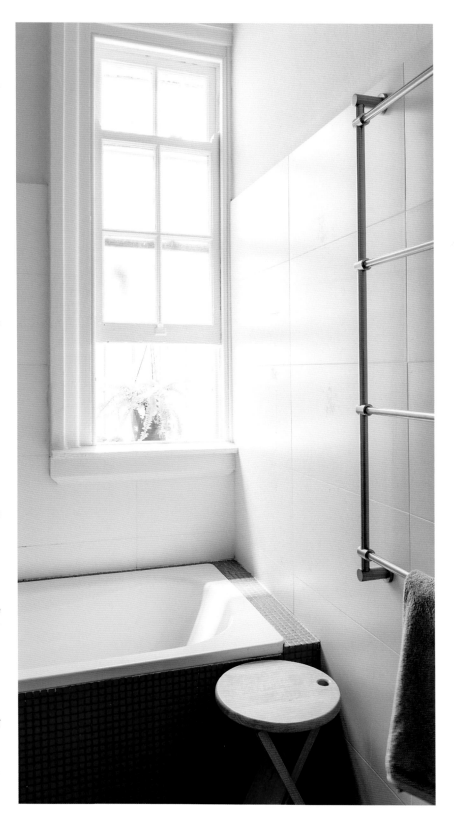

▶ Mix your glazing from fixed to louvres in the bathroom to give options for airflow and light. The airflow from the louvres in this ensuite has also been harnessed to cross-ventilate the adjoining bedroom.

shutters that allows light through when you need it. A beautifully lit bathroom can become a lovely background to a bedroom. This technique of borrowing light can also be used in other parts of the house. For example, you could open up the vanity part of your family bathroom to a hallway and share light. In the middle of a family get-up-and-go there is no issue with having these spaces connected as it is just a communal washing area. However, a sliding cavity door or otherwise is advised so that you can shut it off when required.

MIRRORING

Mirror is a great aid to the feeling of light in your bathroom. Often the opportunity to get natural light into a bathroom is not great: they are usually small rooms and well down the list in terms of placement for the house's best orientation to the sun. But if you have gone to great effort to get natural light into your bathroom despite this, now is the time to make the most of it. Use mirror, and don't be afraid to use more than you think you may need. Apart from the sense of space that it gives, a big mirror reflects the light that you have and gives a strong sense that you have more. I often create vanity benches 2 metres (78 in) or more long and then fill the wall above them with mirror up to the ceiling. The amount of light that it bounces around is amazing and mirror has the added benefits of being cost-effective and easy to clean.

SMART HOME

LIGHTING IS IMPORTANT FOR BALANCING CIRCADIAN RHYTHMS. THE BATHROOM IS THE PLACE YOU VISIT IMMEDIATELY AFTER OR BEFORE BED, SO LIGHTING SEQUENCES CAN BE DESIGNED TO HELP YOU WAKE UP OR RELAX FOR SLEEP. BEING IN AN OVERBRIGHT BATHROOM JUST BEFORE BED IS NOT THE BEST WAY TO CALM DOWN.

TASK LIGHTING

Always start with positioning your task lighting. Good task lighting is imperative in the bathroom, not only for making yourself presentable to the world, but also as one of the few places where you have the privacy and time to properly check yourself out. Good task lighting over the vanity is key. Make sure you place light in the middle of the bench between the front bench edge and the mirror. This ensures you not only light up the bench and everything on it, but also your face. If the light is further into the room, it will only light

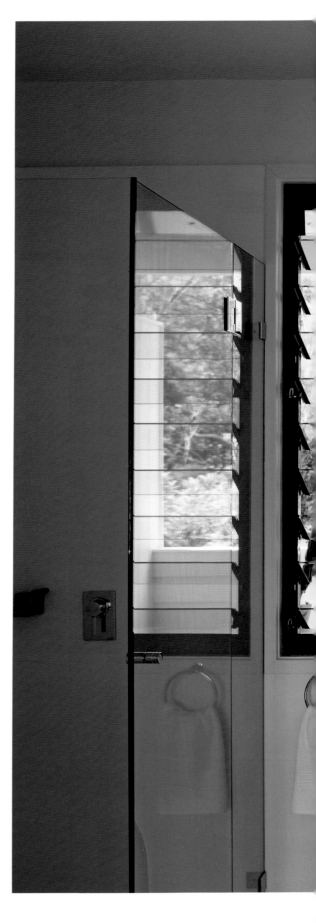

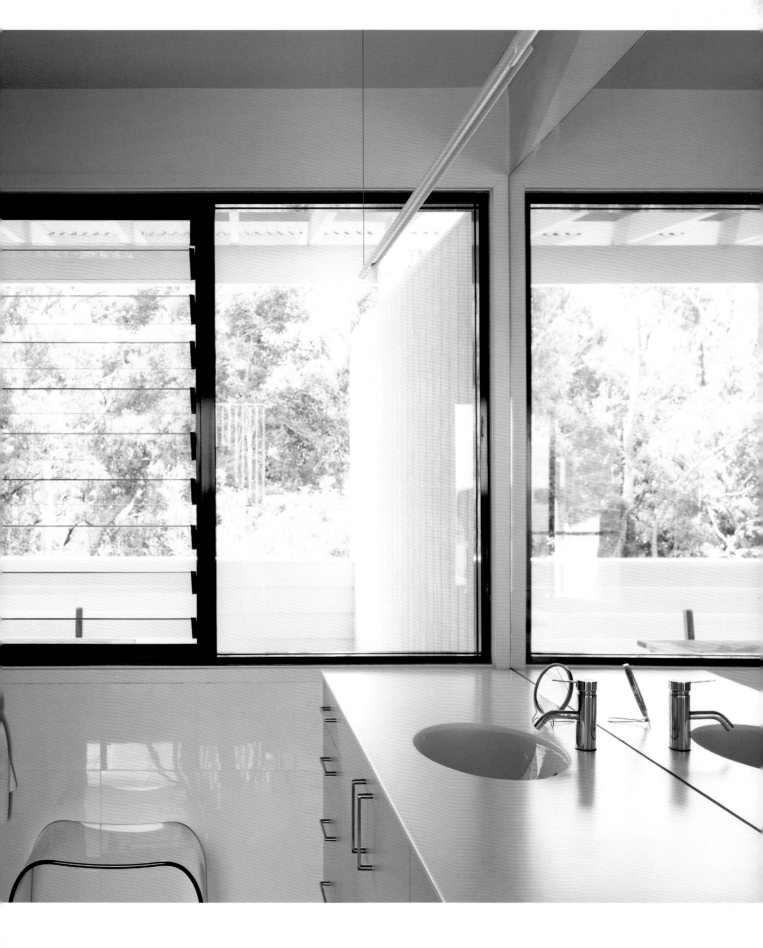

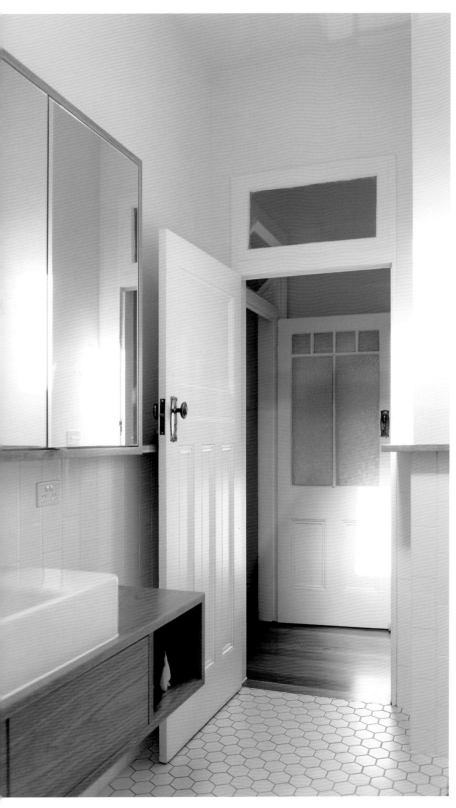

the top of your head as you stand at the basin and that will cast a shadow forward over your face.

Hollywood lights around a mirror are a great way to bring even light to your face and it is no accident that these are used by professional make-up artists. There are many updated versions on the market now, so you don't have to have the big bulbs surrounding the mirror. Be careful to check them out before you buy: I have found that some simply don't work and are more for room aesthetics than actual lighting.

Consider also using strip lighting under the vanity for the wow factor. Sometimes a bathroom needs a lift and placing some LED under the vanity can do just that, even making the vanity appear to float.

SHOWER LIGHTING

I like to place a waterproof task light in the shower. It is incredibly useful to have a good-quality light in there so that you can see yourself properly if you need to. It should not be in a spot where you look into it as you raise your face to the shower, and it must be on a separate switch or dimmable, so that if you find the bright light intrusive you can remove or soften it, especially when you are relaxing ready for bed at night. Interestingly enough, a recent trend has been LEDs in showerheads. Some are gimmicky, but I think they will move beyond this and start to represent more clinical solutions.

SPOTLIGHT A FEATURE

If you have a large and well-ventilated bathroom, I am a big believer in bringing in art or photography so that you have something to contemplate while you spend time there. Whether it's a painting or photograph, make sure you introduce a spotlight that will focus and make the feature pop. Don't be afraid to introduce sculpture into your bathroom – there is a long history of humans connecting sculpture and water. Just ensure that it is properly lit.

AMBIENT LIGHTING

I use wall wash lighting in a bathroom, especially if I have a feature wall to show off. A wall wash light brings a textured wall to life with a play of light and shade. Wall-mounted uplights work well

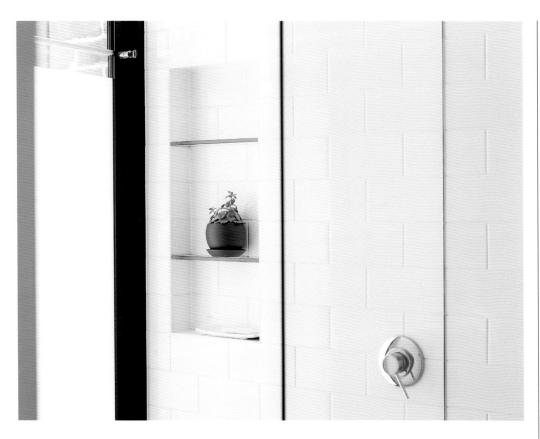

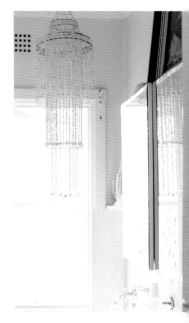

in a bathroom off a white ceiling, as they can have a big impact in a relatively small room. Ensure they are dimmable, so that you can get the light down to a really low glow if you are trying to relax in the bath.

THE ULTIMATE LUXURY

And, speaking of sleep and rest, there can be no better and more relaxing light in your bathroom in the evening than firelight. If you are soaking in the bath, candlelight is a lovely luxury. The warm light is relaxing, as are the flickering shadows that move across the room. If you can couple this with seeing stars through a window or skylight as you sit back in the bath then you have a truly great room. A scented candle can bring in a practical aspect: it looks beautiful while other less desirable scents are burnt off.

More extravagant again is to locate a fireplace in your bathroom. This harks back to times when we used fire to heat our water for bathing. A wonderful idea for a separating wall between a bedroom and ensuite is to put in a two-way

fireplace. It needs to be carefully and professionally fitted for safety, but imagine a fire adding ambience to both the bedroom and the bathroom – what a wonderful shared experience.

BRIGHTEN IT UP

For a quick fix, change your bathroom lighting fixture to something more interesting. So many bathrooms are afflicted by downlights or a single lonely oyster. Don't be afraid to introduce a game changer like a sophisticated Scandinavian pendant or even a chandelier. Create a minimum of three lighting effects in the bathrooms, depending on the activity you are doing: task lighting for washing and applying cosmetics, general ambient lighting for moving around your bathroom and then a relaxing mode of lighting for the evening bath or shower. Make your lighting fixtures work with your taps and accessories – they should be in a companion style.

▲ A chandelier is an unexpected and charming highlight in this otherwise simple bathroom.

◀ Translucent film on the exterior glass lets in a lot of sunlight while maintaining privacy. Such a nice touch to have a plant on the recessed shower shelf.

◀◀ There is not a huge amount of sunlight getting into this bathroom; however, the most is made of it with the clever placement of the mirror.

▶▶ These bright green shutters fully open on hinges for those occasions when the bathroom needs a really good airing.

AIR

The enemy of the bathroom is most definitely stinky air. The primary battle in the bathroom is to combat this and ensure your room always smells fresh as a daisy.

EXTRACTOR FANS

A proper extraction system direct to the outdoors is your most potent and effective weapon against both smelly air and damp, and there are many types on the market. Make sure it is placed either in the ceiling or high on the wall – the most efficient models extract to the outdoors either through your wall or through your roof. You can get extractor fans with filters but these do not handle moisture well. Also make sure you have your fan and lights on separate switches – it is an inefficient waste of energy to have your extractor fan switched with the light, as there are many activities in the bathroom that don't require the removal of smell or steam. An extractor fan should be quiet, but not so quiet that it gets left on all day.

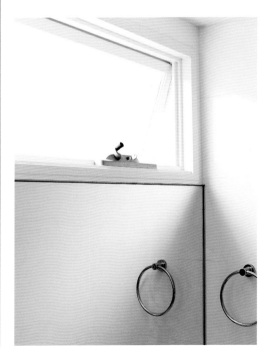

▶ High-level windows and skylights are a great way to get air and light into a bathroom and still ensure the space is private.

If steam is not removed quickly and efficiently it tends to gather on the ceiling. If the bathroom is not well aired then it can create pockets of moisture that never dry out and can lead to mould. With wetness and mould come nasty smells and even potential health problems. So a well-ventilated bathroom is a key step in a bathroom for a better life.

An extractor fan can come in handy in winter – you can extract air without opening windows and letting in cold air. In terms of cooling a summer bathroom, a ceiling fan never hurts. There is something quite holiday-like about a fan in the bathroom and it can aid a great deal with airflow and ventilation out of the windows.

SKYLIGHT VENTILATION

Another form of ventilation is the trusty and beautiful skylight. Steam rises and an open skylight is perfect for catching the breeze. Remember, if you want air movement in a room then you need to give the air a pathway with a different entry and exit; for example, a skylight in the ceiling that opens to the sky and a set of louvre windows in the wall.

LOUVRE WINDOWS

Louvres are great in a bathroom as you can open or close them very quickly and also leave them ajar: perfect to allow airflow throughout the day and night if it is warm. Louvre designs have improved a lot over the years and many are now very secure and can be fitted with flyscreens. They can also help in terms of privacy, as they're available in opaque materials such as timber, and translucent to opaque glass. You can, of course, have regular windows such as sliding, awning or double hung. I would advise fitting them all with flyscreens for two reasons: flies can be attracted to the occasional smells of a bathroom; and it is nice to be able to leave the window open all night in summer without finding a whole lot of insects in there in the morning.

PROBLEMS?

If you have to use air freshener in your bathroom, then you may be covering up a problem that really needs to be fixed rather than just masked. Make sure there is not a permanent problem creating long-term smells in your bathroom. It could be some plumbing that has gone awry, such as a dry drain, which is often easily fixed by a bucket of water down the drain. Or it could be a more insidious problem like mould. A clean, fresh and well-ventilated bathroom should be able to handle the daily goings on of a family and you shouldn't need air fresheners. Consider instead candles, or bring in some nature in the form of plants or flowers. It is well worth seeking out good-quality natural cleaning products. Not only are these better for the environment but some of them also have wonderful scents.

NOT JUST HOT AIR

In winter a bathroom can be a pretty horrible place because of its usually hard cold surfaces. So, if you can warm the air then you can start to improve those early mornings. If possible, orientate the bathroom to the morning sun so that you catch the early rays. Even a sense of sunlight can be warming.

Introduce warm timbers to areas that you touch, such as a duckboard floor mat for your feet. We use these in winter and they make a big difference, not only in terms of getting you off the cold tiles but also aiding in drying. A simple bathroom rug is also a great addition in winter. Not only does it bring a touch of style and colour to break up the seasons but it also is a welcome relief on those early mornings. (Make sure you have a routine and a location for airing and drying the bathroom rug or mat as they can get unpleasant pretty quickly. Last one out of the bathroom in the morning has to put it in its hanging spot.)

Some people swear by heated towel rails, and I must say that having a dry warm towel is an unexpected and pleasant surprise on a cold morning. Clever people have a timer, so that the rail comes on to warm your towel when you need it in the morning and doesn't waste energy all day.

The most opulent solution is, of course, underfloor heating – no rugs required with this option. The technology is rapidly improving. Properly done with timers, it is a lot more efficient than it used to be; however, it is still a nice-to-have rather than a necessity.

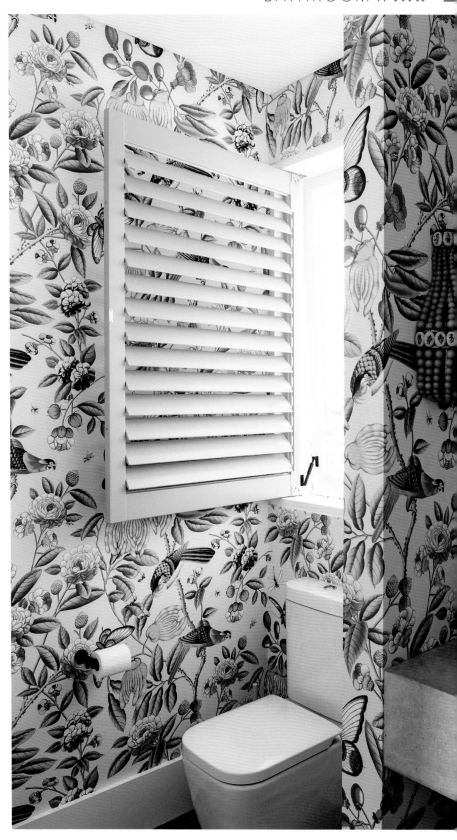

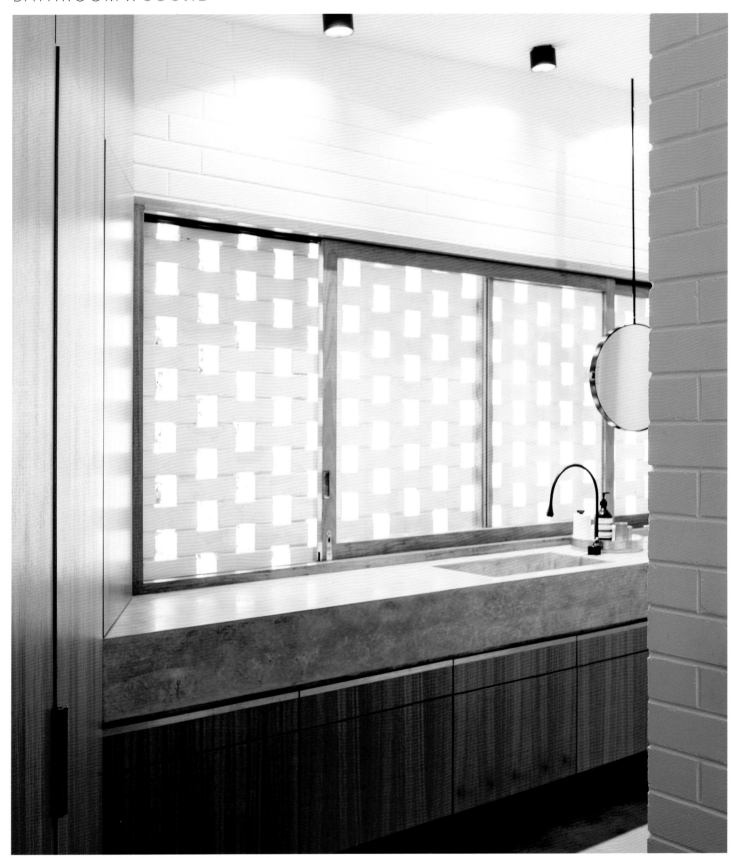

SOUND

Bathrooms can be dreadfully echoey places, and that is not going to put you in a relaxed mood. Usually small boxy rooms made up of hard surfaces, bathrooms seem to be perfectly formed for making sound bounce around, causing potential embarrassment to the occupant. But even the smallest changes can make your bathroom more comfortable: a big batch of fluffy towels on display is not only practical, but will go a long way to helping the acoustics.

SOAK UP THE ECHO

Stop the echo by using sound-absorbing materials. Introduce softer materials, such as timber, particularly jointed timber, to create a natural acoustic that softens and breaks up the sound. Consider a feature wall of wood, for example, that is in a drier area of the bathroom – it will dampen sound and is capable of withstanding steam and condensation, just not constant water contact.

Another, more advanced, solution is to use specially designed ceiling baffles that have been treated to be used in wet areas. These can be painted to match the ceiling so you don't even know they're there, and they do a good job of breaking down the sound reverberation and reducing the echo.

CHECK YOUR DOORS

Maybe even more uncomfortable than the echo is the thought of sound escaping from the bathroom into the rest of the house. Particularly in a guest bathroom, you want people to feel at ease and private. This is where a well-fitted door comes in handy. A solid core door, hung properly, will do the job. Be careful with sliding doors and cavity sliding doors; these are right on trend and look great but I have seen some shockers that have huge gaps around them. They are so badly sealed when closed that they are no better than a sheet of paper in terms of sound insulation. So, if you are going to use a sliding door, particularly for more intimate spaces such as an ensuite,

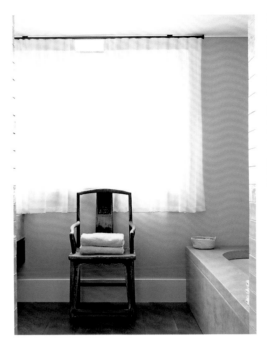

make sure it is solid and well fitted. You could even consider an acoustic seal, which can be supplied as part of the door and also retrofitted if you discover a problem.

CHOOSE YOUR SOUND

Music in the bathroom: now that is a luxury. It is great for waking you up in the morning, or lulling you into a state of relaxation at night. An integrated speaker system in the bathroom is the ideal. There are plenty of waterproof speakers available these days, but get them properly fitted and remember to NEVER mix electrics and water.

When I lived in London I lodged for a while with a friend who got up early every morning to have a bath. He always had a small transistor radio going in the bathroom, as he got ready, to listen to the BBC. It was a ritual he went through every morning, washing and getting ready physically for the day, but at the same time catching up on the news, the markets and what was happening in the world so he could attack it mentally. His bathroom was designed to enhance his day. It suited his habit of bathing; you can't hear the radio very well in the shower!

◀◀ The use of a number of different surfaces, including timber, disrupts sound waves and reduces echo.

◀ The soft translucent curtain and fluffy towels help dampen the sound in this bathroom.

MUST DON'T

ENSURE A GUEST BATHROOM IS FITTED WITH A SOLID, WELL-FITTED DOOR. IF NECESSARY, ADD ACOUSTIC SEALS TO MAKE IT PROPERLY SOUND-PROOF. IT IS ALL ABOUT YOUR GUESTS' PRIVACY AND COMFORT. NEVER LEAVE GAPS AROUND A POWDER ROOM DOOR.

VIEW

A sanctuary demands privacy from outsiders and a bathroom is the space in the house that demands the most visual privacy. No view *into* the bathroom when it is not wanted is a rule that should never be broken. So, when designing your space, make sure that you give great control to the occupant so that they can inhibit any views from within or outside the house. Doors and screens can be used to provide privacy, as can thoughtfully placed high windows.

I always try to design a bathroom to be very private but still let in light and air, and high-level windows or skylights are a perfect response to this brief. Remember though that the private times are reasonably limited and there are many activities conducted in the bathroom that are semi-private or not private at all. During these times it can be an absolute joy to be able to open a bathroom up and let in the sunshine and fresh air.

LOOKING IN

Externally fitted metal or timber screens can be vital for creating privacy from outside while allowing light and air to flow in. The fantastic thing about screens is that they can be laid in the horizontal or vertical depending on where the potential overlooking is coming from.

In terraced housing, where you might have close overlooking from neighbours, vertical screens can work wonderfully. By fitting vertical external screens to your windows, you can stop anyone looking in from the horizontal, effectively putting blinkers on; so you can look out to a view but the cross view is blocked. This means you can see out over your garden, for example, but any horizontal view from the neighbour into your bathroom is blocked. In the same way, horizontal shutters can be used to stop anyone seeing in from above or below – if you have a big building next to you, for example.

Shutters can be attached on the inside or the outside and can be adjustable or fixed. Opaque louvres in effect become horizontal shutters and so can be very useful for privacy as well as letting in light and air.

LOOKING OUT

Bathrooms are usually not large spaces and by their definition are often enclosed and boxy rooms. That's even more reason to generate a view to lift the soul. The best bathrooms are those that have a fantastic view to the outside, yet are completely private. In a new build, this is what you are aiming for – there are few better treats than gazing over a garden or landscape while soaking in the bath.

FRAME A VIEW

I try to design windows to let in light and air, but then I will also design a window to capture a particular view. For example, think about where you stand when you are brushing your teeth or where you look when you are sitting on the loo.

▼ Mirrors are an asset when it comes to surprising with unexpected views. As bathrooms are often small, large areas of mirror can create an illusion of space.

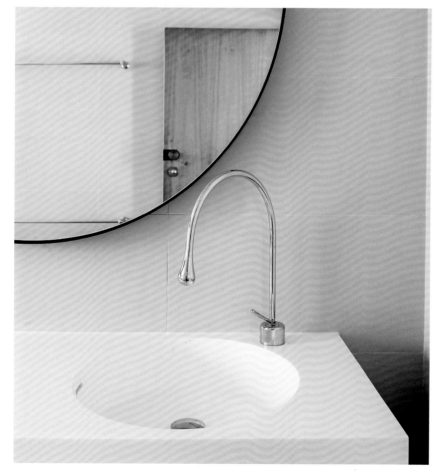

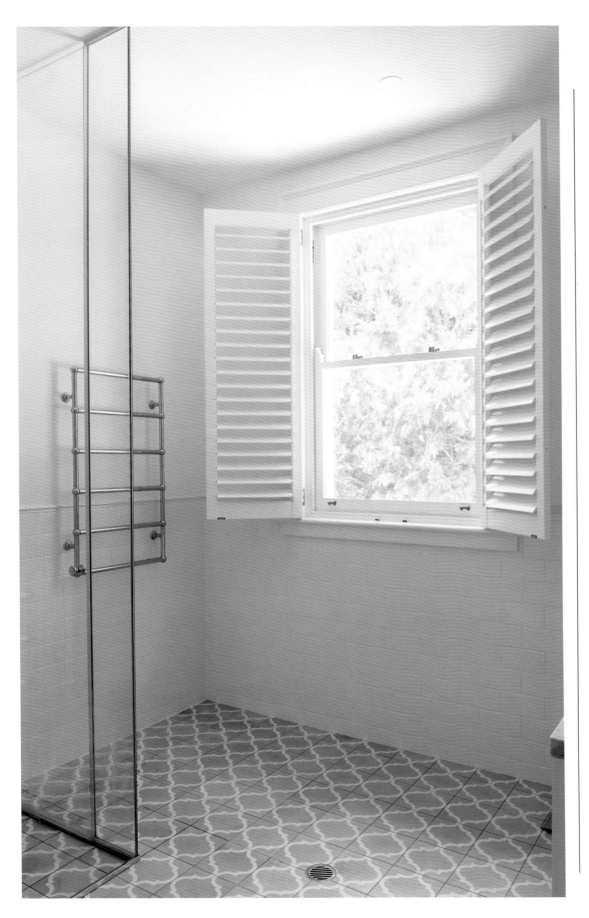

◄ When privacy is not required these shutters are flung open to let in not only sunshine and air, but also the uplifting view of green foliage.

Try to consider what view you will be capturing. Make sure you shut out the neighbours and that ugly chimney. But perhaps try to frame the crown of the flowering tree next door. If you are concerned about privacy, screen the lower part of your window with opaque vinyl or glass.

Make sure you bring a window down to a height where you can see out of it while you're in the bath. This is where horizontal screens can make all the difference; they channel your view into the garden, yet block out any potential overlooking from neighbours higher or lower.

BATHROOM DECK

Knowing that a bathroom is often a limited internal space, look for opportunities to expand the view beyond the room. I designed a house for a woman whose only time to herself was in the morning in the bathroom before the kids got up. So I created a small east-facing deck off her bathroom where she could go outside in privacy and dry her hair and even catch some morning sun. In many ways a view from your bathroom is more important than from your bedroom, and incorporating an outdoor deck is a true luxury.

If you can't have a deck, make sure you keep plants on the window ledge or the vanity (and there is no excuse for not watering them).

STEALING BEAUTY

Look internally to borrow a view as well, especially if you don't have the opportunity for outside views. In an ensuite, extend the view from your vanity out into the master bedroom. Why enclose yourself in a box when you could expand the sense of view? Most of us spend more waking hours in the bathroom than in the bedroom, so you might as well share the spaces. By fitting the bath in the bedroom you can create a view from your bath that is very different than if it were in a bathroom, and most likely a lot more spacious.

▼ This relatively small bathroom feels bigger due to the use of clear shower blades and frameless fittings that maximise internal views.

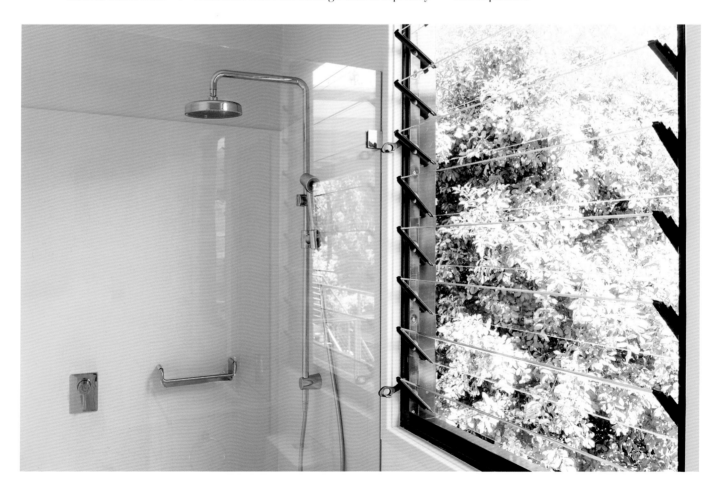

If you can, position the loo so that your outlook is as long as possible within the room, rather than directly at a wall less than a metre away. Perhaps fit it at the end of a long horizontal vanity that allows your eye to follow the edge to meet a beautiful textured feature wall with the sun falling across it so it changes throughout the day.

REFLECT IT BACK

A bathroom by its very nature needs a mirror, so take this practical requirement, expand it and get creative with it. Use mirror for the whole wall above your vanity, or a section of wall, so that the room reflects itself to give another dimension.

If you only have high windows, align the mirror next to them on the adjacent ninety-degree wall so that you extend the sky into the room and therefore the view. Make sure the mirror catches more than just the reflection of your mug. Ensure that it brings in a sense of the sky and the outdoors.

Making a whole wall of mirror makes the room feel bigger and more glamorous and it is relatively cheap. Add a surprise with mirror by putting it at the back of your bathroom cabinet; it gives an unexpected view and also reveals products that you didn't know you had, hidden behind others.

SHOWER BLADES

A glass shower blade – a piece of glass with minimal fittings, set into the floor and wall (and the ceiling if it reaches) – can be a great modern addition to a bathroom. One of its greatest assets is that glass doesn't inhibit the longest possible view in a relatively small bathroom, particularly in comparison to framed shower screens. Suddenly the shower is part of the overall space – the room feels bigger and the views are more substantial.

If you spend a bit extra, you can have your shower blade made out of Starphire glass, which is clearer than standard green-tinged glass and lets the light bounce around. You will be surprised by the way this glass disappears in your peripheral vision and causes no interruption in the view of the room.

If, however, you have a larger bathroom and no issues with light then you could consider introducing a material such as stone or marble as a shower blade. Or, if you have the room and a

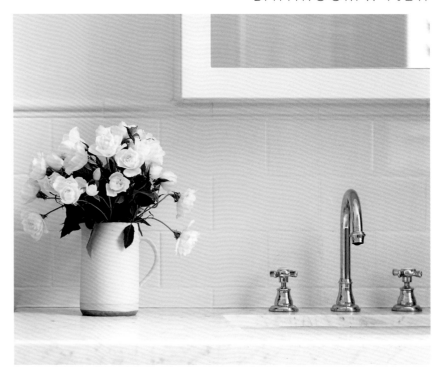

good enough fall in your bathroom floor to aid drainage, you could do away with shower blades altogether – now that is an uninhibited view!

THE QUICKEST OF FIXES

And as a quick fix, if there really is no view available to you, why not introduce a decal on a wall? It could be a beach scene, the bright lights of the city or an artwork. Remember, decals don't always have to be big. In a bathroom there are often small, finicky twists and turns: place a floral decal in these small spots and surprise with the unexpected. Sometimes the little views are more satisfying and intriguing than the bigger ones.

In the same way, don't underestimate the power of a perfectly placed vase of flowers becoming the focus of a bathroom that doesn't have a view; once again you have created your own solution and ensured the room has risen above the mundane.

Or you could consider your shower curtain as a blank canvas – an opportunity for a statement work of art. As a shower curtain needs to be drawn to dry, it becomes a great opportunity for a splash of colour or landscape. Change the look of your bathroom in an instant by drawing the statement curtain closed.

So simple — but a perfectly placed vase of flowers instantly lifts your bathroom above the ordinary.

A LAST WORD

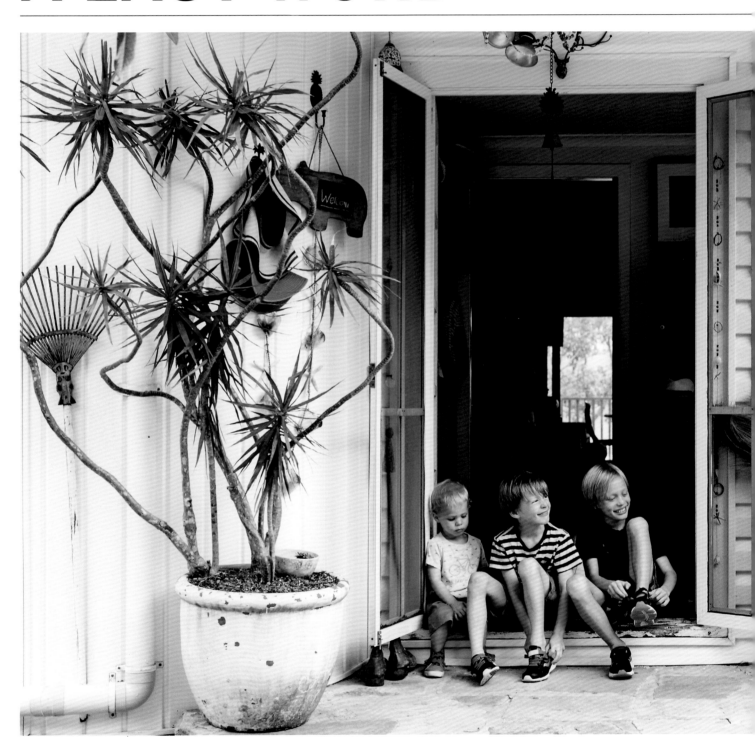

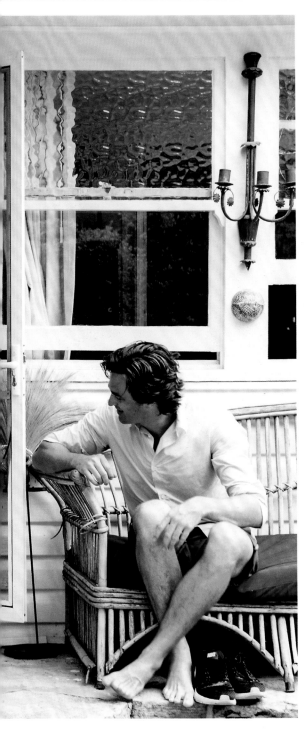

Everyone deserves to live in excellent shelter. It is a fundamental element of human survival and after thousands of years of development we should have it down pat. However, sometimes I think we forget the basics. Sometimes we put the cart before the horse and get carried away with pursuing a particular style or fashion, when we have not invested in the part of the home that really matters: the bones. The beauty is that if we get the bones right, our style and our fashion will never look better.

So, in your current or next home, apply the 5x5 Design Steps to improve those important bones of your house or apartment. Have the confidence to create a healthy, nourishing and inspiring shelter that, coupled with your unique style and taste, will create your best home.

ACKNOWLEDGMENTS

FOR KEVIN SNELL. Thank you for introducing me to architecture, its meaning and qualities, from day one. I often think of the Armidale kid, being so inspired by the majestic John Horbury Hunt buildings in the local area that he decided he should be an architect; now that is a vision. And thanks to Jillian, for putting up with another architect in the family!

Thank you to Laura, Asger, Bjorn and Peter, who have supported me while I disappeared for many hours to write this book.

And thanks also to the Snell Architects office for your great work.

To Murdoch Books: Wow, that was a ride! Thank you for your belief and support. Diana, Jane and Vivien, and everyone else: thanks for your intelligence, style and commitment – it made all the difference.

Thanks to Phu Tang for creating simply beautiful photographs that bring this book to life – it is not easy to capture concepts such as light, air and sound, and you did an amazing job. I enjoyed our many hours together.

Thanks also to 6 Degrees Management, Titus and the crew, for all your support and helping make this book happen.

I'd like to say thanks to Channel Seven and the *House Rules* team for a fantastic four seasons. For bringing me onto the team and guiding me, thanks to Maxine, Rikkie and Deb. As well, big hugs to Johanna for your guidance and support, and also Carolyn; lots of laughs, you two! And to Wendy: did we spend some hours travelling Australia or what? Loved it – thanks for all those long chats, your support and friendship.

And finally, to the very talented architects and home owners who welcomed Phu and me into their homes and creations – thank you so much for your generosity and for sharing your way of life in the home.

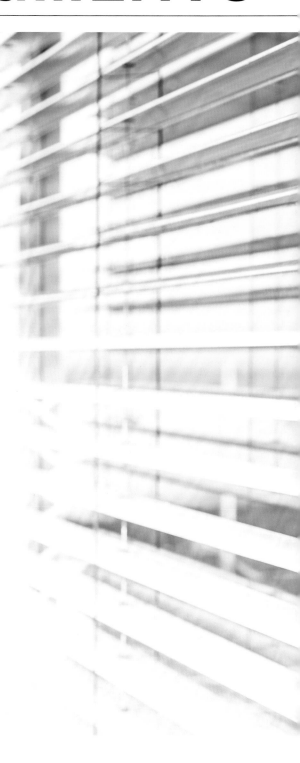

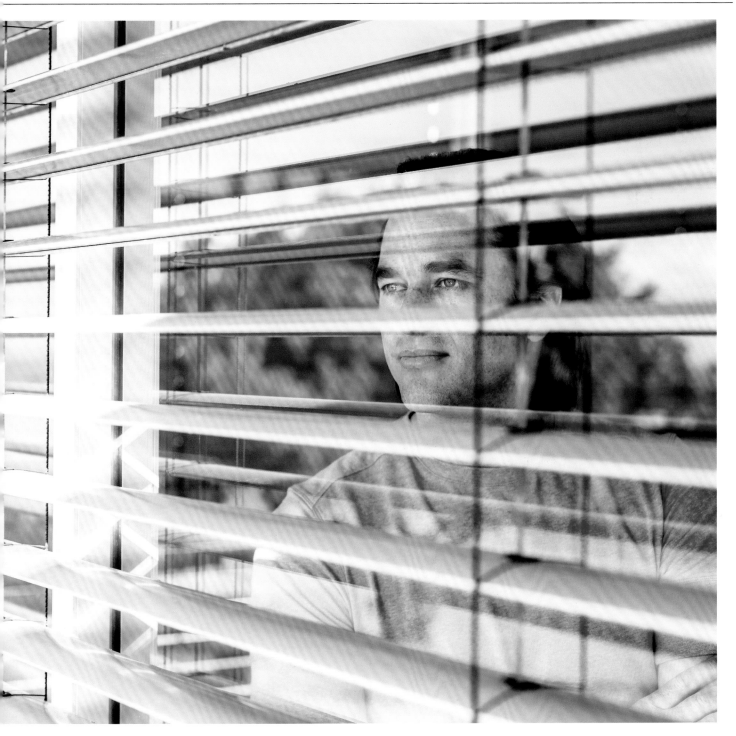

INDEX

Published in 2017 by Murdoch Books, an imprint of Allen & Unwin

Murdoch Books Australia
83 Alexander Street, Crows Nest NSW 2065
Phone: +61 (0)2 8425 0100
murdochbooks.com.au
info@murdochbooks.com.au

Murdoch Books UK
Ormond House, 26–27 Boswell Street,
London WC1N 3JZ
Phone: +44 (0) 20 8785 5995
murdochbooks.co.uk
info@murdochbooks.co.uk

For corporate orders and custom publishing contact our business development team at
salesenquiries@murdochbooks.com.au

Publisher: Diana Hill
Editor: Jane Price
Design Manager: Vivien Valk
Design concept: Lauren Camilleri
Design layout: Vivien Valk; Jacqui Triggs
Photographer: Phu Tang
Production Manager: Lou Playfair

ISBN 978 1 74336 915 9 Australia
ISBN 978 1 74336 916 6 UK
A cataloguing-in-publication entry is available from the catalogue of the
National Library of Australia at nla.gov.au
A catalogue record for this book is available from the British Library

Colour reproduction by Splitting Image Colour Studio Pty Ltd, Clayton, Victoria
Printed by C & C Offset Printing, China

The author and publisher would like to thank the following artists whose work appears in the pages of this book.

Page 16-17: Peter Cooley (left); Ali Wood (right)
Page 26: Noel McKenna
Page 37: Brett Coelho
Page 44: Karl Wiebke
Page 47: Peter Booth
Pages 61 and 95: Jock Young
Page 83: Gail English (above sofa); Jenny Sages (above dresser)
Page 84: Zhong Chen
Page 96: Aida Tomescu
Page 97: Darren Gannon

Page 104: Terri Brooks (top left); Amanda Penrose Hart (bottom left); Gloria Petyarre (right)
Page 106-7: Bernard Japanangka Watson; Adrianna Nangala Egan; Paddy Japaljarri Stewart; Deborah Napaljarri Wayne
Page 130: Lyndal Walker
Page 141: Julian Meagher
Page 175: Jung Chen
Page 184: Wary Meyers (left); Adrian Hobbs (right); lamp by Michele de Lucchi for Memphis Milano
Page 196: Patrick Doherty